Pregnancy & Kidney Diseases

Pregnancy & Kidney Diseases

Editors

Priti Meena
MBBS MD DNB (Nephrology) FASN FRCP
Assistant Professor
Department of Nephrology
All India Institute of Medical Sciences
Bhubaneswar, Odisha, India

Arpita Ray Chaudhury (Lahiri)
MD DNB DM (Nephrology)
Nephrology Specialist
Department of Nephrology
North Bengal Medical College and Hospital
Siliguri, West Bengal, India

Manisha Sahay
MD DNB FAMS
Professor and Head
Department of Nephrology
Osmania Medical College and General Hospital
Hyderabad, Telangana, India

Natarajan Gopalakrishnan
MD DM FRCP (London)
Director
Institute of Nephrology
Madras Medical College
Chennai, Tamil Nadu, India

Associate Editor

Vinant Bhargava
DNB (Medicine) DNB (Nephrology) MNAMS FASN FRCP (London) FACP MBA (HCM)
Associate Professor (GRIPMER)
Senior Consultant
Department of Nephrology
Sir Ganga Ram Hospital
New Delhi, India

Foreword

Vivekanand Jha

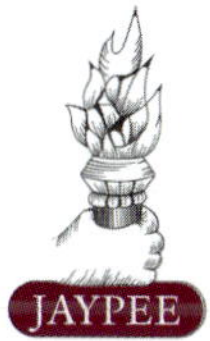

JAYPEE BROTHERS MEDICAL PUBLISHERS
The Health Sciences Publisher
New Delhi | London

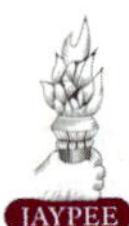

Jaypee Brothers Medical Publishers (P) Ltd

Headquarters
Jaypee Brothers Medical Publishers (P) Ltd
EMCA House, 23/23-B
Ansari Road, Daryaganj
New Delhi 110 002, India
Landline: +91-11-23272143, +91-11-23272703
+91-11-23282021, +91-11-23245672
Email: jaypee@jaypeebrothers.com

Corporate Office
Jaypee Brothers Medical Publishers (P) Ltd
4838/24, Ansari Road, Daryaganj
New Delhi 110 002, India
Phone: +91-11-43574357
Fax: +91-11-43574314
Email: jaypee@jaypeebrothers.com

Overseas Office
JP Medical Ltd
83 Victoria Street, London
SW1H 0HW (UK)
Phone: +44 20 3170 8910
Fax: +44 (0)20 3008 6180
Email: info@jpmedpub.com

Website: www.jaypeebrothers.com
Website: www.jaypeedigital.com

Inquiries for bulk sales may be solicited at: jaypee@jaypeebrothers.com

Pregnancy & Kidney Diseases

First Edition: **2024**

ISBN: 978-93-5696-639-0

Printed in India at Sterling Graphics Pvt. Ltd.

Contributors

Aisha Batool MD
Assistant Professor
Department of Medicine
Medical College of Wisconsin
Brookfield, Wisconsin, USA

Anand Chellappan MD DM (Nephrology)
Assistant Professor and In-Charge
Department of Nephrology
All India Institute of Medical Sciences
Nagpur, Maharashtra, India

Anna Gaddy MD FASN FNKF
Assistant Professor
Department of Medicine
Medical College of Wisconsin
Milwaukee, Wisconsin, USA

Anuja Java MD
Associate Professor of Medicine
Department of Nephrology
Washington University School of Medicine
St Louis, Missouri, USA

Arpita Ray Chaudhury (Lahiri)
MD DNB DM (Nephrology)
Nephrology Specialist
Department of Nephrology
North Bengal Medical College and Hospital
Siliguri, West Bengal, India

Arunkumar S DM (Nephrology)
Assistant Professor
Department of Nephrology
All India Institute of Medical Sciences
New Delhi, India

Corina Gabriela Teodosiu MD
Nephrologist
Carol Davila University of Medicine and Pharmacy
Bucharest, Romania

Dhanin Puthiyottil MBBS MD DM
Assistant Professor
Department of Nephrology
Government Medical College
Kannur, Kerala, India

Dilip Kumar Pal MCh (Urology)
Professor and Head
Department of Urology
Institute of Postgraduate
Medical Education and Research
and SSKM Hospital
Dean, Faculty of Modern Medicine
West Bengal University of Health Sciences
Kolkata, West Bengal, India

Dipankar Bhowmik DM (Nephrology)
Professor and Head
Department of Nephrology
All India Institute of Medical Sciences
New Delhi, India

Divya Bajpai
MD (Med) DM (Nephrology)
Professor
Department of Nephrology
Seth Gordhandas Sunderdas Medical College
and KEM Hospital
Mumbai, Maharashtra, India

Jayasurya R MBBS MD DM (Nephrology)
Consultant
Department of Nephrology
Apollo Multispeciality Hospital
Kolkata, West Bengal, India

Kapil Navin Sejpal
MBBS MD DM (Nephrology)
Assistant Professor
Department of Nephrology
Jawaharlal Nehru Medical College
Wardha, Maharashtra, India

Kayan Siodia
MBBS DNB (Med) DNB (Cardiology)
Interventional Cardiologist
Department of Cardiology
SL Raheja Hospital
Mumbai, Maharashtra, India

Kiran Munir MD
Fellow in Nephrology
Division of Kidney Diseases and Hypertension
Northwell Health System
Great Neck, New York, USA

Mala Sachdeva MD
Professor of Medicine
Hofstra Northwell School of Medicine
Division of Kidney Diseases and Hypertension
Northwell Health System
Great Neck, New York, USA

Manish Rathi DM (Nephrology)
Professor
Department of Nephrology
Postgraduate Institute of
Medical Education and Research
Chandigarh, India

Manisha Sahay
MD DNB FAMS
Professor and Head
Department of Nephrology
Osmania Medical College and
General Hospital
Hyderabad, Telangana, India

Manjusha Yadla DM FISN
Professor and Head
Department of Nephrology
Gandhi Medical College
Hyderabad, Telangana, India

Manuel Urra MD
Department of Nephrology
Renal Medicine and Hypertension
University of Colorado
Aurora, Colorado, USA

Mayuri Trivedi
DNB (Medicine) DM (Nephrology)
Head
Department of Nephrology
Lokmanya Tilak Municipal General Hospital
Mumbai, Maharashtra, India

Namrata Parikh MD DNB (Nephrology)
Transplant Fellow
Division of Transplantation
Mayo Clinic
Jacksonville, Florida, USA

Narayan Prasad MD DNB (Med) DM DNB MNAMS
FISN FASN (Nephro) FRCP (London)
Professor and Head
Department of Nephrology
Sanjay Gandhi Postgraduate
Institute of Medical Sciences
Lucknow, Uttar Pradesh, India

Natarajan Gopalakrishnan
MD DM FRCP (London)
Director
Institute of Nephrology
Madras Medical College
Chennai, Tamil Nadu, India

Partha Pratim Sinha Roy MCh (Urology)
Senior Resident
Department of Urology
Institute of Postgraduate
Medical Education and Research
and SSKM Hospital
Kolkata, West Bengal, India

Prasoon Verma MD
Assistant Professor
Department of Pediatrics
University of Cincinnati College of Medicine
Cincinnati, Ohio, USA

Priti Meena
MBBS MD DNB (Nephrology) FASN FRCP
Assistant Professor
Department of Nephrology
All India Institute of Medical Sciences
Bhubaneswar, Odisha, India

Priyamvada PS
MBBS MD DM (Nephrology)
Professor
Department of Nephrology
Jawaharlal Institute of Postgraduate Medical Education and Research
Puducherry, India

Rajesh Jhorawat MBBS MD DM
Associate Professor
Department of Nephrology
All India Institute of Medical Sciences
Jodhpur, Rajasthan, India

Renu Singh MS
Department of Obstetrics and Gynecology
Queen Marys Hospital
King George's Medical University
Lucknow, Uttar Pradesh, India

Richard Burwick
Maternal Fetal Medicine MD MPH
Clinical Associate Professor
Western University of Health Sciences
Obstetrics and Gynecology
San Gabriel Valley Perinatal Medical Group
Pomona Valley Hospital Medical Center

S Jayalakshmi MD DM
Professor
Institute of Nephrology
Madras Medical College
Chennai, Tamil Nadu, India

Sabarinath S
MD DM (Nephrology)
Assistant Professor
Department of Nephrology
Jawaharlal Institute of Postgraduate Medical Education and Research
Puducherry, India

Sabina Yusuf
MD DM (Nephrology)
Associate Professor
Department of Nephrology
Christian Medical College
Vellore, Tamil Nadu, India

Sakthi Rajagopal MD
Final Year Resident
Department of Nephrology
Osmania Medical College
Hyderabad, Telangana, India

Sanjeev Nair
MD DM (Nephrology)
Senior Consultant
Department of Nephrology
Institute of Kidney Disease, Urology, and Organ Transplant
Madras Medical Mission
Chennai, Tamil Nadu, India

Shannon Lyons
Division of Renal Diseases and Hypertension
University of Colorado School of Medicine
Aurora, Colorado, United States

Silvi Shah MD MS
Associate Professor
Department of Nephrology
University of Cincinnati
Cincinnati, Ohio, USA

Smita Subhash Divyaveer
DM (Nephrology)
Associate Professor
Department of Nephrology
Postgraduate Institute of Medical Education and Research
Chandigarh, India

Sreejith Parameswaran
MBBS MD DNB DM
Professor and Head
Department of Nephrology
Jawaharlal Institute of Postgraduate Medical Education and Research
Puducherry, India

Subhajit Malakar MCh (Urology)
Senior Resident
Department of Urology
Institute of Postgraduate Medical Education and Research and SSKM Hospital
Kolkata, West Bengal, India

Suceena Alexander
DM (Nephrology) FRCP (Lon) FASN PhD
Professor
Department of Nephrology
Christian Medical College
Vellore, Tamil Nadu, India

Urmila Anandh MBBS MD DNB DM DNB FRCP (Glasgow) FASN FISN (Fellow International Society of Nephrology) FISN (Fellow Indian Society of Nephrology)
Senior Consultant and Head
Department of Nephrology
Amrita Hospitals
Faridabad, Haryana, India
WCN Social Media Team
2019/2020/2021/2022/2023
Member, International Society of Nephrology CME Committee
Member, South Asia Regional Board, International Society of Nephrology
Member, Dialysis Working Group, International Society of Nephrology
Mentor, ISN Mentorship Program
Member, ISN-ACT Committee
President, Women in Nephrology-India
President, Society of Renal Nutrition and Metabolism (Southern Chapter)

Vaibhav Tiwari
DM (Nephrology)
Consultant
Department of Nephrology
Sir Ganga Ram Hospital
New Delhi, India

Vaishnavi Venkatasubramanian
DM (Nephrology)
Senior Resident
Department of Nephrology
Postgraduate Institute of Medical Education and Research
Chandigarh, India

Vinant Bhargava
DNB (Medicine) DNB (Nephrology) MNAMS FASN FRCP (London) FACP MBA (HCM)
Associate Professor (GRIPMER)
Senior Consultant
Department of Nephrology
Sir Ganga Ram Hospital
New Delhi, India

Foreword

Pregnancy is a profound and transformative experience for most women. It is marked by significant physiological changes and emotional milestones. For women with kidney disease, this journey is fraught with unique challenges and complexities that require specialized medical attention and care. *Pregnancy & Kidney Diseases* finds its purpose within this intricate intersection of nephrology and obstetrics.

This comprehensive guide is a compilation of the massive knowledge accumulated over years of clinical expertise and scholarly rigor, distilled by a group of eminent and expert authors and editors. The book is designed to be a thorough and detailed resource covering the entire spectrum of kidney disorders in pregnancy.

The chapters are meticulously crafted to offer a lucid and comprehensive perspective on the complex interactions between pregnancy and kidney function. Chapters are enriched with clinical vignettes, diagnostic algorithms, and therapeutic paradigms, ensuring that no aspect of this multifaceted subject is left unexamined. The book has a combination of clear explanations, plain language summaries, and crisply presented practice points for practical application. The integration of visual aids, including expressive diagrams and infographics accompanying each chapter, further enhances the clarity and accessibility of the content.

The contributors are experts in their respective fields and provide a nuanced understanding of the specific issues related to kidney health and pregnancy. A note must be made of the focus on India, reflecting the composition of the editorial team. This regional focus is helpful, as it addresses the unique challenges healthcare providers face in this part of the world. The lessons learned here are likely applicable in other countries with similar healthcare systems, where the burden of kidney disease is particularly high and access to specialized care and advanced medical technologies is limited. Women in these settings face compounded challenges, including delayed diagnosis, limited access to therapies, including dialysis, and higher rates of pregnancy-related complications such as preeclampsia and acute kidney injury. Women with preexisting kidney disease face particular, even unsurmountable, difficulties in regions with weak healthcare systems. The book covers recent advances, in the understanding of pathogenesis and early diagnosis of preeclampsia and pregnancy-induced atypical hemolytic uremic syndrome.

The cornerstone of this book is education. I hope the next generation of nephrology trainees and clinicians finds this book useful in acquiring the knowledge and skills required for excellence in caring for women with or at risk of kidney disease. By presenting a tapestry of clinical insights and evidence-based practices, the book aims to enhance the understanding and management of kidney disorders in pregnancy, with the ultimate goal of improving outcomes for both mothers and their babies. I hope the readers will utilize the knowledge to ensure high-quality, equitable access to essential medical services for this population.

We often do not appreciate that pregnancy is a unique entry point into the healthcare system for women. Pregnancy gives the opportunity to uncover hitherto unrecognized health conditions, including kidney disease, and that the care of a pregnant woman does not end with a successful delivery. For example, we know that pre-eclampsia, gestational hypertension, and gestational diabetes increase the lifetime risk of development of hypertension, diabetes, cardiovascular disease, and kidney diseases. Similarly, acute kidney injury during pregnancy increases the lifetime risk of development of chronic kidney disease. The health system, therefore, should ensure that all women have the opportunity to receive appropriate care throughout their lives.

There remains an unfinished public health agenda and a pressing need for robust research to better understand and manage kidney health during pregnancy in a resource-sensitive and patient-centered manner. Research priorities should include not only improved understanding of pathobiology but also the development of comprehensive risk assessment tools to identify those at risk of adverse outcomes during pregnancy and the exploration of effective interventions to mitigate the risks associated with kidney diseases and pregnancy.

I congratulate and thank the contributors and editors who have dedicated their time and expertise to this project. Their relentless pursuit of knowledge and commitment to patient care are evident in every page of this book. It will be an invaluable tool for nephrology trainees, practitioners, gynecologists, and other healthcare professionals caring for pregnant women with or at risk of developing kidney disease.

As you delve into the chapters of this book, I hope you find the information both enlightening and practical. May it serve as a beacon of knowledge, guiding you in the complex yet rewarding task of caring for pregnant women with kidney disease.

Vivekanand Jha
MD DM FRCP FAMS
Executive Director, The George Institute for Global Health, India
Chair of Global Kidney Health
Faculty of Medicine, Imperial College, London
Conjoint Professor of Medicine, University of New South Wales, Sydney
Past President, International Society of Nephrology

Preface

Kidney disorders in pregnancy present a complex clinical challenge that necessitates careful evaluation and management. Nephrologists and gynecologists must understand the physiological changes in the kidneys during pregnancy to identify and address abnormal phenomena. There are numerous diagnostic challenges, including the effective use of noninvasive serological markers, determining when to perform renal biopsies, managing current medications, and understanding teratogenic risks.

This book serves as a comprehensive and detailed guide, comprising the entire spectrum from diagnosis to prognosis. Written by eminent experts in the discipline, this book represents a collective endeavor that gathers their professional proficiency into a useful reference.

The primary aim of the book is educational, equipping clinicians with the knowledge and skills necessary for excellence in patient care. Each chapter is meticulously crafted, featuring clinical vignettes, diagnostic algorithms, and therapeutic paradigms. Key aspects, ranging from fundamental principles of diseases to detailed therapeutic methods, are clearly explained.

Illustrations are essential components of the book's structure. Illustrative diagrams elucidate dense concepts, while concise one-page infographics effectively communicate essential insights into complex knowledge. In addition, each chapter contains a concise synopsis to facilitate easy understanding of the content.

This book is primarily intended for nephrology trainees preparing for entry and exit nephrology superspecialty examinations. Additionally, nephrologists, general practitioners, and obstetricians-gynecologists will gain enriching insights in this book, which will enhance their comprehension and help them stay up-to-date with their clinical practices.

Vinant Bhargava

Acknowledgments

We extend heartfelt gratitude to all our mentors and teachers for generously imparting their knowledge and wisdom.

"to our colleagues for their unwavering support and camaraderie throughout this journey.....
....our sincere gratitude to our patients for entrusting us with their care and allowing us to serve them".

We deeply appreciate our family members for their constant support and understanding, enabling us to pursue our passions and aspirations.

Contents

CHAPTER 1

Renal Physiological Adaptation in Pregnancy

Kapil Navin Sejpal, Dhanin Puthiyottil, Priyamvada PS

HIGHLIGHTS

- Substantial structural, functional, and hemodynamic changes occur during normal pregnancy.
- Understanding these changes is crucial for recognizing normal values and abnormal mechanisms to identify disorders during pregnancy.
- Kidneys typically increase in size by up to 30%, with a 1–1.5 cm increase in length.
- In early pregnancy, renal plasma flow (RPF) exceeds glomerular filtration rate (GFR), leading to a lower filtration fraction compared to nonpregnant individuals.
- All renal changes normalize 4–6 weeks after delivery.

INTRODUCTION

A normal kidney plays an integral role in completing a successful pregnancy. Pregnancy acts as a "physiologic cardio-metabolic stress test". Maternal systemic vascular resistance (SVR) starts falling around 4–6 weeks, leading to reduced mean arterial pressures, reaching a nadir between 18 and 24 weeks of gestation. The low SVR leads to a reduced afterload, resulting in increased cardiac output. The increased cardiac output, low SVR, and the hormonal changes of pregnancy alter the renal hemodynamics, tubular handling of electrolytes, and body's acid–base status.

ANATOMIC CHANGES

The bipolar length of the kidney increases by approximately 1–1.5 cm, and the volume increases by 30% compared to nonpregnant levels. These changes revert to nonpregnant levels by around 6 months postpartum. The increments in kidney size are attributed to changes in the interstitial and renovascular volumes rather than true hypertrophy. Ultrastructurally, the glomerulus, tubulo-interstitial, and vascular compartments appear similar to the nonpregnant stage.

Marked morphological changes occur in the collecting system—the pelvicalyceal system and upper two-thirds of the ureters dilate, more pronounced on the right side, stopping short at the pelvic brim. The dilation starts in the first trimester; up to 15% first-trimester ultrasound reveal hydronephrosis, that becomes more evident as pregnancy progresses. Primi gravidas are prone to developing hydronephrosis. Serial ultrasound measurements have reported a peak incidence of hydronephrosis around 28 weeks of gestation. This dilatation is often called the "physiological hydronephrosis of pregnancy", as some degree of hydronephrosis can be observed in >80% of pregnant women by the third trimester.

The hydronephrosis is attributed to the progesterone-mediated relaxation of the ureteric smooth muscles. However, the progesterone effect cannot explain the right-sided preponderance; instead, an obstructive cause might be responsible. The sigmoid colon tends to push the gravid uterus to the right side; the gravid uterus may compress the ureter as it crosses the pelvic brim. The other proposed reasons include compression of the right ureter by the iliac and ovarian vessels; the right ureter crosses these vessels at an acute angle, while the left ureter runs parallel to ovarian vessels.

PHYSIOLOGIC CHANGES

Renin–Angiotensin–Aldosterone System

The components of the renin–angiotensin–aldosterone system (RAAS) play an integral role in placentation as well as the maintenance of pregnancy. In pregnancy, almost all components of the RAAS are upregulated. As early as 4 weeks, systemic vasodilatation and decreased SVR are seen, presumably due to angiotensin 1 (AT1)-mediated vasodilator effects. Due to systemic vasodilatation, RAAS gets activated. The uteroplacental unit also contributes to RAAS activation. Renin levels are increased due to extrarenal synthesis by ovaries and the maternal decidua. The circulating estrogen increases the hepatic angiotensinogen levels, leading to high AT and increased aldosterone levels. The elevated RAAS components are essential for maintaining the enhanced intravascular volumes needed for the smooth completion of pregnancy. Despite the overall upregulation of RAAS, the maternal vasculature remains refractory to the pressor effects. The increased progesterone and prostacyclin levels due to pregnancy reduce the AT receptor sensitivity and upregulate the vasodilatory AT2 receptors. Also, there is a predominance of monomeric AT1 receptors that are more labile to oxidative stress, resulting in a reduced sensitivity to AT. In pathological conditions like preeclampsia, the maternal vasculature loses its refractoriness to RAAS. In pregnancy, the blood pressure decreases by about 10 mm Hg by the second trimester, with an average value of around 105/60 mm Hg.

Renal Plasma Flow, Filtration Fraction, and Glomerular Filtration Rate

As early as 5 weeks of gestation, there is increased cardiac output and reduced SVR. The vasodilatation of pregnancy is attributed to the effects of relaxin and nitric oxide. Relaxin is a peptide hormone produced by the corpus luteum and placenta in response to human chorionic gonadotropin (hCG). Relaxin increases endothelial nitric oxide production, leading to generalized renal vasodilation and decreased renal arteriolar resistance. As a result of these adaptive changes, the renal plasma flow increases up to 80% in pregnancy by the end of the first trimester.[1] The renal plasma flow remains around 30% higher than prepregnancy values between weeks 21 and 30; beyond 30 weeks, there is a relatively rapid fall, reducing below prepregnancy levels in early postpartum.

During the luteal phase of regular menstrual cycles, there is a marginal increase in glomerular filtration rate (GFR); in the case of conception, the GFR continues to increase. A 20% increment in GFR might be evident as early as 4 weeks after conception and reaches around 45% of the baseline by week 16. The GFR remains elevated, achieving a maximum increase of 40–50% above the

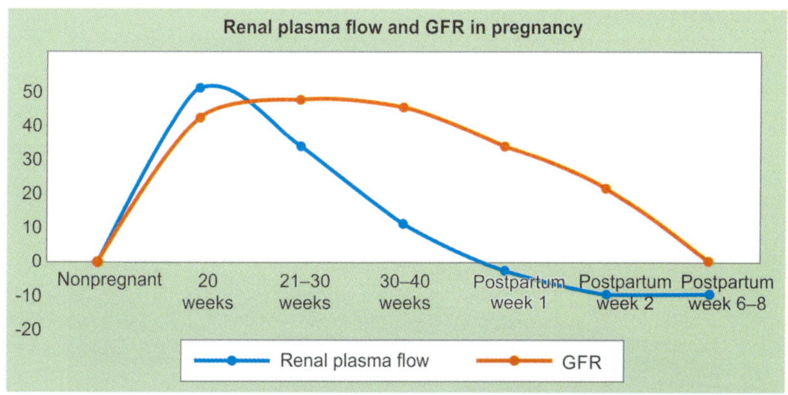

Fig. 1: Relationship between renal plasma flow and glomerular filtration rate (GFR).

baseline in the second trimester.[2] GFR and renal plasma flow exhibit a somewhat linear relationship until around 20 weeks of gestation **(Fig. 1)**. Despite the relative reductions in renal plasma flow in the third trimester and postpartum, the increment in GFR is sustained throughout. Immediate postpartum, the hyperfiltration continues at a 20% higher value than baseline and returns to prepregnant levels by 4 weeks. The compensatory increase in GFR is demonstrated in solitary kidneys and renal allografts despite already undergoing structural and functional hypertrophy.

The reasons for the increased GFR in pregnancy are poorly elucidated. Traditionally, the enhanced GFR in pregnancy had been solely attributed to the increased renal plasma flow. However, in early pregnancy, the increase in GFR (40–60%) always lags behind the observed increments in renal plasma flow (60–80%). Also, despite a rapid decline in renal plasma flow in the third trimester, the GFR elevations remain sustained, implying additional physiologic mechanisms. The forces determining the glomerular filtration are the same as those operating across other capillary beds. The forces affecting the GFR can be written as follows:

$GFR = K_f \times$ Net filtration pressure

- Net filtration pressure $= (P_{GC} - P_{BC}) - \pi_{GC}$

K_f: Ultrafiltration coefficient

P_{GC}: Capillary hydrostatic pressure

P_{BC}: Bowman's capsule hydrostatic pressure

π_{GC}: Glomerular capillary oncotic pressure

K_f is directly proportional to the glomerular capillary hydraulic conductivity and surface area. The capillary hydrostatic pressure favors ultrafiltration (UF), whereas the capillary oncotic pressure and Bowman's capsule hydrostatic pressure oppose UF. As the filtrate is protein-free, the contribution of Bowman's capsule oncotic pressure is negligible. Filtration continues till the net filtration pressure becomes zero (filtration equilibrium). As renal blood flow rates increase, the site of filtration equilibrium shifts distally toward the efferent arteriolar end.

Further, the hemodilution-induced reductions in capillary oncotic pressure ensure a higher net filtration pressure across the capillary bed **(Figs. 2A to C)**. Modest changes in K_f resulting from the increased capillary surface area and increased hydraulic permeability of capillaries also contribute. The contribution of the

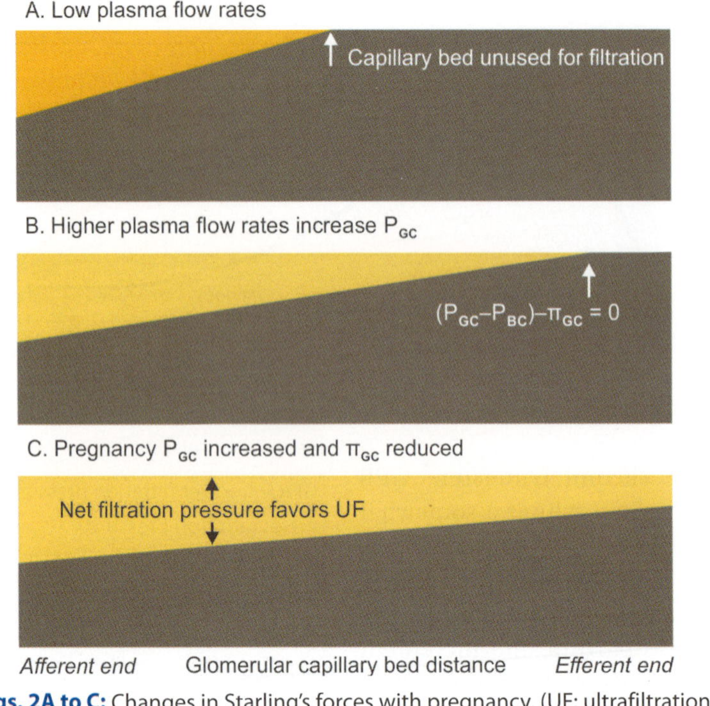

Figs. 2A to C: Changes in Starling's forces with pregnancy. (UF: ultrafiltration)

hydrostatic pressure gradient ($P_{GC} - P_{BC}$) is controversial due to a lack of experimental data. In a human study involving postpartum females, it has been demonstrated that changes in transcapillary hydrostatic pressure gradients account for 16% of enhanced GFR.[3]

Kidney Function Tests in Pregnancy

Glomerular filtration rate: The increase in the GFR leads to enhanced clearance of urea, uric acid, and serum creatinine. GFR estimating equations like modification of diet in renal disease study (MDRD) and chronic kidney disease epidemiology collaboration (CKD-EPI) underestimate the GFR in pregnancy. Also, serum cystatin C to estimate GFR has not been validated in pregnant females. Endogenous creatinine clearance, measured by 24-hour urine collection, is the standard technique for estimating GFR during pregnancy. However, it may be cumbersome for the patient; over- or undercollection is frequent; urinary stasis due to lower tract dilatation may compromise the results. Serum creatinine in pregnancy falls to around 86% or less of the nonpregnant upper normal limit. Hence, a serum creatinine of >0.8 mg/dL in a pregnant female should lead to an evaluation for an underlying renal disease.

Changes in Urinary Protein Excretion

There is an increase in proteinuria in pregnancy, especially after 20 weeks. The increased protein excretion is mainly attributed to increased GFR and consists mainly of Tam Horsfall protein with small amounts of albumin and other proteins.[4] Proteinuria continues to increase even after GFR starts falling in late pregnancy.[5] The potential reasons include elevated soluble antiangiogenic factors, alterations in glomerular charge, and defective tubular reabsorption contribute to protein excretion in pregnancy. During normal pregnancy, proteinuria can reach 200–260 mg/day by the end of the third trimester. The accepted cutoff to define significant proteinuria during pregnancy is >300 mg/24 hours. Even though the gold standard is 24-hour urine protein estimation, a urine protein creatinine ratio >0.3 is also considered significant.[6]

Changes in Water and Electrolytes

Water: Pregnancy is associated with reduced serum osmolality by 10 mOsm/kg and serum sodium by 4–5 mmol/L.[5] The fall in osmolality and serum sodium starts after conception and reaches a nadir by the 8th to 10th week of gestation. Multiple mechanisms increase the antidiuretic hormone (ADH)-mediated water reabsorption, amounting to reabsorption of an additional 6–8 L/day. The increased relaxin levels stimulate the posterior pituitary to release ADH. A downward reset of the hypothalamic osmoreceptors, mediated by hCG and relaxin in early pregnancy also contributes to enhanced water reabsorption.

Similarly, the thirst center is reset to respond to a lower threshold of serum osmolality. Towards peripartum, other non-osmotic stimuli like pain during delivery and sympathetic activation also contribute to higher arginine vasopressin (AVP) release high levels of oxytocin, secreted at parturition, can stimulate the V2 receptors in the kidney, facilitating water retention. On the other hand, toward the latter half of pregnancy, placental secretion of the ADH-metabolizing enzyme vasopressinase is increased by three to four times the basal values, creating a transient diabetes insipidus-like scenario.

Sodium: Pregnancy is associated with net sodium retention amounting to 1,000 mEq. The vasodilatation of pregnancy activates the sympathetic system and RAAS via the arterial baroreceptors; enhanced sympathetic and RAAS activity leads to elevated aldosterone levels. The placental/ovarian production of renin and increased angiotensinogen production by the liver also contribute to increased aldosterone levels. Deoxycorticosterone, a metabolite of progesterone, can stimulate the mineralocorticoid receptors in the kidney. Despite all these sodium-retaining mechanisms, fractional sodium excretion is higher than in nonpregnant states. Progesterone is a potent aldosterone antagonist, preventing the enhanced sodium reabsorption in the distal nephron. The rise in GFR leads to increased distal sodium delivery, potentiating renal excretion of sodium. The enhanced plasma volumes lead to a 40% increment in the atrial natriuretic peptide in the third trimester, facilitating sodium excretion. As a result of these changes, the outcome will be preferential water retention over sodium, leading to mild hyponatremia.[7]

Potassium: Pregnancy is associated with a net potassium gain of approximately 300 mEq/L. A third of this potassium is in the products of conception. The renal mechanisms responsible for potassium retention remain poorly defined. The progesterone acts as an aldosterone antagonist, reducing renal potassium excretion. However, the plasma levels fall despite potassium retention due to overall volume expansion.

Other divalent ions: Ionized calcium and phosphate levels are normal in pregnancy. The total calcium levels are low due to hypoalbuminemia-related reductions in the bound fraction and volume expansion.

The placenta secretes parathyroid hormone (PTH)-related peptides (PTHrPs) that stimulate 1α-alpha hydroxylase activity in the kidney. The placenta also secrete active vitamin D_3. This increases calcium absorption from the gut and finally leads to calciuria.[8] Total and ionized serum magnesium levels are marginally lowered due to hemodilution.

Changes in the Acid–base Balance

Progesterone increases the sensitivity of the medullary respiratory center to carbon dioxide, increasing the respiratory minute volume, leading to respiratory alkalosis. It also has an inhibitory effect on smooth muscle tone of the airways. The pressure on the diaphragm by the gravid uterus also contributes to hyperventilation and reduced pCO_2, eventually tilting the blood's pH toward the alkalotic side (7.4–7.47). Usually, $PaCO_2$ is reduced to 27–32 mm Hg, and a normal value should alert an early respiratory decompensation.[9] There will be a compensatory increase in bicarbonate excretion by the kidneys to maintain the body's pH around the normal range. The mild alkaline shift in pH shifts the oxygen dissociation curve rightward, facilitating more oxygen extraction in the placenta and peripheral tissues. Pregnancy does not contribute to acidosis; however, patients are prone to starvation ketosis due to insulin resistance with increased counter-regulatory hormones.[10] Vomiting or reduced oral intake, particularly during the third trimester, can precipitate starvation ketosis, resulting in high anion gap metabolic acidosis. Other acid–base abnormalities like respiratory acidosis and metabolic alkalosis are rare and need evaluation for specific causes, as in a nonpregnant state. The serum albumin tends to fall in pregnancy, with the lowest values observed in the third trimester. Since albumin is a weak acid, a proportionate reduction in the serum anion gap is observed in pregnancy.

Changes in Tubular Function

There are alterations in the tubular functions of the kidney during pregnancy. Normoglycemia with glucosuria in pregnancy is observed due to increased GFR, causing increased filtered glucose load and defective tubular reabsorption.[11] Glucosuria is found at some point in about 50% of pregnant women, making it an insensitive marker of gestational diabetes mellitus. There is decreased fractional reabsorption of uric acid, amino acids, and β-microglobulin, which increases the excretion of these substances in the urine.

Endocrine changes during pregnancy: In healthy pregnancy, the levels of erythropoietin (EPO) increase by roughly two to four times during the early first trimester.[12] This increase is a response to the adaptive 40% increase in plasma volume and is directed at increasing the mass of red blood cells. PTH is suppressed to the lower range or slightly below the normal reference range in the first trimester, while the levels of PTHrP increase.[13] PTHrP, mostly derived from the placenta, is the primary hormonal regulator of calcium balance during pregnancy, reaching its highest levels in the third trimester. PTHrP replicates the impact of PTH on the kidneys and bone. The levels of 25-hydroxyvitamin D remain unaffected, while the levels of 1,25(OH)2 vitamin D increase due to the stimulation of 1-alpha hydroxylase by PTHrP and estrogen.[14] **Figure 3** shows physiological changes during pregnancy.

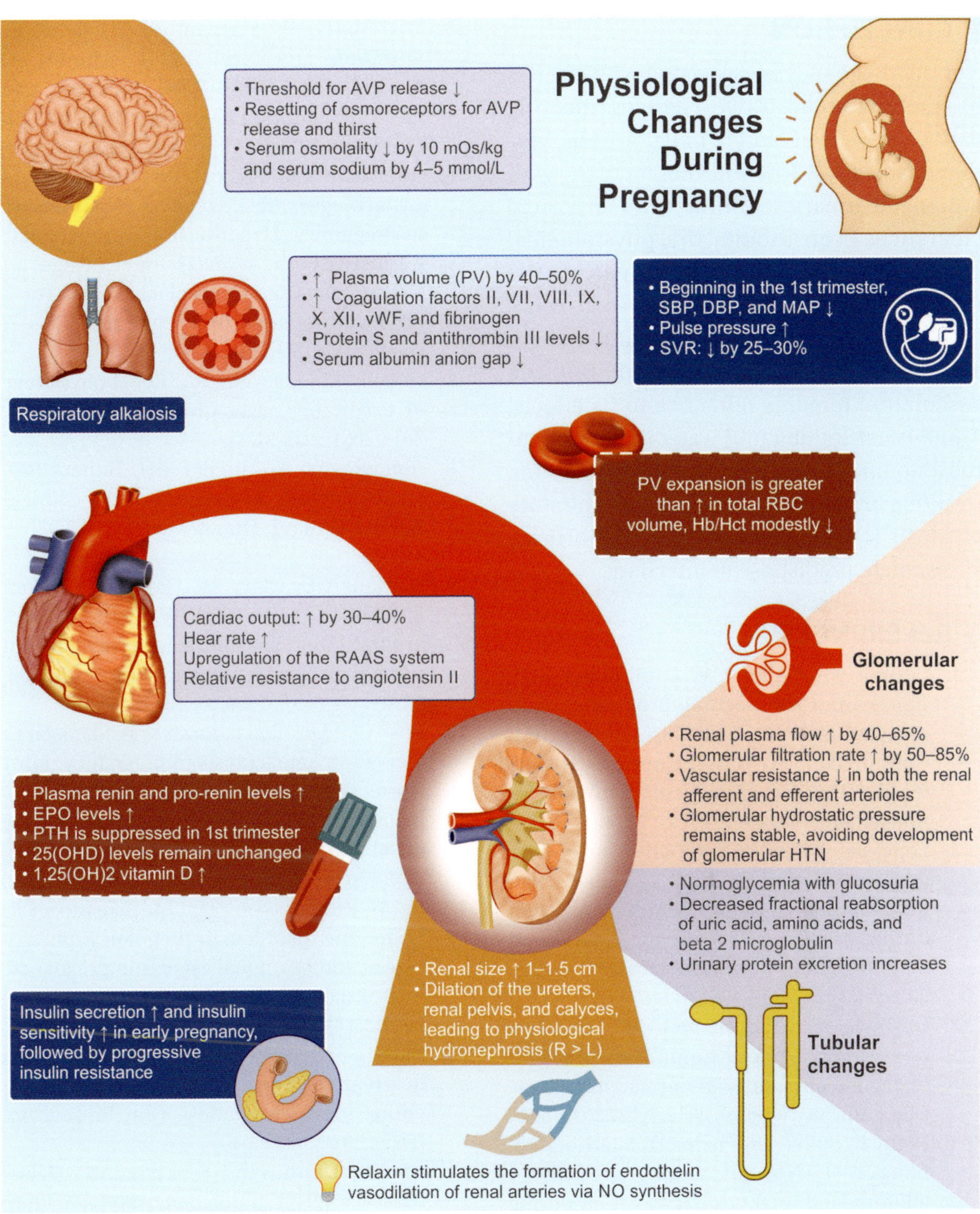

Fig. 3: Physiological changes during pregnancy. (AVP: arginine vasopressin; BP: blood pressure; DBP: diastolic blood pressure; EPO: erythropoietin; Hb: hemoglobin; HCT: hematocrit; HTN: hypertension; MAP: mean arterial pressure; NO: nitric oxide; PTH: parathyroid hormone; PV: plasma volume; RAAS: renin–angiotensin–aldosterone system; RBC: red blood cell; SBP: systolic blood pressure; SVR: systemic vascular resistance; vWf: von Willebrand factor)

Courtesy: Dr Priti Meena.

CONCLUSION

Normal pregnancy is associated with a series of carefully orchestrated changes affecting various aspects of kidney function **(Fig. 3)**—the renal plasma flow and GFR increase, with enhanced urea, creatinine, and uric acid clearance. Even though the physiological changes associated are delineated, the mechanisms behind the increased renal blood flow and GFR are poorly understood. The RAAS system is activated, but the vasculature remains refractive to its effects. There is net sodium and water retention, but the amount of water tends to surpass sodium, resulting in hyponatremia. A mild respiratory alkalosis is seen in pregnancy. The urinary stasis might predispose to infections.

REFERENCES

1. Conrad KP, Gaber LW, Lindheimer MD. The kidney in normal pregnancy and preeclampsia. In: Taylor RN, Roberts JM, Cunningham FG (Eds). Chesley's Hypertensive Disorders in Pregnancy, 4th edition. Amsterdam: Academic Press; 2014.
2. Lopes van Balen VA, van Gansewinkel TAG, de Haas S, Spaan JJ, Ghossein-Doha C, van Kuijk SMJ, et al. Maternal kidney function during pregnancy: systematic review and meta-analysis. Ultrasound Obstet Gynecol. 2019;54(3):297-307.
3. Odutayo A, Hladunewich M. Obstetric nephrology: renal hemodynamic and metabolic physiology in normal pregnancy. Clin J Am Soc Nephrol. 2012;7(12):2073-80.
4. Higby K, Suiter CR, Phelps JY, SilerKhodr T, Langer O. Normal values of urinary albumin and total protein excretion during pregnancy. Am J Obstet Gynecol. 1994;171: 984-9.
5. Yoshimatsu J, Matsumoto H, Goto K, Shimano M, Narahara H, Ahmed A. Fetomaternal Acid-Base Balance and Electrolytes during Pregnancy. Indian J Crit Care Med. 2021;25(Suppl 3):S193-9.
6. American College of Obstetricians and Gynecologists. Task Force on Hypertension in Pregnancy. Hypertension in pregnancy. Report of the American College of Obstetricians and Gynecologists' Task Force on Hypertension in Pregnancy. Obstet Gynecol. 2013;122:1122-31.
7. Cheung KL, Lafayette RA. Renal physiology of pregnancy. Adv Chronic Kidney Dis. 2013;20(3):209-14.
8. Almaghamsi A, Almalki MH, Buhary BM. Hypocalcemia in Pregnancy: A Clinical Review Update. Oman Med J. 2018;33(6): 453-62.
9. Hankins GD, Clark SL, Harvey CJ, Uckan EM, Cotton D, Van Hook JW. Third-trimester arterial blood gas and acid base values in normal pregnancy at moderate altitude. Obstet Gynecol. 1996;88(3):347-50.
10. Frise CJ, Mackillop L, Joash K, Williamson C. Starvation ketoacidosis in pregnancy. Eur J Obstet Gynaecol Reprod Biol. 2013;167:1-7.
11. Bishop JH, Green R. Glucose handling by distal portions of the nephron during pregnancy in the rat. J Physiol. 1983;336(1):131-42.
12. Feldt-Rasmussen U, Mathiesen ER. Endocrine disorders in pregnancy: physiological and hormonal aspects of pregnancy. Best Pract Res Clin Endocrinol Metab. 2011;25(6):875-84.
13. Morton A, Teasdale S. Physiological changes in pregnancy and their influence on the endocrine investigation. Clin Endocrinol (Oxf). 2022;96(1):3-11.
14. Ali DS, Dandurand K, Khan AA. Hypoparathyroidism in pregnancy and lactation: Current approach to diagnosis and management. J Clin Med. 2021;10:1378.

CHAPTER 2

Electrolyte and Metabolic Abnormalities in Pregnancy

Aisha Batool, Anna Gaddy

HIGHLIGHTS

- Management of metabolic and electrolyte disorders during pregnancy requires the clinician to differentiate physiologic changes of pregnancy from pathologic processes.
- The renin–angiotensin–aldosterone system (RAAS) is typically upregulated in a normal pregnancy via increase in renin, angiotensin, and aldosterone levels; however, blood pressure does not rise due to downregulation of angiotensin II receptors, reduced sensitivity of arterial smooth muscle, and secretion of vasodilatory mediators.
- The balance of several natriuretic and antinatriuretic factors results in sodium and water retention, with net result of lower serum sodium around 130 mmol/L.
- During pregnancy, a rise of hematocrit and serum albumin from baseline is strongly indicative of volume contraction.

INTRODUCTION

Pregnancy is a state of many physiologic changes to meet the requirements of the gravida and fetus. While many of these changes are of survival benefit, metabolic and electrolyte disorders outside the range of normal during pregnancy affect fetal and maternal outcomes. It is of prime importance to differentiate physiologic changes from pathological illnesses for best patient management and outcomes.

HEMODYNAMIC CHANGES AND UPREGULATION OF THE RENIN–ANGIOTENSIN–ALDOSTERONE SYSTEM

With the start of pregnancy, progesterone, prostaglandins and nitric oxide exert their vasodilatory effects leading to peripheral vasodilation and decreased systemic vascular resistance (SVR). Peripheral vasodilation is also responsible for decrease of blood pressure early in pregnancy, an effect which reaches its peak of physiologic hypotension by 20–24 weeks of gestation.[1-2] Simultaneously, sympathetic activity increases, and an increased heart rate leads to a 20% increase in cardiac output. These physiologic changes lead to an underfilled intravascular compartment, causing a compensatory increase in plasma volume via the upregulation of the renin–angiotensin–aldosterone system (RAAS) **(Fig. 1)**.

This activation of the RAAS system happens in a series of steps. Firstly, estrogen produced by the placenta increases the synthesis of angiotensinogen by the liver, which results in an increase in circulating angiotensin II. Secondly, renin is released

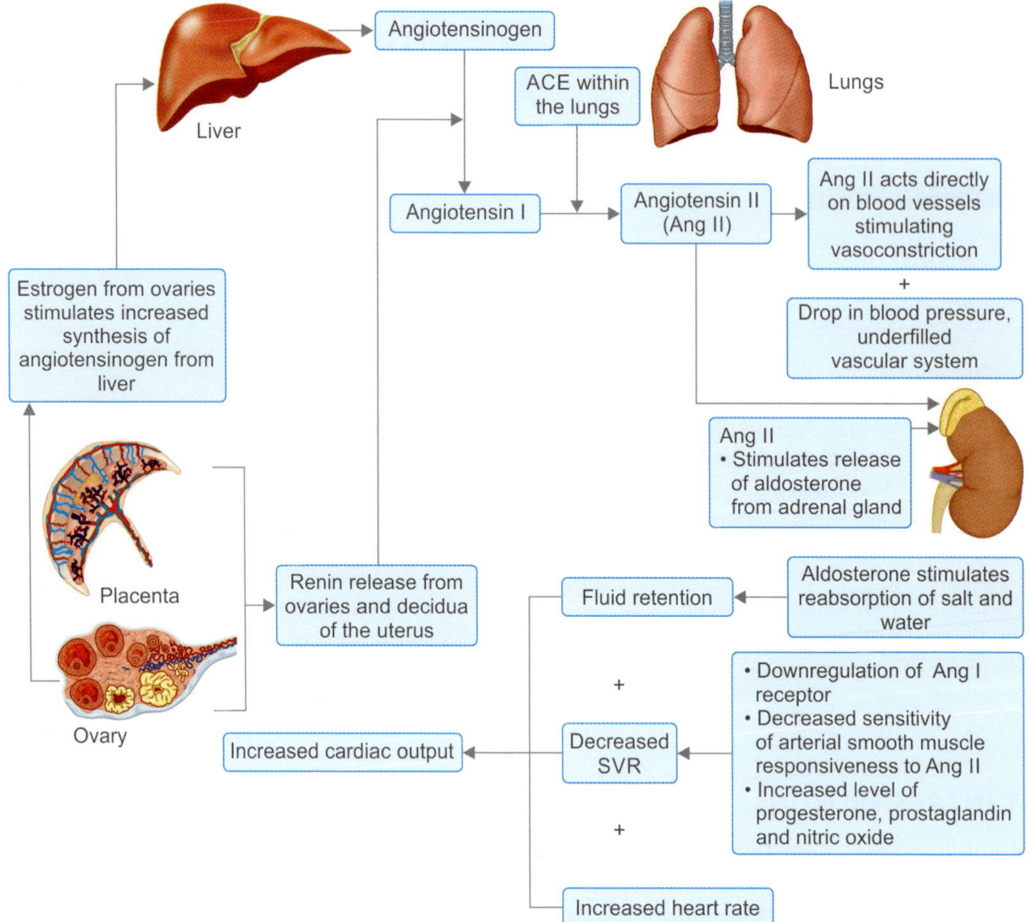

Fig. 1: Upregulation of the renin–angiotensin–aldosterone system (RAAS) during pregnancy. (ACE: angiotensin converting enzyme; Ang: angiotensinogen; SVR: systemic vascular resistance)

from the ovaries and decidua of the uterus. Thirdly, renin is released from the juxtaglomerular apparatus in response to the underfilled vascular system as described above. The aldosterone level can start rising as soon as 8 weeks of gestation and can reach three to six times the upper limit of normal in the third trimester. All these physiologic changes result in an increase in plasma volume by at least 1.5 L approximately (40–50% above nonpregnant volume). These mechanisms protect against pathologic hypotension but do not typically result in hypertension during pregnancy. A healthy pregnancy is associated with the downregulation of angiotensin I receptors, reduced sensitivity of arterial smooth muscles, and hence reduced responsiveness to angiotensin II. Clinically, this has been noted in pregnant patients requiring dramatically higher doses of angiotensin infusions when in shock.[4]

An increase in plasma volume is evident in a "dilutional" reduction in sodium concentration (135–138 mEq/L rather than 135–145 mEq/L in a nonpregnant state), hence mildly reducing serum osmolarity

TABLE 1: List of natriuretic and antinatriuretic factors affecting sodium and water homeostasis during pregnancy.

Natriuretic factors	*Antinatriuretic factors*
Increased GFR	Decreased blood pressure
Progesterone	Aldosterone
ANP	Angiotensin II
Nitric oxide	Estrogen
Prostaglandins	Deoxycorticosterone
	Placental shunting
	Upregulation of ENaC

(ANP: atrial natriuretic peptide; ENaC: epithelial sodium channels; GFR: glomerular filtration rate)

as well (approximately 280 mOsm/L).[3-7] There is also dilutional anemia, stimulating increased maternal erythropoietin production and an increase in RBC mass by up to 30% approximately. This compensation ameliorates but does not eliminate physiologic/dilutional anemia of pregnancy.

Table 1 shows a list of natriuretic and antinatriuretic factors affecting sodium and water homeostasis during pregnancy.

EFFECT ON GLOMERULAR FILTRATION RATE

Vasodilation of afferent and efferent arterioles along with increased cardiac output leads to increased renal plasma flow by approximately 80% (thereby resulting in a decreased filtration fraction). Despite increased renal plasma flow, there is no change in glomerular pressure because of equal dilation of the preglomerular and postglomerular resistance vessels.[4,5] This leads to at least a 50% increase in glomerular filtration rate (GFR) and subsequent decrease in serum creatinine. It has been proposed that serum creatinine of >0.8 mg/dL in a pregnant patient may indicate an underlying renal dysfunction. The increase in clearance has a significant effect on the elimination of renally cleared medications and also is reflected in increased urinary glucose and protein.

Progesterone, atrial natriuretic peptide (ANP), and prostaglandins all promote natriuresis, which is balanced by the upregulation of RAAS favoring sodium and water retention.[7-10] Given the underestimation of true GFR by both Modification of Diet in Renal Disease (MDRD) and Chronic Kidney Disease Epidemiology Collaboration (CKD-EPI) formulae, it remains challenging to conventionally estimate renal clearance in a pregnant woman. Other biomarkers, such as cystatin C, have not been validated for use in pregnancy. The use of inulin or creatinine clearance remains the only reliable method to measure true GFR, and the change in $eGFR_{Cr}$ or trend of $eGFR_{Cr}$ remains the most useful predictor of renal function as pregnancy advances.

EFFECT ON RENAL VOLUME AND COLLECTING SYSTEM

During pregnancy, there is a physiological increase in kidney volume by 30% and size by 1–1.5 cm. This is thought to be secondary to increased vascular volume and not nephron mass. The combined effects of progesterone and relaxin on smooth muscles are also seen in the urinary collecting system (postulated impaired peristalsis). This combined effect leads to dilation of the collecting system, causing stasis of urine (the dilated urinary system can hold up to 200–300 mL of urine) and thereby predisposing to urinary tract infections. This change is responsible for the recommendation to treat asymptomatic bacteriuria in pregnant patients. Dilation of the urinary collecting system is observed more on the right side and is attributed to the physiologic uterine position of dextrorotation and compression by iliac vessels.[2-6]

SODIUM AND WATER HOMEOSTASIS

Sodium and water homeostasis in pregnancy is a balance of several natriuretic and antinatriuretic factors as described below. Filtered solute load increases as a result of increased GFR; however, tubular reabsorption is also increased. As a result, serum sodium starting early in normal pregnancy is 4–5 mmol/L below nonpregnant levels, reflected by a decrease in serum osmolality by 10 mOsm/kg (270 mOsm/kg).[6] This is not corrected by intake due to altered thirst mechanism during pregnancy. It is proposed that β-human chorionic gonadotropin (β-hCG) and relaxin may play a role in resetting osmotic and thirst mechanisms. Systemic vasodilation and thereby underfilled state result in the release of arginine vasopressin (AVP), resulting in decreased serum sodium. At the same time, increase in GFR and elevated progesterone cause natriuresis. This is balanced by increased sodium reabsorption via angiotensin II, aldosterone, increased deoxycorticosterone, and upregulation of epithelial sodium channel (ENaC). The balance of these factors is such that there is a gradual net gain in total body sodium of about 900–1,000 mmol and a much larger water gain resulting in a net decrease in serum sodium level.[11-15]

During pregnancy, an adequate intravascular volume plays an essential role in preserving GFR. Due to vasodilatory state and later compression by gravid uterus, peripheral edema is seen in a normal pregnancy and hence this finding should not be utilized for assessing volume status. In patients with preexisting chronic kidney disease (CKD), baseline hematocrit and serum albumin should be measured in the first trimester. A relative rise of either value from the baseline is strongly indicative of volume contraction. However, a decrease in either value is not a predictor of volume expansion. **Figure 2** shows sodium and water homeostasis during pregnancy.

OSMOREGULATION AND STIMULATION OF ARGININE VASOPRESSIN

Arginine vasopressin release is decreased by serum osmolality and increased by nonosmotic stimuli such as arterial vasodilation-mediated neurohormonal and sympathetic system activation. Later, during delivery, pain and sympathetic stimulation further increases AVP secretion. There is also secretion of the enzyme vasopressinase by placental trophoblasts, which leads to increased degradation of AVP. The balance between these factors of increased release and increased degradation is such that serum sodium remains between 130 and 135 mmol/L. If serum sodium falls below 130, clinicians should identify a pathological cause.[11-15]

DISORDERS OF WATER AND SODIUM HOMEOSTASIS DURING PREGNANCY

Hyponatremia

Pregnant patients are prone to developing hyponatremia (defined as serum sodium <130 mmol/L during pregnancy). Major factors are poor intake during the first trimester due to nausea and vomiting; during the third trimester, pain-mediated AVP release plays a role as well. During delivery, excessive use of hypotonic saline and oxytocin (oxytocin is structurally similar to AVP and can stimulate AVP R2 receptors in renal collecting ducts, hence promoting fluid retention).[9-12] Sometimes, pregnancy can unmask prior subclinical hyponatremia due

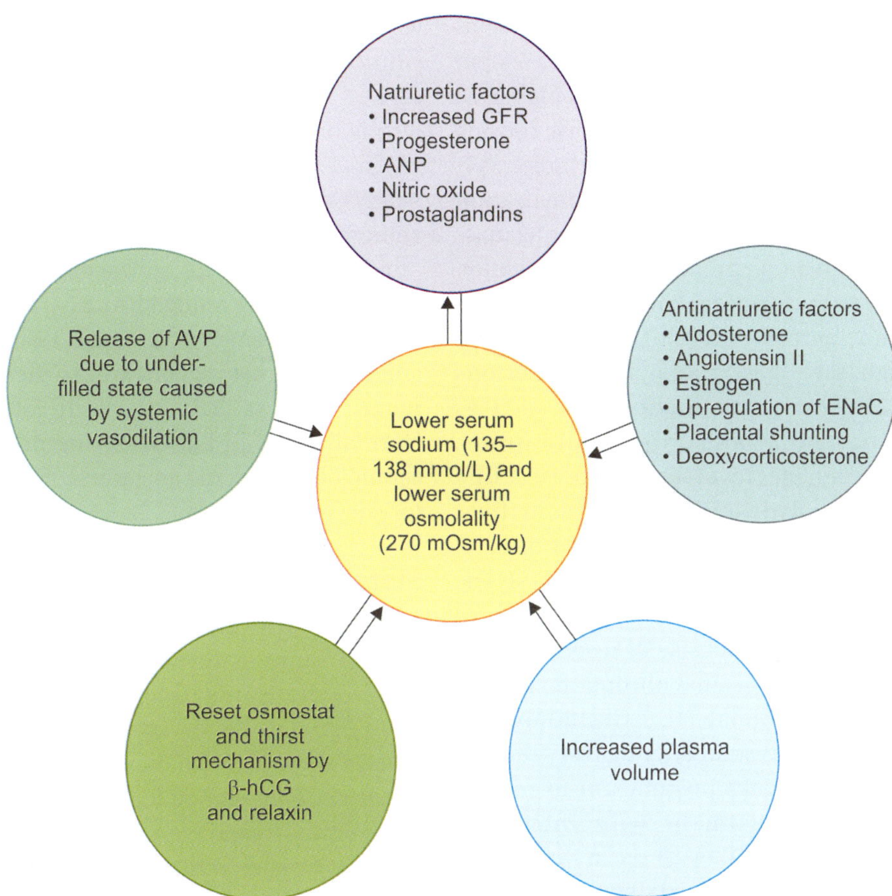

Fig. 2: Sodium and water homeostasis during pregnancy. (ANP: atrial natriuretic peptide; AVP: arginine vasopressin; ENaC: epithelial sodium channel; GFR: glomerular filtration rate; β-hCG: β-human chorionic gonadotropin)

to preexisting causes completely unrelated to the pregnant state; hence, the approach to hyponatremia during pregnancy should be in the standard protocol as in nonpregnant patients. Extra caution should be taken when restricting fluids in a pregnant patient who has euvolemic hypotonic hyponatremia [syndrome of inappropriate antidiuretic hormone (SIADH)]. This might put them at risk of dehydration and the fetus at risk as well, due to oligohydramnios. Therefore, water intake should be at least 1.5 L daily with close monitoring of ultrasound-guided amniotic fluid index.[16] However, acute hyponatremia below 120 mmol/L should be managed by hypertonic saline infusion, due to the high risk of convulsions. Serum sodium correction should not exceed 8–10 mEq/L in 24 hours. Babies born in these circumstances should be expected to have neonatal hyponatremia.[5,8,10]

Hypernatremia

Hypernatremia during pregnancy is uncommon and if present is typically iatrogenic, related to intravenous infusions (such as sodium bicarbonate infusion) or unmasking of preexisting etiologies such as central or nephrogenic diabetes insipidus (DI). Gestational DI is rare, occurring in 2–6 cases per 100,000 pregnancies. It is caused by increased secretion of placental vasopressinase causing increased degradation of the hormone AVP, causing polyuria resulting in dehydration and hypernatremia. Increased placental mass such as in twin pregnancies and conception via in vitro fertilization are associated with an increased risk of gestational DI. Though rare, gestational DI has serious fetal and maternal implications such as hypernatremia and oligohydramnios. Vasopressinase level can also rise due to decreased degradation seen in liver dysfunction such as in chronic liver disease, preeclampsia, and HELLP (hemolysis, elevated liver enzymes, low platelet count) syndrome. Sudden release of vasopressinase as seen during placental abruption can also result in gestational DI.[17] Gestational DI typically resolves soon after delivery but can take up to 6 weeks postpartum to resolve completely. Treatment with intranasal desmopressin (DDAVP is a synthetic analog of AVP and is usually referred to as desmopressin) is effective because DDAVP is resistant to placental vasopressinase. DDAVP also lacks vasopressor activity and hence does not result in increased blood pressure or preeclampsia. Even though it has structural similarity to oxytocin, intranasal desmopressin is 75 times less potent than oxytocin and hence is not implicated in causing uterine contractions.[4-6]

ACID–BASE DISORDERS IN PREGNANCY

Respiratory Alkalosis

Respiratory alkalosis is a normal physiological response in pregnancy. During pregnancy, stimulation of the respiratory center by progesterone results in hyperventilation, which increases minute ventilation (Minute ventilation = Tidal volume × respiratory rate).[18,19] Minute ventilation increases during pregnancy mainly by increasing tidal volume, whereas respiratory rate remains nearly constant. The kidneys respond to this change by increasing bicarbonate excretion. An overall result of the above changes is that $PaCO_2$ is reduced to 27–32 mm Hg, serum bicarbonate level is 17–19 mmol/L, and resulting pH remains within the normal range (however slightly alkalotic 7.40–7.45). Normalization of $PaCO_2$ during pregnancy should be considered an early sign of respiratory decompensation.[5]

Metabolic Acidosis

Metabolic acidosis etiologies in pregnancy are the same as in nonpregnant patients; hence, the same diagnostic algorithm should be utilized. However, starvation ketosis during pregnancy requires special attention. Pregnant patients demonstrate an exaggerated response to fasting, since the metabolic milieu during pregnancy favors an insulin resistance state. Placental glucagon and placental lactogen act as counter-regulatory hormones resulting in increased degradation of fatty acids. This leads to an increased production of ketone bodies and a high anion gap metabolic acidosis.[20-25]

Metabolic Alkalosis

In pregnant patients, the etiologies of metabolic alkalosis are similar to nonpregnant patients. The most commonly seen causes are gastrointestinal or renal loss of acid- and chloride-rich fluid from vomiting or diuretics, respectively, which should be corrected with volume replacement with chloride-containing solution. Occasionally, alkalosis is the result of elevated aldosterone levels as discussed previously which should be corrected with potassium repletion as well as addressing the etiology of high aldosterone levels.[5,18-20]

Respiratory Acidosis

The most common cause of respiratory acidosis during pregnancy and the postpartum period is residual effects of anesthetics used during general anesthesia (uncommon) in patients undergoing cesarean section. Central nervous system (CNS) depression can occur from drugs (such as antiepileptics), respiratory muscle fatigue in patients with increased work of beathing, hypermagnesemia, or neurological disorders such as stroke or cerebral venous thrombosis.[18,19]

POTASSIUM HOMEOSTASIS

Pregnancy is a state of increased aldosterone levels, which together with mild alkalosis causes serum potassium to be at the lower limit of normal. Despite these changes, overt hypokalemia is uncommon in pregnancy. Progesterone is responsible for keeping potassium in the normal range partly due to antimineralocorticoid effects and partly due to progesterone-mediated inhibition of potassium excretion by renal tubules. In patients with hyperemesis gravidarum and starvation ketosis, careful supplementation of thiamine along with electrolytes and gradual increase in calorie intake should be followed given the risk of refeeding syndrome.[5,6,22,25]

CALCIUM HOMEOSTASIS (FIG. 3)

Serum ionized calcium is unchanged during pregnancy. However, total serum calcium is slightly decreased due to a decrease in serum albumin levels and also due to volume expansion. In pregnancy, calcium metabolism undergoes significant changes to promote fetal growth and skeletal development. The main factor affecting calcium metabolism is elevated 1,25-hydroxyvitamin D levels (active form of vitamin D) which results

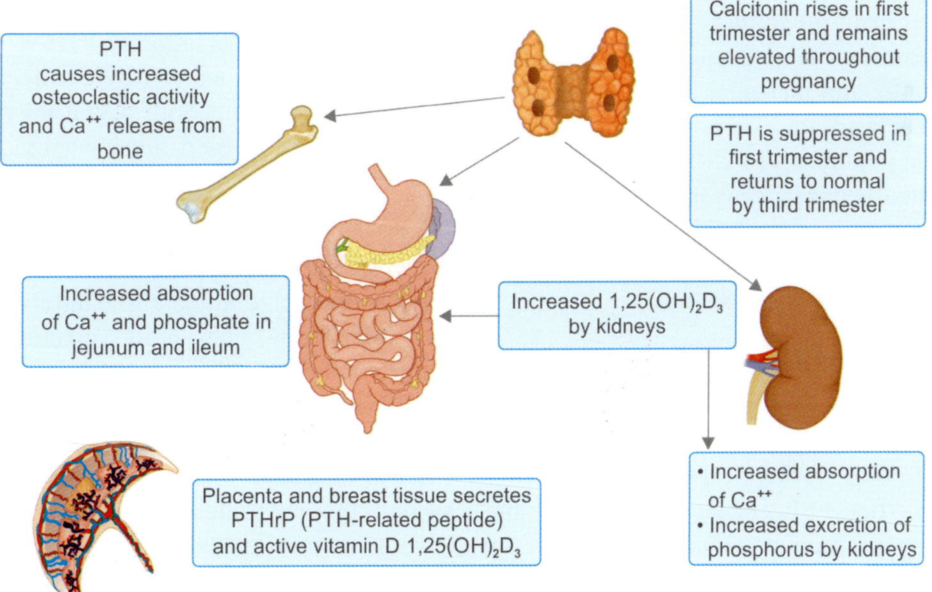

Fig. 3: Calcium homeostasis during pregnancy. (Ca: calcium; PTH: parathyroid hormone)

in increased calcium and phosphorous absorption in the gut. There is also increased 1,25-hydroxyvitamin D production in the kidneys of pregnant patients resulting in increased calcium absorption from the gut and increased urinary calcium excretion, commonly referred to as "absorptive calciuria of pregnancy".[26] This results in urinary calcium supersaturation; however, there is also increased urinary excretion of citrate, acidic glycoproteins, and nephrocalcin that help prevent calcium oxalate stone formation.[27]

Calcitonin also rises in the first trimester and remains elevated throughout pregnancy, as it is secreted by breasts and placenta during pregnancy. It prevents calcium release and bone remodeling of the maternal skeleton throughout pregnancy. Parathyroid hormone (PTH) is suppressed in the first trimester and returns to the mid-normal range by the third trimester. This results in increased calcium content of maternal bones in the first trimester, which will be utilized by the fetal skeleton later during pregnancy. Neither PTH nor calcitonin crosses the placenta. Estradiol, prolactin, and placental lactogen influence breasts and placenta to secrete PTH-related peptide and 1,25-hydroxyvitamin D. Elevated levels of both these factors result in calcium transport to the fetus against the concentration gradient (fetal calcium is higher than maternal calcium).

Hypocalcemia

The required daily calcium allowance in a nonpregnant state is 1 g/day, which increases to 1.2 g/day during pregnancy and further to 1.3 g/day during lactation. Hypocalcemia during pregnancy is mainly caused by low dietary calcium and vitamin D intake which results in lower fetal calcium levels, stimulating fetal PTH. This results in a cascade and many changes in fetal bony skeleton such as subperiosteal bone resorption. If maternal hypocalcemia is left untreated, intrauterine fracture of fetal ribs and limbs, bowing of long bones, and low birth weight can occur. Treatment is supplementation of calcium and vitamin D during pregnancy and postpartum.[27-30]

Hypercalcemia

Hypercalcemia during pregnancy, though rare, is a very serious condition causing adverse maternal–fetal outcomes. It usually presents with nonspecific symptoms such as nausea, vomiting, and generalized aches and often causes lethargy and depression, with or without anxiety. The mainstay of treating hypercalcemia during pregnancy remains hydration and calcitonin. Primary hyperparathyroidism which was previously undiagnosed can unmask itself during pregnancy. Parathyroidectomy, if indicated, is usually performed during the second trimester. During lactation, there is increased secretion of PTH-related peptide which can worsen hypercalcemia, especially in patients with primary hyperparathyroidism. These patients need to seek expert advice if planning to breastfeed.[31]

MAGNESIUM HOMEOSTASIS

Magnesium is predominantly an intracellular ion, and serum magnesium concentration is not a reliable marker of magnesium deficiency. It is an essential element for many enzymatic reactions and helps regulate vascular vasomotor tone. Magnesium homeostasis is poorly understood in pregnancy. Serum magnesium level is slightly lower in the pregnant state, attributed mainly to volume expansion leading to hemodilution.

Magnesium infusion is commonly utilized during preterm labor due to its effect of antagonizing calcium-induced uterine contractions. Infusions are also given for preeclampsia, during which it acts to inhibit endothelin I- and angiotensin II-mediated vasoconstriction as well as via less well-defined immunomodulatory action.[32]

Hypomagnesemia

Hypomagnesemia during pregnancy is usually associated with other coexisting electrolyte abnormalities due to either poor nutritional intake or hyperemesis gravidarum. Other common etiologies and presentations are similar to nonpregnant states and are managed in a similar manner.

Hypermagnesemia

Hypermagnesemia during pregnancy is exclusively iatrogenic due to the use of intravenous magnesium infusion during preterm labor or preeclampsia. Therapeutic level is usually kept in a range of 1.8–3.0 mmol/L, as higher levels can result in neurological complications. For example, serum magnesium levels higher than 3.5 mmol/L result in impaired deep tendon reflexes, and levels higher than 5 mmol/L can result in respiratory paralysis. Extremely high levels can lead to conduction abnormalities and cardiopulmonary arrest. Maternal magnesium infusion can sometimes lead to fetal hypermagnesemia as well, which is usually asymptomatic; however, extremely high levels can result in fetal hypotonia and CNS depression.

Uric Acid

Early in pregnancy, serum uric acid level usually falls to 2.0–3.0 mg/dL, attributed to volume expansion. In the later part of the second trimester, there is increased uric acid production due to placental trophoblast breakdown, ischemia, and release of cytokines. There is also increased renal tubular absorption of urates. By the end of the third trimester, serum uric acid is usually normalized to the nonpregnant state.[5]

Table 2 shows comparison of common laboratory parameters during pregnancy and nonpregnant state.

TABLE 2: Comparison of common laboratory parameters during pregnancy and nonpregnant state.

Laboratory parameter	*Nonpregnant state*	*During pregnancy*
Arterial pH	7.40	7.44
Arterial PCO_2 (mm Hg)	40	30
Serum bicarbonate (mmol/L)	24	20
Serum sodium (mmol/L)	140	135
Serum osmolality (mOsm/kg)	285	275
Serum total protein (g/dL)	7.0	6.0
Serum creatinine (mg/dL, µmol/L)	0.8 (73)	0.5 (45)
Blood urea nitrogen (mg/dL)	12.7	9.3
Serum uric acid (mg/dL)	4	Early: 3.2 Late: 4.3
Hematocrit (%)	41	33

REFERENCES

1. Poisner AM. The human placental renin-angiotensin system. Front Neuroendocrinol. 1998;19(3):232-52.
2. Langer B, Grima M, Coquard C, Bader AM, Schlaeder G, Imbs JL. Plasma active renin, angiotensin I, and angiotensin II during pregnancy and in preeclampsia. Obstet Gynecol. 1998;91(2):196-202.
3. Brown MA, Gallery ED, Ross MR, Esber RP. Sodium excretion in normal and hypertensive pregnancy: a prospective study. Am J Obstet Gynecol. 1988;159(2):297-307.
4. Gant NF, Worley RJ, Everett RB, MacDonald PC. Control of vascular responsiveness during human pregnancy. Kidney Int. 1980;18(2):253-8.
5. Teasdale S, Morton A. Changes in biochemical tests in pregnancy and their clinical significance. Obstet Med. 2018;11(4):160-70.
6. Wiles K, Chappell L, Clark K, Elman L, Hall M, Lightstone L, et al. Clinical practice guideline on pregnancy and renal disease. BMC Nephrol. 2019;20(1):401.
7. Belzile M, Pouliot A, Cumyn A, Côté AM. Renal physiology and fluid and electrolyte disorders in pregnancy. Best Pract Res Clin Obstet Gynaecol. 2019;57:1-14.
8. Brunton PJ, Arunachalam S, Russel JA. Control of neurohypophysial hormone secretion, blood osmolality and volume in pregnancy. J Physiol Pharmacol. 2008;59(Suppl 8):27-45.
9. Pazhayattil GS, Rastegar A, Brewster UC. Approach to the diagnosis and treatment of hyponatremia in pregnancy. Am J Kidney Dis. 2015;65(4):623-7.
10. Sutton RA, Schonholzer K, Kassen BO. Transient syndrome of inappropriate antidiuretic hormone secretion during pregnancy. Am J Kidney Dis. 1993;21:444-5.
11. Roberts TJ, Nijland MJM, Williams L, Ross MG. Fetal diuretic responses to maternal hyponatremia; contribution of placental sodium gradient. J Appl Physiol. 1999;87(4):1440-7.
12. Razavi AS, Chasen ST, Gyawali R, Kalish RB. Hyponatraemia associated with preeclampsia. J Perinat Med. 2017;45:467-70.
13. Sandhu G, Ramaiah S, Chan G, Meisels I. Pathophysiology and management of pre-eclampsia-associated severe hyponatremia. Am J Kidney Dis. 2010;55(3):599-603.
14. Joo KW, Jeon US, Kim GH, Park J, Oh YK, Kim YS, et al. Antiduiuretic action of oxytocin is associated with increased urinary excretion of aquaporin-2. Nephrol Dial Transplant. 2004;19:2480-6.
15. Knight S, Snellen H, Humphreys M, Baylis C. Increased renal phosphodiesterase-5 activity mediates the blunted natriuretic response to ANP in the pregnant rat. Am J Physiol Renal Physiol. 2007;292:F655-9.
16. Moen V, Brudin L, Rundgren M, Irestedt L. Hyponatraemia complicating labour - rare or unrecognised? A prospectional observational study. BJOG. 2009;116:552-61.
17. Ananthakrishnan S. Gestational diabetes insipidus: Diagnosis and management. Best Pract Res Clin Endocrinol Metab. 2020;34(5):101384.
18. Bobrowski RA. Pulmonary physiology in pregnancy. Clin Obstet Gynecol. 2010;53(2):285-300.
19. Barta V, Koncicki H. Electrolyte Disorders in Pregnancy. Obstet Gynecol Nephrol. 2019;11:113-27.
20. Lain K, Catalano PM. Metabolic changes in pregnancy. Clin Obstet Gynecol. 2007;50:938-48.
21. Frise CJ, Mackillop L, Joash K, Williamson C. Starvation ketoacidosis in pregnancy. Eur J Obstet Gynecol Reprod Biol. 2013;167(1):1-7.
22. Boelig RC, Barton SJ, Saccone G, Kelly AJ, Edwards SJ, Berghella V. Interventions for treating hyperemesis gravidarum: a Cochrane systematic review and meta-analysis. J Matern Fetal Neonatal Med. 2018;31(18):2492-505.
23. Chauhan SP, Perry KG, McLaughlin BN, Roberts WE, Cullivan CA, Morrison JC. Diabetic ketoacidosis complicating pregnancy. J Perinatol. 1996;16:173-5.

24. Sibai BM, Viteri OA. Diabetic ketoacidosis in pregnancy. Obstet Gynecol 2014;123: 167-78.
25. Owen OE, Caprio S, Reichard GA Jr, et al. Ketosis of starvation: a revisit and new perspectives. Clin Endocrinol Metab. 1983;12:359-79.
26. Cross NA, Hillman LS, Allen SH, Krause GF, Vieira NE. Calcium homeostasis and bone metabolism during pregnancy, lactation, and postweaning: a longitudinal study. Am J Clin Nutr. 1995;61(3): 514-23.
27. Semins MJ, Matlaga BR. Management of urolithiasis in pregnancy. Int J Womens Health. 2013;5:599-604.
28. Rosenberg E, Sergienko R, Abu-Ghanem S, Wiznitzer A. Nephrolithiasis during pregnancy: characteristics, complications, and pregnancy outcome. World J Urol. 2011; 29(6):743-47.
29. Hatswell BL, Allan CA, Teng J, Wong P, Ebeling PR, Wallace EM, et al. Management of hypoparathyroidism in pregnancy and lactation - A report of 10 cases. Bone Rep. 2015;3:15-9.
30. Bilezikian JP, Khan A, Potts JT, Jr, Brandi ML, Clarke BL, Shoback D, et al. Hypoparathyroidism in the adult: epidemiology, diagnosis, pathophysiology, target-organ involvement, treatment, and challenges for future research. J Bone Miner Res. 2011;26(10):2317-37.
31. Appelman-Dijkstra NM, Ertl DA, Zillikens MC, Rjenmark L, Winter EM. Hypercalcemia during pregnancy: management and outcomes for mother and child. Endocrine. 2021;71(3):604-10.
32. Dalton LM, Ní Fhloinn DM, Gaydadzhieva GT, Mazurkiewicz OM, Leeson H, Wright CP. Magnesium in pregnancy. Nutr Rev. 2016; 74(9):549-57.

CHAPTER 3

Hypertensive Disorders of Pregnancy

Manisha Sahay, Sakthi Rajagopal

HIGHLIGHTS

- Hypertensive disorders of pregnancy (HDP) are associated with significant risk of adverse maternal and fetal outcomes.
- Hypertensive disorders of pregnancy are categorized into four types: (1) preeclampsia, (2) gestational hypertension, (3) superimposed preeclampsia, and (4) chronic hypertension.
- Preeclampsia is diagnosed by hypertension after 20 weeks of gestation accompanied by proteinuria, organ damage, or uteroplacental dysfunction.
- Home blood pressure monitoring aids in managing chronic hypertension and is essential for white coat hypertension management.
- Severe hypertension (>160/110 mm Hg) in any HDP necessitates urgent treatment in a monitored setting using agents like oral nifedipine, intravenous labetalol, or hydralazine.
- The presence of chronic hypertension, gestational hypertension, or preeclampsia is associated with long-term maternal cardiovascular risks.

INTRODUCTION

Hypertensive disorders of pregnancy (HDP) complicate 10% pregnancies each year and are a major cause of maternal and fetal morbidity and mortality worldwide.

The physiological decrease in systemic vascular resistance during pregnancy results in a decline in blood pressure, reaching its nadir at 16–18 weeks of gestation and gradually returns to pre-pregnancy levels by the third trimester. This decrease primarily affects diastolic blood pressure, with reductions of up to 20 mm Hg being more pronounced compared to systolic blood pressure.

Hypertensive disorders are characterized by a BP ≥140/90 mm Hg on two occasions at least 4 hours apart.

American College of Obstetrics and Gynecology (ACOG), International Society for the Study of Hypertension in Pregnancy, and National Institute of Clinical Excellence (NICE) have published updated guidance on the diagnosis and management of HDP.[1-3] As per the guidelines, the hypertensive disorders can be classified as under.

CLASSIFICATION (FIG. 1)

- *Chronic hypertension (CHTN):*
    - Chronic hypertension with superimposed preeclampsia (PE)
- Gestational hypertension (GHTN)
- *Preeclampsia:*
    - Without severe features
    - With severe features

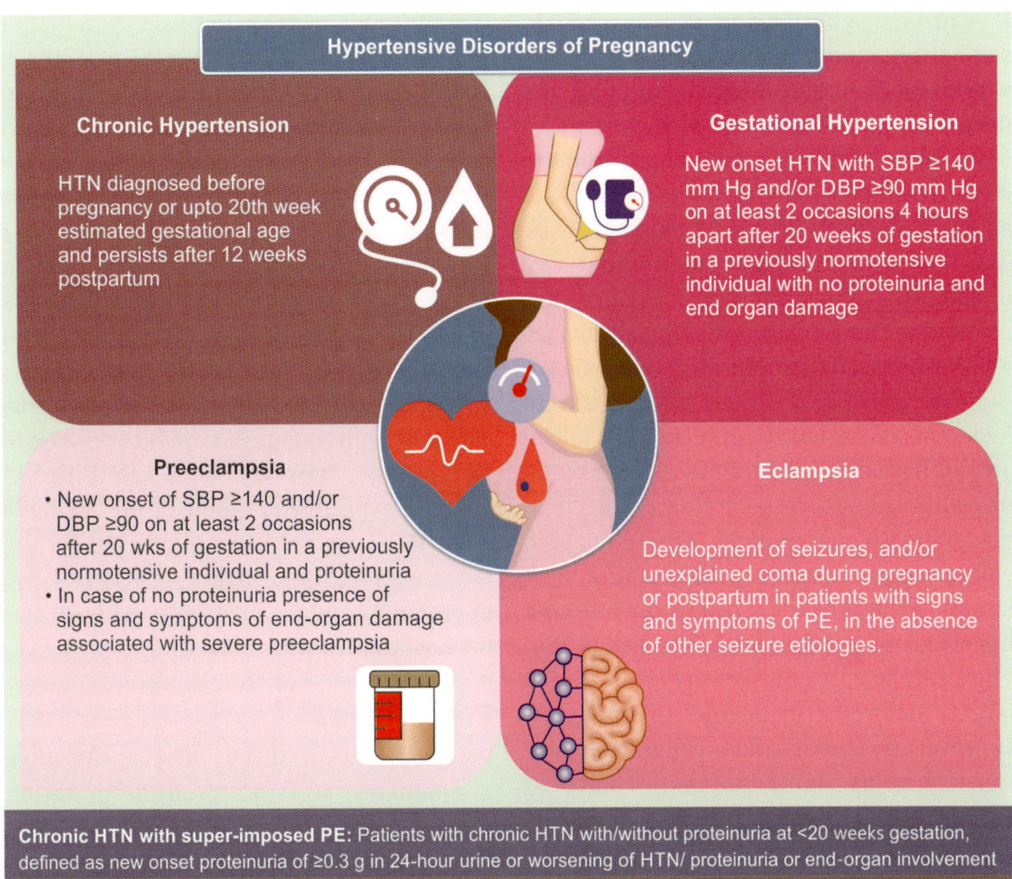

Fig. 1: Classification of hypertensive disorders of pregnancy. (DBP: diastolic blood pressure; GHTN: gestational hypertension; HELLP: hemolysis, elevated liver enzymes, and low platelets; HTN: hypertension; PE: preeclampsia; SBP: systolic blood pressure)

- Eclampsia
- Hemolysis, elevated liver enzymes, and low platelets (HELLP)

Chronic Hypertension

Chronic hypertension is defined as blood pressure exceeding 140/90 mm Hg before pregnancy or before 20 weeks' gestation. Chronic hypertension is a primary disorder in 90–95% of cases or may be secondary to some identifiable underlying disorder in 10% cases. Secondary hypertension is usually suspected where maternal age is <35 years, hypertension is severe or unresponsive to treatment, there is an absence of familial hypertension history, or laboratory findings suggest hypokalemia, elevated creatinine, or albuminuria in early course of pregnancy. Additionally, the rising prevalence of obesity among women of reproductive age underscores the potential significance of obstructive sleep apnea in contributing to secondary hypertension during pregnancy.

Chronic hypertension in nonpregnant state also includes white coat hypertension where blood pressure is high in the clinic and normal at home and masked hypertension when BP is higher at home and normal in clinic. White coat hypertension is linked with an elevated risk of PE. Home blood pressure monitoring (HBPM) becomes imperative in managing white coat hypertension, as it is prudent to refrain from initiating antihypertensive therapy when home BP measurements indicate normalcy. Unless there is severe hypertension (≥160/110 mm Hg), it is advisable to base decisions on the average blood pressure readings over several days rather than reacting to isolated readings. When compared with pregnant women with gestational or chronic hypertension, those with white coat hypertension exhibited a lower risk of PE.[4] The prevalence of masked hypertension is largely unknown in normal pregnancies. However, the identification of masked hypertension holds significant importance in pregnant women at high risk, as it can serve as a robust and independent indicator for the onset of PE and adverse neonatal outcomes.[5] Diagnosis typically involves HBPM or ambulatory blood pressure monitoring (ABPM) initiated upon detecting evidence of hypertensive-related organ damage in the mother [such as unexplained chronic kidney disease (CKD) or left ventricular hypertrophy] or uteroplacental dysfunction despite no apparent hypertension during clinical visits. Thus, the use of ABPM in pregnancy has added value in diagnosis of white coat hypertension and masked hypertension.

Gestational Hypertension

Gestational hypertension refers to hypertension (≥140 mm Hg systolic or 90 mm Hg diastolic on two separate occasions at least 4 hours apart) with onset in the latter part of pregnancy (>20 weeks' gestation). Alternately, a patient with systolic blood pressure >160 mm Hg or diastolic blood pressure >110 mm Hg can be confirmed to have GHTN if she has a similar pressure after a short interval. GHTN occurs without any other features of PE and followed by normalization of the blood pressure postpartum. It occurs in 6% of all pregnancies. Of women who initially present with apparent GHTN, about one-third may develop preeclampsia. The pathophysiology of GHTN is unknown. GHTN may, however, be a harbinger of chronic hypertension later in life. Patients with HDP have a 2.4-fold higher risk for the development of new hypertension 10 years later, compared with patients who do not have such a history.

Preeclampsia[6-10]

Preeclampsia specifically affects 2–8% of all pregnancies, and 14% multiple gestation pregnancies. It also recurs in 18% of cases. PE presents as a multifaceted medical condition. It is essentially hypertension accompanied by proteinuria or other organ damage such as maternal acute kidney injury, liver abnormalities, neurological manifestations, hemolysis or low platelet count, or fetal growth restriction. Mostly PE stems from placental issues as there is rapid alleviation of clinical symptoms following placental delivery. Details of PE pathogenesis, diagnosis, and treatment are provided in Chapters 4 and 5.

Preeclampsia superimposed upon chronic hypertension is diagnosed when PE occurs in a patient with pre-existing chronic hypertension. It is characterized by worsening or resistant hypertension (especially acutely), the new onset of proteinuria or a sudden increase in proteinuria, and/or significant new end-organ dysfunction after 20 weeks of gestation or postpartum in a patient with chronic hypertension.

DIFFERENTIAL DIAGNOSIS

Hypertension before pregnancy or before 20 weeks gestation is chronic HTN, GHTN occurs after 20 weeks but without end-organ damage while PE occurs after 20 weeks but is accompanied by end-organ damage.

Other conditions such as acute fatty liver of pregnancy, thrombotic thrombocytopenic purpura (TTP), hemolytic uremic syndrome (HUS), and exacerbation of systemic lupus erythematosus (SLE) or pre-existing renal disease can manifest as hypertension and should be considered and ruled out in the differential diagnosis **(Table 1)**.

BIOMARKERS AND EARLY PREDICTION OF PE

In GHTN or women with chronic hypertension, "triple test" [comprising maternal factors, mean arterial pressure, uterine artery pulsatility index, and placental growth factor (PlGF)] may be a useful tool for diagnosis of superimposed PE.

The updated NICE guideline on hypertension in pregnancy recommends a single PlGF-based test at the time of presentation

TABLE 1: Differential diagnosis of hypertension in peripartum period.

	Onset	*HTN*	*Low platelets*	*Elevated liver enzymes*	*Coagulopathy*	*Course*
PE	80% antepartum, 20% post-partum	100%	15%	10%	23%	Improves by 3rd day of postpartum
HELLP	Postpartum 92%	98%	78%	73%	56%	Improves by 3–5 days postpartum
APH	Antepartum	10%	2%	7%	2%	
PPH	Postpartum	2%	3%	11%	3%	
Acute fatty liver of pregnancy (AFLP)	3rd trimester	20%	5%	High bilirubin, and liver enzymes	Yes	Improves after delivery
Lupus nephritis	Any time	60%	20%	20%	10%	Urine RBC+, low complement Improves with steroids
Sepsis	Postpartum 79%	20%	17%	32%	36%	Antibiotics
Hemolytic uremic syndrome (HUS)	Majority post-partum	98%	65%	2%	2%	Worsens after delivery, plasmapheresis, eculizumab for Rx

(APH: antepartum hemorrhage; HELLP: hemolysis, elevated liver enzymes and low platelets; HTN: hypertension; PE: preeclampsia; PPH: postpartum hemorrhage)

with suspected preterm PE between 20 and 34 + 6 weeks' gestation.[10] Prediction of short-term outcome in pregnant women with suspected preeclampsia (PROGNOSIS) study showed that sFlt-1:PlGF ratios of 38 or lower have a high negative predictive value for diagnosing superimposed PE within 1 week.[11]

MANAGEMENT OF HYPERTENSIVE DISORDERS OF PREGNANCY

The goal of management is to maintain a safe blood pressure and diagnose superimposed PE early and maternal safety with delivery of healthy newborn.

Antenatal Care

There are very few indications for immediate delivery in chronic hypertension or GHTN (listed down). Expectant management is indicated for majority of women with chronic HTN, GHTN, or even superimposed PE without severe features. Expectant management can be as an outpatient (OP) or inpatient (IP).

Outpatient Management

This can be done if there are no severe features of superimposed PE. The patient should reside near the hospital and should have some attendants at home. In May 2023, US-FDA approved sFlt-1:PlGF test for ruling out PE. If ratio is <40, and patient is stable, and she can be managed at home with careful follow-up as the risk of developing PE with severe features in the next 2 weeks is <5%. Management of patients with a ratio >40 is unclear since the PPV is only 65%; decision-making depends on patient's clinical scenario. Patients should be made aware of features of severe PE.

Outpatient management includes:

Regular maternal surveillance: BP measurements should be done twice a day at home (and twice a week in clinic). Laboratory assessments (platelet count, serum creatinine, and liver enzymes) should be done twice a week. Though other blood tests may be abnormal, i.e., lactate dehydrogenase, hemoglobin, schistocytes, these are not routinely advised for OP management. Urine protein-creatinine ratio (UPCR) is used for diagnosis of superimposed PE but is not repeated as it has no prognostic value.

Regular fetal surveillance: Fetal kick count should be done daily. Fetal testing, i.e., nonstress test (NST) or biophysical profile (BPP) which is NST plus ultrasound are used to assess body movements, muscle tone, breathing movements, amniotic fluid, and heartbeat and should be performed at diagnosis and then every 2–4 weeks. Fetal testing should be performed promptly if there is an abrupt change in maternal condition or decreased fetal activity.

Evaluation of umbilical artery Doppler velocimetry indices is useful if fetal growth restriction is suspected.

Management of hypertension: Strict bed rest is not recommended. Lateral decubitus position while lying down is recommended as it improves blood flow.

Blood pressure targets: The debate surrounding the optimal blood pressure thresholds for initiating and titrating antihypertensive therapy during pregnancy remains unresolved, with differing recommendations from various medical societies approach. While the American College of Obstetricians and Gynecologists (ACOG) suggests initiating therapy at higher blood pressure levels, other organizations such as the International Society for the Study of Hypertension

TABLE 2: Recommendations from various guidelines about management of hypertension in pregnancy.

Guidelines	*Treatment threshold*	*Targets*
ACOG	• Treatment threshold ≥160/105 with diagnosis of chronic hypertension • ≥160/110 if acute chronic hypertension • A lower treatment threshold for chronic hypertension if comorbidities or renal failure is present	120–160/80–110 mm Hg
2021 International Society for the Study of Hypertension in Pregnancy	Severe hypertension of ≥160 mm Hg or diastolic blood pressure of ≥110 mm Hg requires urgent antihypertensive therapy	Antihypertensive therapy should aim to achieve a diastolic blood pressure target of 85 mm Hg, irrespective of systolic blood pressure as indicated by the CHIPS trial. Emphasizing this simplified focus on DBP led to effective control of SBP as well, resulting in a mean blood pressure of 133/85 mm Hg from randomization to delivery

(ACOG: American College of Obstetricians and Gynecologists; DBP: diastolic blood pressure; SBP: systolic blood pressure)

in Pregnancy (ISSHP) and the National Institute for Health and Care Excellence (NICE) advocate for a more aggressive stance, recommending treatment at lower thresholds. This is an important change from previous practice when treatment was recommended if blood pressure exceeded 150/100 mm Hg and reflects evidence from CHIPS (Control of Hypertension in Pregnancy Study)[12] **(Table 2)**. There are arguments that aggressive blood pressure control can mitigate severe hypertension and neurological complications associated with PE, potentially extending pregnancies and reducing the incidence of preterm births. This approach may be particularly crucial for women with multiple pregnancies, who face prolonged exposure to uncontrolled hypertension and heightened risks of immediate and postpartum complications. However, despite these arguments, there is a lack of conclusive evidence supporting the benefits of treating nonsevere hypertension during pregnancy, especially in young women without underlying cardiovascular risks. Moreover, concerns arise regarding potential fetal risks from aggressive maternal blood pressure control, such as reduced uteroplacental circulation and exposure to antihypertensive medications. Once antihypertensive treatment has been started, the target blood pressure is 135/85 mm Hg. Newer trials such as OPTIMUM and BUMP trial are exploring the impact of self-monitoring of BP during pregnancy.[13,14]

The revised NICE guidance recommends labetalol as the first-line treatment for hypertension in pregnancy, with nifedipine recommended if labetalol is not suitable and methyldopa recommended if neither labetalol or nifedipine is suitable or tolerated (anti-hypertensive therapy is discussed in the section under use of anti-hypertensives in pregnancy in this chapter). Sodium restriction below the recommended daily intake is not advised in GHTN while in chronic hypertension, salt restriction is recommended (NICE 2019). Diuretics have no role in routine therapy of hypertension and are indicated only for pulmonary edema. Volume expansion is not indicated.

Use of aspirin: Aspirin may have far-reaching effects in reducing both early onset PE and preterm birth and should be used in those with chronic hypertension from 12th week onward.

Inpatient Management

Hospitalization is recommended for those with severe features or those who are non-adherent to monitoring. Even in a hospital, the management can be expectant and immediate delivery may not be required unless indications for imminent delivery are present as listed below.

Fetal and maternal assessment: An initial assessment is conducted to determine eligibility for expectant management. Maternal stabilization, continuous monitoring of BP and symptoms, and laboratory evaluations are performed. Fetal ultrasound for estimated fetal weight is conducted, and continuous fetal monitoring is done until stability and eligibility for expectant management are confirmed.

The timing of delivery is based on specific indications:

- *Chronic hypertension controlled on medications:* 37–40 weeks
- *Gestational hypertension:* 37 weeks
- *PE without severe features:* 37 weeks (level A recommendation)
- *PE and GHTN with severe features and stable maternal and fetal conditions:* 34 weeks (level B recommendation)
- *PE with severe features, unstable or complicated, or before viability:* Delivery as soon as possible after maternal stabilization

Delivery should not be postponed beyond 37 weeks. Antenatal steroids are indicated if delivery is expected <1 week and gestation age is <34 weeks. Expectant management should be terminated if there is any indication for imminent delivery as listed below.

Indications for imminent delivery: Criteria for immediate delivery (within 48–72 hours) in PE are determined based on maternal and fetal factors.

- Development of PE with severe features at or beyond 34 weeks
- *Irrespective of gestation age:* Maternal indications include uncontrolled severe hypertension, eclampsia, persistent cerebral symptoms or abdominal pain refractory to treatment, pulmonary edema, placental abruption, HELLP syndrome, renal failure, stroke, or myocardial infarction. Fetal indications include persistent nonreassuring fetal status, lethal fetal anomalies, fetal death, or a previable fetus (<22 weeks). Delivery timing may be individualized based on maternal stability. The fullPIERS model[15] and PREP-S prediction model may be used to predict adverse outcomes and time the delivery.[16-20]

Intrapartum management: involves monitoring of blood pressure, neurologic examination, pulse oximetry, and fluid status in the mother and continuous fetal monitoring.

Postpartum management: Monitoring of blood pressures and symptoms is important. Those with superimposed preeclampsia or HELLP syndrome have regular monitoring of CBC and LFT every 12 hours at least till 3 days or till improvement. Antihypertensive medication is continued till hypertension persists. Patients should be called for follow-up visit in 3 days for those on medication and 7 days for those without medications. Methyldopa should be stopped in 2 days and if needed other anti-hypertensives should be used. If hypertension persists beyond 12 weeks postpartum, the diagnosis of chronic hypertension should be considered, and the patient should be referred to their primary care physician.

COMPLICATIONS

HELLP Syndrome

It is characterized by hemolysis [evidenced by schistocytes or helmet cells on peripheral smear, lactate dehydrogenase (LDH) >600 U/L, or bilirubin >1.2 mg/dL], elevated liver enzyme levels (twice normal values), and low platelets (platelet count <100,000/mm^3). The patient should be managed as severe PE.

Eclampsia

The aim is to provide supportive care and prevent maternal injury. Magnesium sulfate is used to prevent recurrent seizures (level A recommendation). Delivery should be performed after maternal stabilization. Eclampsia itself is not an indication of cesarean delivery. The method of delivery depends on factors such as gestational age, fetal presentation, and cervical examination. Head imaging and intubation may be considered in cases that are refractory to magnesium sulfate.

USES OF ANTIHYPERTENSIVE DRUGS DURING PREGNANCY

Initial antihypertensive therapy during pregnancy can involve monotherapy with a first-line drug, commonly either labetalol or methyldopa, as widely established. Some societies advocate for the use of nifedipine as an alternative initial therapy. Numerous clinical trials have compared various short-acting antihypertensives in cases of acute, severe hypertension during pregnancy. These trials often focus on parenteral hydralazine, parenteral labetalol, and oral nifedipine (in short-, intermediate-, or long-acting formulations).[21] See **Tables 3 and 4** for various drugs used in management of

TABLE 3: Drugs used in management of severe hypertension in pregnancy.

Drug	*Dose*	*Comments*	*Onset of action*
Labetalol	10–20 mg IV, then 20–80 mg every 10–30 minutes to a maximum cumulative dosage of 300 mg; or constant infusion 1–2 mg/min IV	• Tachycardia is less common with fewer adverse effects • Avoid in women with asthma, preexisting myocardial disease, decompensated cardiac function, and heart block and bradycardia	1–2 minutes
Hydralazine	5 mg IV or IM, then 5–10 mg IV every 20–40 minutes to a maximum cumulative dosage of 20 mg; or constant infusion of 0.5–10 mg/hour	Higher or frequent dosage associated with maternal hypotension, headaches, and abnormal fetal heart rate tracing; may be more common than other agents	10–20 minutes
Nifedipine (immediate release)	10–20 mg orally, repeat in 20 minutes if needed; then 10–20 mg every 2–6 hours; maximum daily dose is 180 mg	May observe reflex tachycardia and headaches	5–10 minutes

(IM: intramuscular; IV: intravenous)

TABLE 4: Drugs used in management of hypertension in pregnancy.

Drug	*Dosage*	*Comments*
Labetalol	• 200–2,400 mg/day orally in two to three divided doses • Commonly initiated at 100–200 mg twice daily	• Potential bronchoconstrictive effects • Avoid in women with asthma, pre-existing myocardial disease, decompensated cardiac function, and heart block and bradycardia
Nifedipine	• 30–120 mg/day orally of an extended-release preparation • Commonly initiated at 30–60 mg once daily (extended-release)	Do not use sublingual for immediate-release formulation should generally be reserved for control of severe, acutely, elevated blood pressures in hospitalized patients. Should be avoided in tachycardia
Methyldopa	• 500–3,000 mg/day orally in two to four divided doses • Commonly initiated at 250 mg twice or three times daily	Safety data up to 7 years of age in offspring. May not be as effective as other medications, especially in control of severe hypertension. Use limited by side effect profile (sedation, depression, and dizziness)
Hydrochlorothiazide	12.5–50 mg daily	Second-line or third-line agent

hypertension in pregnancy. A multicenter, parallel-group, open-label, randomized controlled trial compared nifedipine retard, methyldopa, and labetalol where they found that nifedipine retard demonstrated a higher frequency of reaching the primary outcome compared to labetalol or methyldopa.[22] In resource-limited settings, methyldopa, nifedipine, and labetalol are all considered viable initial options for treating severe hypertension. Limited data are available on the use of amlodipine or nicardipine in pregnancy.

Diuretics should be used cautiously in women with PE due to concerns about exacerbating volume depletion and promoting reactive vasoconstriction. However, recent guidelines suggest that diuretics may be safely used, albeit at lower doses, in women with salt-sensitive chronic hypertension or CKD and reduced glomerular filtration rate. NICE guidelines advise against the use of thiazide diuretics.

Regarding beta-blockers, metoprolol and pindolol are acceptable alternatives to labetalol based on limited data in pregnant patients, while atenolol and propranolol are generally avoided.

For resistant hypertension, additional agents such as clonidine and furosemide may be considered, although data on their efficacy are limited. Nitroprusside use is restricted in pregnancy due to limited clinical experience and the risk of fetal cyanide poisoning.

Intravenous hydralazine is an acceptable antihypertensive drug for acute severe hypertension during pregnancy, but its hypotensive response is less predictable than that of labetalol. However, its oral use is limited due to reflex tachycardia and fluid retention.

Safety profile of renin-angiotensin system blockers: Avoidance of renin-angiotensin-aldosterone system blockers (RAASB)[23,24] is advised during pregnancy, particularly in the second and third trimesters, as inhibiting the fetal renin-angiotensin system can disrupt kidney development and function. However, pregnancy is not necessarily contraindicated if someone is already taking these medications. While there is a well-established link between maternal use of RAASB in the later stages of pregnancy and fetopathy, the association with first-trimester use is less consistent and thus less certain. For individuals planning pregnancy while on RAASB, early detection of pregnancy is crucial to minimize embryonic exposure. If patients present in early pregnancy while on angiotensin-converting enzyme (ACE) inhibitors or angiotensin receptor blockers (ARBs), immediate discontinuation is recommended, with an alternative agent initiated if necessary. Common issues associated with exposure to ACE inhibitors or ARBs in the second and third trimesters include impaired fetal/neonatal kidney function, leading to oligohydramnios during pregnancy as well as anuria and kidney failure after birth. Histological lesions indicative of renal tubular dysgenesis have been observed in affected neonates. ACE inhibitors are excreted into breast milk, but levels in the milk are minimal. Captopril and enalapril are not expected to cause adverse effects in breastfed infants.

PROGNOSIS OF GESTATIONAL HYPERTENSION

Women with GHTN often have a positive prognosis; however, it is incorrect to assume that GHTN is simply less concerning than PE.[25] Studies indicate that GHTN is linked to adverse pregnancy outcomes and may not be entirely distinct from PE. It is noted that up to half of women with GHTN may eventually develop proteinuria or other signs of end-organ dysfunction consistent with PE, especially if hypertension is diagnosed before 32 weeks of gestation. It is recommended that women with GHTN presenting with severe blood pressure elevations should be managed similarly to those with severe PE. Furthermore, there is evidence suggesting that GHTN and PE may share similar long-term cardiovascular risks, including the development of chronic hypertension.

PROGNOSIS OF CHRONIC HYPERTENSION

It depends on the efficacy of control of hypertension and the underlying etiology. Chronic hypertension with superimposed PE can worsen the fetal and maternal prognosis as discussed above.

LONG-TERM FOLLOW-UP

Long-term follow-up is essential as CKD or recurrence of hypertension in next pregnancy can occur. Also gestation hypertension complicated by PE can be associated with CV disease, cognitive impairment. Children born to GHTN mothers with superimposed PE are often small for date (SFD) at risk of CKD and metabolic syndrome and need observation.

Hypertension is found to develop at higher frequencies among the women with HDP, with diagnosis occurring up to a decade earlier compared to those who experienced normotensive pregnancies. However, the exact timing necessitates further investigation. **Figure 2** shows maternal and fetal complications of HDP.

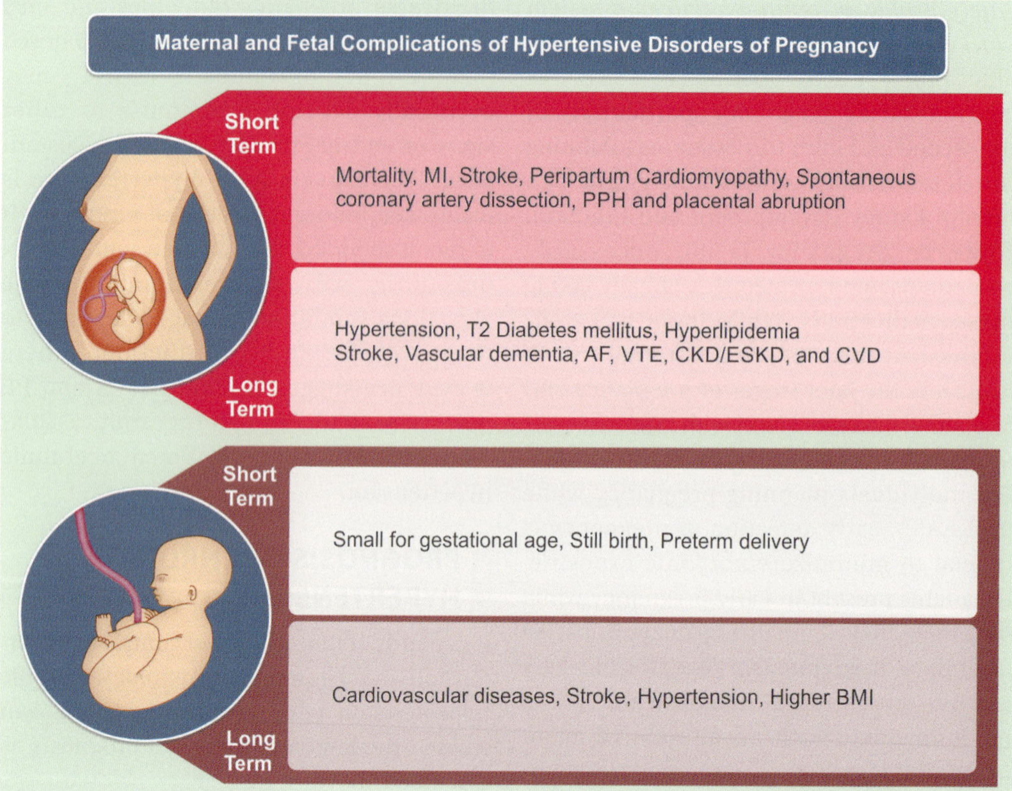

Fig. 2: Maternal and fetal complications of hypertensive disorders of pregnancy. (AF: atrial fibrillation; BMI: body mass index; CKD: chronic kidney disease; CVD: cardiovascular disease; ESKD: end-stage kidney disease; MI: myocardial infarction; PPH: postpartum hemorrhage; VTE: venous thromboembolism)

CONCLUSION

Hypertensive disorders of pregnancy are an important cause of maternal and fetal morbidity and mortality. GHTN may be a harbinger of chronic hypertension in later life. Women who develop superimposed PE over GHTN or chronic hypertension have reduced life expectancy, with increased risks of stroke, cardiovascular disease, and diabetes, while babies from a preeclamptic pregnancy have increased risks of preterm birth, perinatal death, neurodevelopmental delay, and cardiovascular and metabolic disease later in life. Angiogenic biomarkers accelerate diagnosis and minimize adverse maternal outcomes when used in the assessment of suspected disease. Their use will enable risk stratification and appropriate resource redistribution, and these are similarly recommended in updated national guidelines. New evidence is awaited regarding the impact of HBPM on severe hypertension and adverse outcomes. The CHIPS trial demonstrated better outcomes with tight blood pressure control in pregnancy hypertension, and this has been incorporated into national guidance. There is evidence regarding timing of delivery at 37 weeks' gestation in GHTN or chronic hypertension and between 34 and

37 weeks if superimposed PE, and shared decision-making with women regarding anti-hypertensive medication and timing of delivery is vital. Aspirin may have far-reaching effects in reducing both early onset PE and preterm birth.

REFERENCES

1. Brown MA, Magee LA, Kenny LC, Karumanchi SA, McCarthy FP, Saito S, et al. The hypertensive disorders of pregnancy: ISSHP classification, diagnosis and management recommendations for international practice. Pregnancy Hypertens. 2018:13;291-310.
2. Magee LA, Brown MA, Hall DR, Gupte S, Hennessy A, Karumanchi SA, et al. The 2021 International Society for the Study of Hypertension in Pregnancy classification, diagnosis & management recommendations for international practice. Pregnancy Hypertens. 2022;27:148-69.
3. Sinkey RG, Battarbee AN, Bello NA, Ives CW, Oparil S, Tita ATN. Prevention, diagnosis, and management of hypertensive disorders of pregnancy: a comparison of international guidelines. Curr Hypertens Rep. 2020;22:66.
4. Hadizadeh S, Shahmohamadi E, Khezerlouy-Aghdam N, Heidary L, Tarafdari A, Hantoushzadeh S, et al. Development of preeclampsia in pregnant women with white-coat hypertension: a systematic review and meta-analysis. Arch Gynecol Obstet. 2024;309(3):929-37.
5. Espeche WG, Salazar MR. Ambulatory Blood Pressure Monitoring for Diagnosis and Management of Hypertension in Pregnant Women. Diagnostics (Basel). 2023;13(8):1457.
6. American College of Obstetricians and Gynecologists. ACOG Practice Bulletin No. 203: Chronic Hypertension in Pregnancy. Obstet Gynecol. 2019;133:e26-50.
7. American College of Obstetricians and Gynecologists. ACOG practice bulletin No 202: gestational hypertension and pre-eclampsia. Obstet Gynecol. 2019;133:e1-e25.
8. Waugh J, Hooper R, Lamb E, Robson S, Shennan A, Milne F, et al. Spot protein-creatinine ratio and spot albumin-creatinine ratio in the assessment of pre-eclampsia: A diagnostic accuracy study with decision-analytic model-based economic evaluation and acceptability analysis (DAPPA). Health Technol Assess. 2017;21(61):1-90.
9. Phipps EA, Thadhani R, Benzing T, Karumanchi SA. Pre-eclampsia: pathogenesis, novel diagnostics and therapies. Nat Rev Nephrol. 2019;15(5):275-89.
10. Karumanchi SA. Angiogenic factors in pre-eclampsia: from diagnosis to therapy. Hypertension. 2016;67:1072-9.
11. Gray KJ, Saxena R, Karumanchi SA. Genetic predisposition to preeclampsia is conferred by fetal DNA variants near FLT1, a gene involved in the regulation of angiogenesis. Am J Obstet Gynecol. 2018;218:211-8.
12. Chappell LC, Duckworth S, Seed PT, Griffin M, Myers J, Mackillop L, et al. Diagnostic accuracy of placental growth factor in women with suspected preeclampsia: a prospective multicenter study (PELICAN). Circulation. 2013;128(19):2121-31.
13. Zeisler H, Llurba E, Chantraine F, Vatish M, Staff AC, Sennström M, et al. Predictive Value of the sFlt-1:PlGF Ratio in Women with Suspected Preeclampsia (PROGNOSIS). N Engl J Med. 2016;374(1):13-22.
14. Magee LA, von Dadelszen P, Rey E, Ross S, Asztalos E, Murphy KE, et al. Less-tight versus tight control of hypertension in pregnancy (CHIPS). N Engl J Med. 2015;372(5):407-17.
15. Pealing L. (2016). OPTIMUM Trial Protocol: Optimising titration and monitoring of maternal blood pressure. [online] Available from: https://www.isrctn.com/ISRCTN16018898. [Last accessed May, 2024]
16. University of Oxford. (2017). Blood Pressure Monitoring in High Risk Pregnancy to Improve the Detection and Monitoring of Hypertension (BUMP). [online] Available from: https://classic.clinicaltrials.gov/ct2/show/NCT03334149. [Last accessed May, 2024]

17. Ukah UV, Payne B, Karjalainen H, Kortelainen E, Seed PT, Conti-Ramsden FI, et al. Temporal and external validation of the fullPIERS model for the prediction of adverse maternal outcomes in women with pre-eclampsia. Pregnancy Hypertens. 2019;15:42-50.
18. Thangaratinam S, Allotey J, Marlin N, Mol BW, Von Dadelszen P, Ganzevoort W, et al. Development and validation of Prediction models for Risks of complications in Early-onset Pre-eclampsia (PREP): a prospective cohort study. Health Technol Assess. 2017; 21(18):1-100.
19. Webster K, Fishburn S, Maresh M, Findlay SC, Chappell LC; Guideline Committee. Diagnosis and management of hypertension in pregnancy: summary of updated NICE guidance. BMJ. 2019;366:l5119.
20. Broekhuijsen K, van Baaren GJ, van Pampus MG, Ganzevoort W, Sikkema JM, Woiski MD, et al. Immediate delivery versus expectant monitoring for hypertensive disorders of pregnancy between 34 and 37 weeks of gestation (HYPITAT-II): an open-label, randomised controlled trial. Lancet. 2015;385(9986):2492-501.
21. Awaludin A, Rahayu C, Daud NAA, Zakiyah N. Antihypertensive medications for severe hypertension in pregnancy: a systematic review and meta-analysis. Healthcare (Basel). 2022;10(2):325.
22. Easterling T, Mundle S, Bracken H, Parvekar S, Mool S, Magee LA, et al. Oral antihypertensive regimens (nifedipine retard, labetalol, and methyldopa) for management of severe hypertension in pregnancy: an open-label, randomised controlled trial. Lancet. 2019; 394(10203):1011-21.
23. Buawangpong N, Teekachunhatean S, Koonrungsesomboon N. Adverse pregnancy outcomes associated with first-trimester exposure to angiotensin-converting enzyme inhibitors or angiotensin II receptor blockers: a systematic review and meta-analysis. Pharmacol Res Perspect. 2020;8(5): e00644.
24. Karthikeyan VJ, Ferner RE, Baghdadi S, Lane DA, Lip GY, Beevers DG. Are angiotensin-converting enzyme inhibitors and angiotensin receptor blockers safe in pregnancy: a report of ninety-one pregnancies. J Hypertens. 2011;29(2): 396-9.
25. Saudan P, Brown MA, Buddle ML, Jones M. Does gestational hypertension become pre-eclampsia? Br J Obstet Gynaecol. 1998;105(11):1177-84.

CHAPTER 4

Preeclampsia: Pathogenesis

Natarajan Gopalakrishnan, S Jayalakshmi

HIGHLIGHTS

- Preeclampsia, the most common hypertensive disease of pregnancy, is a systemic disease with heterogeneous clinical and pathophysiological characteristics.
- Placenta plays a key role in the pathogenesis of preeclampsia. Defective placentation with consequent placental hypoperfusion ensues in the release of antiangiogenic factors causing endothelial dysfunction.
- Generalized endothelial dysfunction is the defining feature of preeclampsia which results in multiorgan dysfunction.
- The persistent residual endothelial dysfunction even after delivery predisposes for cardiovascular and renal risks in the long term.

INTRODUCTION

Preeclampsia is a hypertensive disorder of pregnancy, affecting 2–8% of all pregnancies with a potential for adverse impact on fetal and maternal outcomes and implications on long-term cardiovascular and renal health of the affected women.[1]

Preeclampsia is a systemic disease characterized by endothelial damage, thus having a potential to afflict multiple organs. The pathogenesis of preeclampsia is intriguing with a complex interplay of multiple factors.

PATHOGENESIS

There are two subtypes of preeclampsia with different timelines of occurrence during pregnancy.

Current knowledge indicates that "early" (<34 weeks of gestation) and "late" (>34 weeks of gestation) onset preeclampsias have different pathophysiologies.

In early preeclampsia, also known as "placental preeclampsia", a "two-stage" model is proposed. The first stage involves a defective/abnormal placentation, and the second stage represents the maternal response to placental stress.[2]

The core underlying issue is placental dysfunction occurring due to uteroplacental mismatch resulting either due to increased fetoplacental demand or decreased uteroplacental blood supply. The placental ischemia results in release of antiangiogenic factors like sFLT-1 (soluble *fms*-like tyrosine kinase-1) and soluble endoglin (sEng) with resultant endothelial dysfunction.

In late preeclampsia, also known as "maternal preeclampsia", there is no gross placental hypoperfusion. There is only minimal placental stress. It seems that there is genetic predisposition of the affected mothers for cardiovascular disease which manifests as preeclampsia during the stress of pregnancy.

Early Onset Preeclampsia: Central Role of Placenta

The first stage is characterized by defective placentation due to abnormal remodeling of uterine spiral arteries.

The second stage is the "maternal syndrome" comprising hypertension and varying degrees of multiple organ dysfunction (renal, neurological, cardiac, hepatic, and hematologic abnormalities).

For a successful pregnancy, establishment of a congenial interaction between the villi and the decidua during early stages of pregnancy itself is essential. In normal pregnancy, extravillous trophoblasts (EVTs) with invasive potential arise and migrate into the maternal spiral arteries converting them into high-capacity, low-resistance sinuses which aid in fetal nutrition at the fetomaternal interface. The EVTs invade deep, up to the inner third of myometrium, destroying the smooth muscle cells and elastin of the spiral arteries, replacing with inert fibrinoid material. Such a remodeling of spiral arteries results in dilatation of the terminal portions of the spiral arteries into funnel-shaped structures, increase in the blood flow, and reduction in the velocity and pulsatility of blood flow. These phenomena are essential to ensure adequate nutrition and to prevent damage to the delicate villi. To achieve appropriate spiral artery remodeling, several vasoactive substances, growth factors, proteases and adhesion molecules are secreted by the placenta and the vasculature.

Defective remodeling of spiral arteries, though not specific for preeclampsia, is considered as the crux of its pathophysiology.[3] Suboptimal trophoblast invasion results in narrow spiral arteries with ensuing placental ischemia **(Fig. 1)**.

Decidual Vasculopathy

In addition to being narrow, placental vasculature is afflicted with pathological changes, further compromising placental perfusion.

Decidual vasculopathy (DV) refers to pathological changes in the narrow spiral arteries and uterine radial arteries supplying the decidua, viz., (1) acute atherosis, (2) medial hypertrophy, and (3) perivascular infiltration with lymphocytes. DV is observed in disorders of placental insufficiency including preeclampsia and intrauterine growth restriction.[4] Presence of DV in preeclampsia is associated with higher diastolic blood pressure, severe renal involvement, and poor fetal outcome. It is debatable as to whether DV represents the cause or consequence of preeclampsia.

Genetics

A family history of preeclampsia, especially the early onset form, has been well recognized. But pregnancy also involves maternal–fetal gene interactions.[5] Paternal genetic influence is evident based on some observations. There is increased risk of preeclampsia with fathers born of preeclamptic pregnancy and those who fathered a preeclamptic pregnancy with another woman. This phenomenon is highlighted by the phrase—"dangerous father".[6] However, the maternal influence dominates with variance of heritability of preeclampsia estimated as 35% maternal, 20% fetal, 13% couple effect, and the rest attributed to other effects.

Studies of maternal genome could not succeed in identifying the genes associated with preeclampsia. However, genome-wide association study (GWAS) of fetal genome has identified a variant near the gene encoding Flt-1 (*Fms*-like tyrosine kinase-1), the receptor for vascular endothelial growth

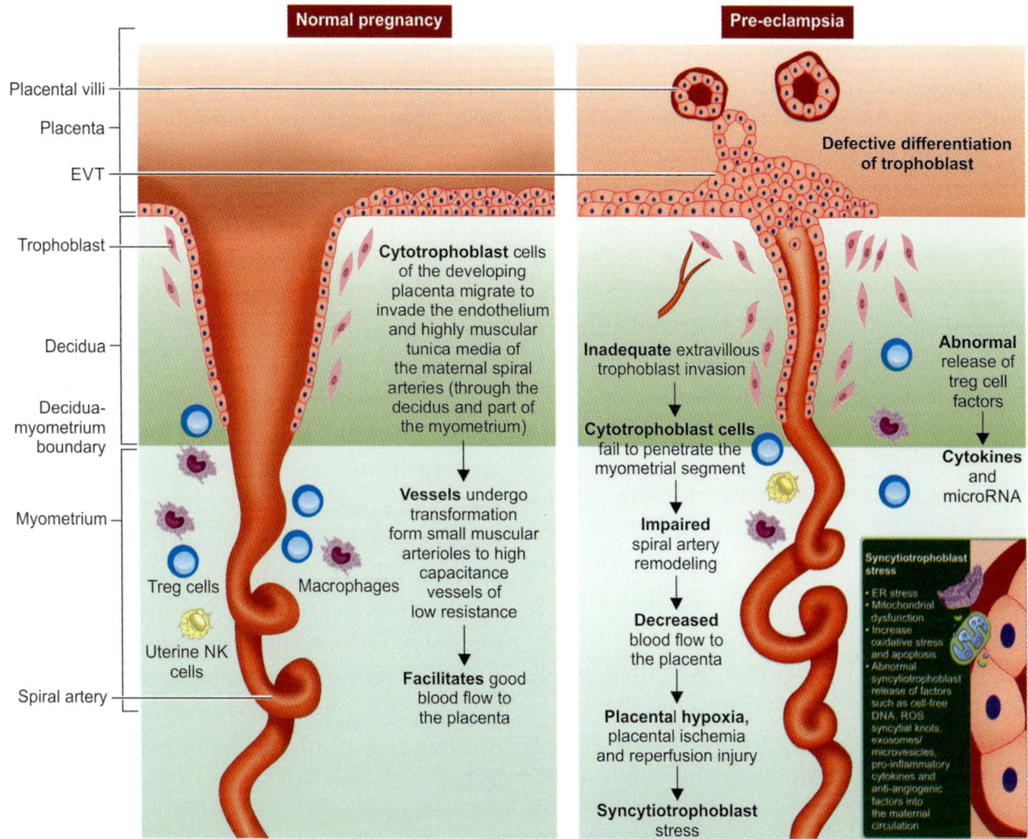

Fig. 1: Central role of placenta in pathogenesis of preeclampsia. (ER: endoplasmic reticulum; EVT: extravillous trophoblasts; NK cells: natural killer cells; ROS: reactive oxygen species; Treg cells: T regulatory cells)

factor (VEGF). The association was strongest with late-onset preeclampsia.[7]

Role of Nature Killer Cells

In immunological point of view, fetus is considered as an allograft. Allorecognition is mediated through interaction between the uterine natural killer cells (uNK cells) and the cytotrophoblast. NK cells, integral component of innate immunity, are potent cytotoxic cells. But uNK cells are not cytotoxic. uNK cells seem to regulate depth of placentation and spiral artery remodeling. Under the influence of progesterone and endometrium-derived interleukin-15, NK cells proliferate in the uterine mucosa during early pregnancy, dwindle in number from mid-gestation and disappear at term. NK cells exhibit KIRs, the killer immunoglobulin-like receptors. The maternal KIRs interact with the fetal human leukocyte antigen-C (HLA-C) molecules of paternal origin on the EVT. Some combinations of KIR and HLA-C are protective against preeclampsia while certain combinations confer risk of preeclampsia. Activation of uNK cells due to nonself HLA-C molecules seems to be essential for normal pregnancy.

Dysregulated Immune System

An abnormal and dysregulated immune system is likely to play a key role in the pathogenesis of preeclampsia. There is a dysregulation in the balance between proinflammatory and anti-inflammatory cytokines. A decrease in the secretion of the cytokine, IL-10, is observed in preeclampsia.[8] IL-10 neutralizes proinflammatory cytokines and mitigates maternal syndrome. IL-10 mediates the differentiation of T-cells into Th2 phenotype. Such a Th2 polarization is characteristic of normal pregnancy. In preeclampsia, an aberrant shift toward Th1 phenotype is observed resulting in insufficient trophoblast invasion.[9]

Complement

There is emerging evidence for the role of complement in preeclampsia. Complement gene abnormalities and/or increased complement activation during early pregnancy predispose for preeclampsia. Mutations in *C3* gene and genes encoding complement regulatory proteins (Factor I, Factor H, and CD46) have been observed in preeclamptic women. Complement gene abnormalities and resultant complement activation are more prominent in HELLP (hemolysis, elevated liver enzymes, and low platelet) phenotype of preeclampsia.[10]

In severe preeclampsia, C5a and soluble C5b-9 are significantly elevated suggesting a critical role for terminal complement pathway activation.[11]

C1q knockout mouse model mimics preeclampsia. C1q is constitutively expressed on the decidual endothelial cells, particularly at the contact sites with the EVT. C1q at the decidual endothelial cells does not seem to get activated. It acts as a molecular bridge between these cells favoring trophoblast invasion and vascular remodeling.[12]

Corin

Corin, a transmembrane enzyme that activates atrial natriuretic peptide, is localized to heart. But it has been found to have a role in trophoblast invasion and spiral artery remodeling also. Significantly decreased expression of corin mRNA in the uterus has been observed in preeclamptic patients.[13]

Hypoxia

Hypoxia plays a central role in the pathogenesis of preeclampsia. Upregulation of hypoxia-inducible transcription factors in the placenta has been noted in preeclampsia. During the early implantation, the gestational sac exists in a low oxygen tension atmosphere favoring trophoblast proliferation. With the formation of sinuses and arrival of maternal blood, there is increasing oxygen tension. The resultant oxidative stress serves as a stimulus for differentiation of trophoblasts from a proliferative to an invasive phenotype which subsequently invades and remodels spiral arteries. Hypoxia-inducible factor 1α and 2α are overexpressed in the proliferative trophoblasts in preeclampsia, indicating hypoxia.[14]

Heme Oxygenase-1

Heme oxygenase-1 (HO-1) plays an anti-inflammatory role and inhibits release of sFLT-1 and sEng via its metabolite, carbon monoxide (CO). In preeclampsia, there is downregulation of HO-1 with resultant augmented inflammatory state and diminution of antioxidant systems.[15]

Oxidative Stress

Low oxygen tension followed by maternal blood flow oxygenation results in normal placentation. Intermittent hypoxia followed by reoxygenation due to abnormal spiral arteries results in oxidative stress. Endoplasmic stress and mitochondrial stress too contribute to oxidative stress. In addition, antioxidant mechanisms are defective in placenta of preeclamptic patients with decreased expression of superoxide dismutase and glutathione peroxidase.

Syncytial Knots

When subjected to stress, syncytiotrophoblasts release "syncytial knots" into maternal circulation. Syncytial knots are nano to microvesicles which comprise exosomes, proinflammatory cytokines, fetal cell-free DNA, and antiangiogenic factors sFLT-1 and endoglin.[16] These factors cause maternal endothelial dysfunction and systemic inflammatory response. Syncytial knots are found in excess in early onset preeclampsia compared to late-onset preeclampsia. Syncytial knots would emerge as significant biomarkers of preeclampsia.

The stressor of trophoblast in early onset preeclampsia is uterine hypoperfusion secondary to defective remodeling of spiral arteries. In late-onset preeclampsia, the mismatch between maternal perfusion and the fetoplacental demand imposes stress on the trophoblasts.[17]

Placental Dysfunction

Placental ischemia and the consequent placental dysfunction result in release of antiangiogenic factors causing an imbalance between angiogenic and antiangiogenic factors **(Fig. 2)**. The major vasoactive substances of interest are VEGF, PlGF (placental growth factor), sFLT-1, and sEng.

Placental Growth Factor

Placental growth factor is expressed by the placenta, particularly by the syncytiotrophoblasts and also by the vascular endothelial cells. PlGF is an important factor for the normal development of placental vasculature. During normal pregnancy, PlGF starts appearing in maternal circulation at about

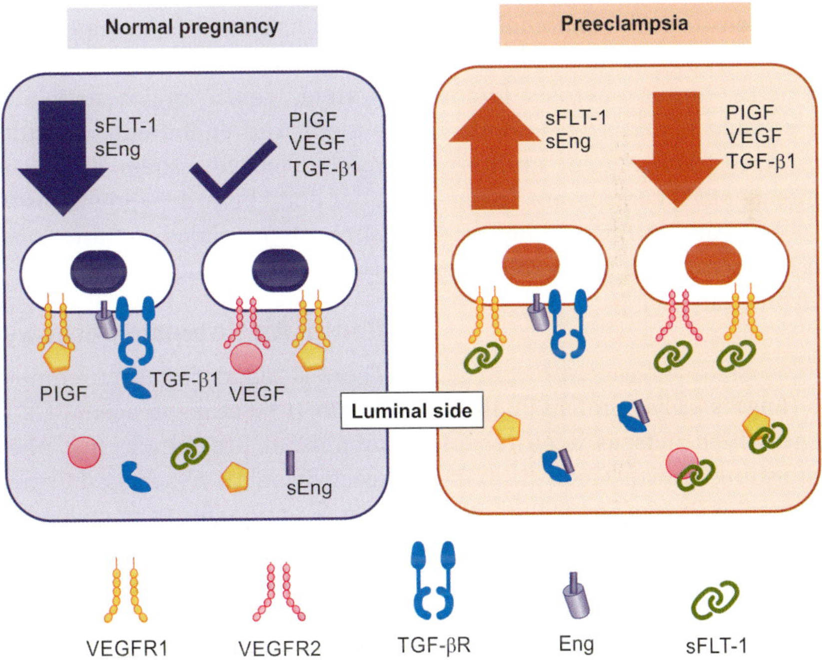

Fig. 2: Imbalance between angiogenic and antiangiogenic factors in preeclampsia. (PlGF: placental growth factor; sEng: soluble endoglin; sFLT-1: soluble fms-like tyrosine kinase 1; TGF: transforming growth factor; VEGF: vascular endothelial growth factor)

8 weeks, reaches a peak at the end of second trimester, and declines thereafter till delivery. In preeclampsia, there is decrease in PlGF levels.

Vascular Endothelial Growth Factor and sFLT-1

Vascular endothelial growth factor is a crucial angiogenic factor for development of placental vasculature and maintenance of normal endothelial function. In preeclampsia, the ischemic placenta liberates sFLT-1, which is a splice variant of VEGF receptor, FLT-1 (fms-like tyrosine kinase-1). sFLT-1 acts as a potent scavenger of VEGF and PlGF, thus preventing their interaction with endothelial receptors leading to endothelial dysfunction.[18]

Indirectly, sFLT-1 prevents the production of VEGF-induced nitric oxide (NO) with resultant exaggerated vasoconstriction and production of reactive oxygen species. Also, sFLT-1 sensitizes the endothelial cells of maternal vasculature to inflammatory cytokines like tumor necrosis factor-α (TNF-α) causing generalized endothelial dysfunction and subsequent multiorgan dysfunction.[19] sFLT-1 levels are found to be elevated as early as 5 weeks before the diagnosis of preeclampsia and correlate with severity of preeclampsia.[20]

Endoglin

Endoglin (Eng) is a glycoprotein on the cell membrane which acts as a co-receptor for transforming growth factor-β (TGF-β) receptor complex. It is expressed on monocytes and endothelial cells, particularly during neoangiogenesis and embryogenesis. The placenta, particularly the syncytiotrophoblast, is an important source of endoglin. The primary physiological roles of endoglin include endothelial cell differentiation and regulation of vascular tone. Proteolytic cleavage of endoglin results in sEng which interferes with TGF-β activity.[21]

Transforming growth factor-β is anti-inflammatory and a vasodilatory cytokine. Hence, disruption of TGF-β activity would result in vasoconstriction and endothelial dysfunction. sEng level in circulation is found to be higher even before clinical manifestations of preeclampsia and decreases after delivery.[22]

Elevated sFLT-1 and sEng act synergistically in severe forms of preeclampsia, the HELLP syndrome.

Autoantibodies to angiotensin II receptor (AT-1) stimulate the release of sEng while HO inhibits its release.

Disordered Vascular Milieu

In preeclampsia, there is generalized vasoconstriction, reduction in blood volume and blood flow to all organs. Systemic vasoconstriction is mediated by activation of neurohormonal systems, viz., sympathetic system, renin–angiotensin–aldosterone system, and endothelin. In addition, as a result of oxidative stress, there is diminution of endothelium-dependent vasodilatation, normally mediated by nitric oxide, VEGF, TGF-β, and prostaglandins.[23]

Renin–Angiotensin Pathway

There is reduced plasma renin and angiotensin II level in preeclampsia compared to normal pregnancy; but, the vascular reactivity to AII is increased in preeclampsia due to antibodies to angiotensin II type-1 receptors (AT-1 AA). These autoantibodies are formed by a subset of B-lymphocytes in response to placental ischemia and systemic inflammation. AT-1 AA induces release of antiangiogenic factors and contributes for hypertension.[24]

Kidney Dysfunction in Preeclampsia

Kidney dysfunction in preeclampsia occurs in very few patients; but the incidence is higher in patients with HELLP syndrome variant of preeclampsia.

There is reduction in the renal blood flow and glomerular filtration rate.[25]

The characteristic pathology is endothelial swelling (endotheliosis). Loss of podocytes, diffuse fibrin deposition, and loss of filtration space are noted.

Pregnancy is a procoagulant state, which gets further enhanced by the inflammatory milieu of preeclampsia. During pregnancy, the tissue factor released from decidua and placenta shifts endothelial cells to a procoagulant balance. Inflammatory cytokines of preeclampsia augment tissue factor expression by the endothelial cells and decrease anticoagulant activity with consequent diffuse microthrombi.

Kidney Involvement in Preeclampsia: Pathomechanism

It is well known that as in all other vascular systems, there is endothelial damage in kidneys too in preeclampsia. But current evidence indicates that there is injury to podocytes and slit diaphragm as well which results in proteinuria. Decrease in proangiogenic factors (VEGF and PlGF) and increase in antiangiogenic factors (sFLT-1—soluble fms-like tyrosine kinase-1, endoglin) result in endothelial dysfunction. The significant consequences of endothelial dysfunction include deficiency of nitric oxide due to downregulation of endothelial nitric oxide synthase, increased production of endothelin-1, and oxidative stress. All these result in structural and functional perturbations of podocytes and slit diaphragm[26] **(Flowchart 1)**.

Slit diaphragm is the most important functional component of glomerular filtration barrier. Nephrin is a critical component protein of the slit diaphragm.

Nephrin has an extracellular domain, transmembrane domain, and an intracellular domain. Nephrin is an important contributor for slit diaphragm network. In addition, with its interaction with other crucial proteins, nephrin plays a pivotal role in passage of information from the slit diaphragm to the contractile apparatus of podocytes. Disordered interaction between the slit diaphragm and the contractile element—actin of the foot process would lead to atrophy of foot process with subsequent

Flowchart 1: Pathogenesis of injury to podocytes and slit diaphragm in preeclampsia.

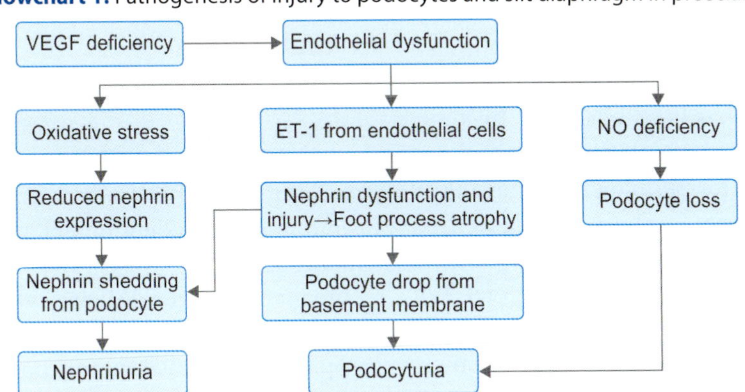

(ET-1: endothelin-1; NO: nitric oxide; VEGF: vascular endothelial growth factor)

detachment from the basement membrane. Nephrin also prevents apoptosis of podocytes.

Increased concentration of nephrin in blood and urine has been documented in preeclampsia. Increase in urinary nephrin level precedes onset of signs of preeclampsia by few days. Podocyturia and decreased expression of nephrin on the excreted podocytes also have been found in preeclampsia. Urinary podocyte and nephrin levels correlate with severity of preeclampsia. An increase in urinary podocin has been documented. Podocin remains bound to podocyte and its presence in the urine is associated with podocyturia.

From these observations, it is clear that there is injury and dysfunction of podocyte and slit diaphragm in preeclampsia. The following is the proposed pathogenic sequence of podocyte injury.

There is interdependence between endothelial cells and podocytes. In preeclampsia, there is increased production of endothelin-1 by endothelial cells. Endothelin, by causing activation of protease which cleaves the extracellular domain of nephrin, causes shedding of nephrin from podocytes.[27]

Some studies have asserted that podocyturia may precede other evidence of preeclampsia as an early marker of preeclampsia with high sensitivity and specificity. Podocyturia can be mechanistically linked to proteinuria and a good correlation between them has been observed. In some, podocyturia may persist after pregnancy and contribute for permanent kidney injury in the long term.[28] There is augmented parietal cell proliferation to compensate for podocyte loss. Defective parietal cell proliferation will lead on to focal segmental glomerulosclerosis which is commonly observed in women who have had preeclampsia.

Late-onset Preeclampsia (Maternal Preeclampsia)

Maternal preeclampsia is not associated with defective placentation and reduced perfusion. Certain maternal characteristics contribute for this form of preeclampsia.

Pregnancy: A Stress Test

Pregnancy, with its metabolic and vascular demands, poses a challenge to the system. The underlying subclinical metabolic and vascular dysfunction as in women with hypertension, diabetes, and obesity is revealed with the challenge of pregnancy. This explains the occurrence of preeclampsia in first pregnancy and the 10–50% increased risk for preeclampsia in subsequent pregnancies in women who had preeclampsia in the first pregnancy.

Prepregnancy vascular dysfunction, such as in chronic hypertension and chronic kidney disease, not only compromises placental perfusion, but also placental response to ischemia. Acute kidney injury episode prior to pregnancy, despite apparent recovery, also is associated with increased risk of preeclampsia.[29] This implies that even subtle renal dysfunction would interfere with hemodynamic adaptation required for successful pregnancy and lead onto placental hypoperfusion.

Animal Models

Spontaneous preeclampsia is unique to humans. Hence, the available animal models do not exhibit all the phenomena of preeclampsia. RUPP (reduced uterine perfusion pressure) rodent model, produced by clipping of abdominal aorta and uterine artery in pregnant Sprague-Dawley rats, develops hypertension, increased vascular reactivity to vasopressors, increased production of reactive oxygen species, sFLT-1, sEng, and AT1-A.

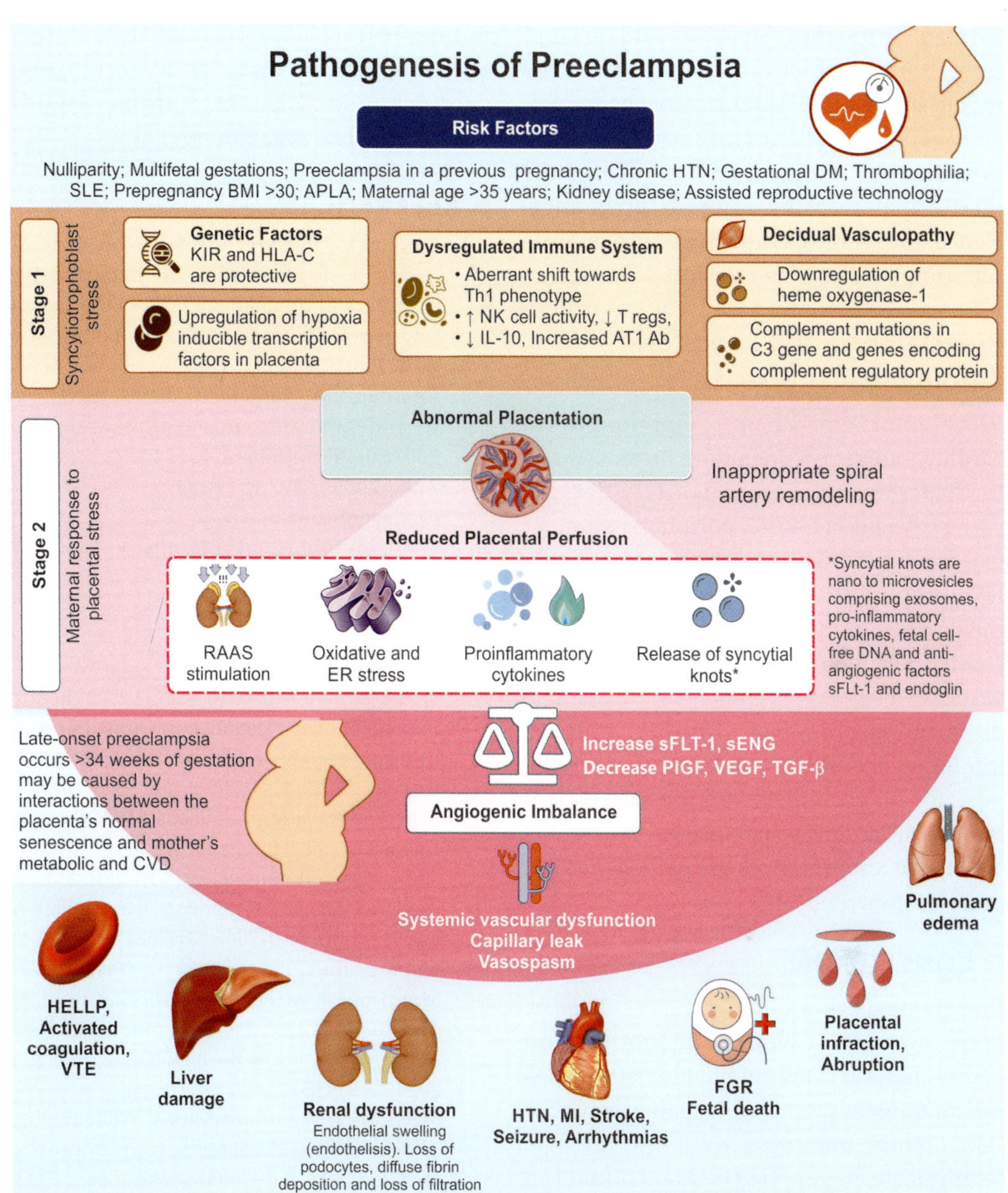

Fig. 3: Pathogenesis of preeclampsia. (APLA: antiphospholipid syndrome; AT1ab: angiotensin II receptor type 1 auto-antibodies; CVD: cardiovascular disease; DM: diabetes mellitus; ER: endoplasmic reticulum; FGR: fetal growth restriction; HELP: elevated liver enzymes and low platelet count; HTN: hypertension; KIR: killer-cell immunoglobulin-like receptor; MI: myocardial infraction; NK: natural killer; OSA: obstructive sleep apnea; PGF: placental growth factor; RAAS: renin-agiotensin-aldosterone system; sENG:sEng: soluble endoglin; sFLT-1: soluble Fms-related receptor tyrosine kinase; SLE: systemic lupus erythematosus; Treg: regulatory T cells; VEGF: vascular endothelial growth factor; VTE: venous thromboembolism)

Courtesy: Dr Priti Meena

C1q knockout mouse and COMT (catechol-O-methyltransferase) knock out rodent and BPH/5 rodents serve as models with expression of varying proportions of preeclamptic features. BPH/5 rodents are mildly hypertensive prior to pregnancy. Hence, they serve as model for preeclampsia superimposed on hypertension.[30]

Preeclampsia and Long-term Cardiovascular Disease

Preeclampsia predisposes for long-term cardiovascular risk, including increased risk for hypertension, coronary artery disease, congestive heart failure, peripheral vascular disease, stroke, vascular dementia, and death. It is proposed that the generalized endothelial damage induced during preeclampsia persists beyond delivery and contributes for vascular disease. Alternatively, the adverse maternal profile, viz., obesity, glucose intolerance, and hypertension may predispose for preeclampsia and the subsequent long-term cardiovascular disease.[31]

Figure 3 summarizes the pathogenesis of preeclampsia.

CONCLUSION

Preeclampsia is a heterogeneous disease, both in terms of clinical phenotype and pathogenesis. It is the culmination of complex interactions between pre-existing maternal risk factors including extremes of age, family history, genetic predisposition and immunologic vulnerability, comorbidities such as obesity, diabetes, hypertension, and chronic kidney disease, and pregnancy-specific factors such as multiple gestation and assisted reproduction, associated with perturbations in pregnancy-relevant phenomena, viz., inflammation, angiogenesis, and coagulation.[32] The ultimate consequence is long-lasting endovascular dysfunction and augmented risk for hypertension, cardiovascular disease, chronic kidney disease, and end-stage kidney failure.

REFERENCES

1. Tooher J, Thornton C, Makris A, Ogle R, Korda A, Hennessy A. All hypertensive disorders of pregnancy increase the risk of future cardiovascular disease. Hypertension. 2017;70(4):798-803.
2. Redman CW, Sargent IL. Latest advances in understanding preeclampsia. Science. 2005;308(5728):1592-4.
3. Zhou Y, Damsky CH, Fisher SJ. Preeclampsia is associated with failure of human cytotrophoblasts to mimic a vascular adhesion phenotype. One cause of defective endovascular invasion in this syndrome? J Clin Invest. 1997;99(9):2152-64.
4. Stevens DU, Al-Nasiry S, Bulten J, Spaanderman MEA. Decidual vasculopathy in preeclampsia: lesion characteristics relate to disease severity and perinatal outcome. Placenta. 2013;34(9):805-9.
5. Skjærven R, Vatten LJ, Wilcox AJ, Rønning T, Irgens LM, Lie RT. Recurrence of preeclampsia across generations: exploring fetal and maternal genetic components in a population based cohort. BMJ. 2005;331(7521):877.
6. Giannubilo SR, Marzioni D, Tossetta G, Montironi R, Meccariello ML, Ciavattini A. The "Bad Father": Paternal Role in Biology of Pregnancy and in Birth Outcome. Biology. 2024;13(3):165.
7. McGinnis R, Steinthorsdottir V, Williams NO, Thorleifsson G, Shooter S, Hjartardottir S, et al. Variants in the fetal genome near FLT1 are associated with risk of preeclampsia. Nat Genet. 2017;49(8):1255-60.
8. Deer E, Herrock O, Campbell N, Cornelius D, Fitzgerald S, Amaral LM, et al. The role of immune cells and mediators in preeclampsia. Nat Rev Nephrol. 2023;19(4):257-70.
9. Saito S, Sakai M. Th1/Th2 balance in preeclampsia. J Reprod Immunol. 2003;59(2):161-73.

10. Regal JF, Burwick RM, Fleming SD. The complement system and preeclampsia. Curr Hypertens Rep. 2017;19(11):87.
11. Burwick RM, Fichorova RN, Dawood HY, Yamamoto HS, Feinberg BB. Urinary excretion of C5b-9 in severe preeclampsia. Hypertension. 2013;62(6):1040-5.
12. Bulla R, Agostinis C, Bossi F, Rizzi L, Debeus A, Tripodo C, et al. Decidual endothelial cells express surface-bound C1q as a molecular bridge between endovascular trophoblast and decidual endothelium. Mol Immunol. 2008;45(9):2629-40.
13. Cui Y, Wang W, Dong N, Lou J, Srinivasan DK, Cheng W, et al. Role of corin in trophoblast invasion and uterine spiral artery remodelling in pregnancy. Nature. 2012;484(7393):246-50.
14. Rajakumar A, Brandon HM, Daftary A, Ness R, Conrad KP. Evidence for the functional activity of hypoxia-inducible transcription factors overexpressed in preeclamptic placentae. Placenta. 2004;25(10):763-9.
15. George EM, Granger JP. Heme oxygenase in pregnancy and preeclampsia. Curr Opin Nephrol Hypertens. 2013;22(2):156.
16. Tannetta D, Collett G, Vatish M, Redman C, Sargent I. Syncytiotrophoblast extracellular vesicles: Circulating biopsies reflecting placental health. Placenta. 2017;52:134-8.
17. Roberts JM, Hubel CA. Is oxidative stress the link in the two-stage model of pre-eclampsia? Lancet. 1999;354(9181):788-9.
18. Maynard SE, Min JY, Merchan J, Lim KH, Li J, Mondal S, et al. Excess placental soluble fms-like tyrosine kinase 1 (sFlt1) may contribute to endothelial dysfunction, hypertension, and proteinuria in preeclampsia. J Clin Invest. 2003;111(5):649-58.
19. Levine RJ, Maynard SE, Qian C, Lim KH, England LJ, Yu KF, et al. Circulating angiogenic factors and the risk of preeclampsia. N Engl J Med. 2004;350(7):672-83.
20. Cindrova-Davies T, Sanders DA, Burton GJ, Charnock-Jones DS. Soluble FLT1 sensitizes endothelial cells to inflammatory cytokines by antagonizing VEGF receptor-mediated signalling. Cardiovasc Res. 2011;89(3):671-9.
21. Powe CE, Levine RJ, Karumanchi SA. Preeclampsia: a disease of the maternal endothelium. Circulation. 2011;123(24):2856-69.
22. Maynard SE, Karumanchi SA. Angiogenic factors and preeclampsia. Semin Nephrol. 2011;31(1):33-46.
23. Rana S, Lemoine E, Granger JP, Karumanchi SA. Preeclampsia. Circ Res. 2019;124(7):1094-112.
24. LaMarca B, Wallukat G, Llinas M, Herse F, Dechend R, Granger JP. Autoantibodies to the angiotensin type I receptor in response to placental ischemia and tumor necrosis factor-α in pregnant rats. Hypertension. 2008;52(6):1168-72.
25. Vikse BE, Irgens LM, Leivestad T, Skjaerven R, Iversen BM. Preeclampsia and the risk of end-stage renal disease. N Engl J Med. 2008;359(8):800-9.
26. Lafayette RA, Druzin M, Sibley R, Derby G, Malik T, Huie P, et al. Nature of glomerular dysfunction in pre-eclampsia1. Kidney Int. 1998;54(4):1240-9.
27. Craici IM, Wagner SJ, Weissgerber TL, Grande JP, Garovic VD. Advances in the pathophysiology of pre-eclampsia and related podocyte injury. Kidney Int. 2014;86(2):275-85.
28. Garovic VD. The role of the podocyte in preeclampsia. Clin J Am Soc Nephrol. 2014;9(8):1337.
29. Tangren JS, Wan Md Adnan WAH, Powe CE, Ecker J, Bramham K, Hladunewich MA, et al. Risk of preeclampsia and pregnancy complications in women with a history of acute kidney injury. Hypertension. 2018;72(2):451-9.
30. Aubuchon M, Schulz LC, Schust DJ. Preeclampsia: animal models for a human cure. Proc Natl Acad Sci. 2011;108(4):1197-8.
31. Berends AL, de Groot CJM, Sijbrands EJ, Sie MPS, Benneheij SH, Pal R, et al. Shared constitutional risks for maternal vascular-related pregnancy complications and future cardiovascular disease. Hypertension. 2008;51(4):1034-41.
32. Garovic VD, Piccoli GB. A kidney-centric view of pre-eclampsia through the kidney-placental bidirectional lens. Kidney Int. 2023;104(2):213-7.

CHAPTER 5

Preeclampsia: Diagnosis and Management

Mayuri Trivedi, Sanjeev Nair, Kayan Siodia

HIGHLIGHTS

- Preeclampsia poses a significant risk to both maternal and neonatal health, contributing to approximately 14% of maternal deaths and 10–25% of perinatal deaths globally.
- It is a complex multisystem disease characterized by sudden-onset hypertension (>20 weeks of gestation) and at least one associated complication such as proteinuria, maternal organ dysfunction, or uteroplacental dysfunction.
- Survivors of preeclampsia face reduced life expectancy and increased risks of stroke, cardiovascular disease, and diabetes. Babies born from preeclamptic pregnancies are at higher risk of preterm birth, perinatal death, neurodevelopmental disability, and later cardiovascular and metabolic diseases.
- Preeclampsia is categorized based on the timing of delivery: preterm (<37 weeks), term (≥37 weeks), and postpartum.
- The maternal syndrome of preeclampsia is driven by dysfunctional placental factors released into maternal blood, leading to systemic inflammation and widespread maternal endothelial dysfunction.

INTRODUCTION

Preeclampsia is a hypertensive disorder of pregnancy unique to human beings characterized by increased risk of mortality and morbidity in both the mother and the child. The adverse effects of preeclampsia extend beyond the period of pregnancy and may lead to increased risk of cardiovascular disease, strokes, hypertension, chronic kidney disease (CKD), and diabetes in the mother. A child of a mother with preeclampsia is at an increased risk for neurodevelopmental disability, perinatal mortality, preterm births, cardiovascular and metabolic diseases. Preeclampsia is a complex multisystem disorder defined by the presence of sudden-onset maternal hypertension (>20 weeks of gestation) with at least one other associated complication including proteinuria, maternal organ dysfunction, or uteroplacental dysfunction.[1] The prerequisite for preeclampsia is the presence of a recent placenta as the pathophysiology of this syndrome is driven by a dysfunctional placenta which secretes factors into the maternal blood and triggers widespread systemic inflammation and endothelial dysfunction.

CLASSIFICATION OF PREECLAMPSIA

As per the International Society for the Study of Hypertension in Pregnancy (ISHPP), preeclampsia is classified based on age of gestation as follows:[1]

- *Preterm preeclampsia:* Delivery <37 weeks of gestation
- *Term preeclampsia:* Delivery ≥37 weeks of gestation
- *Postpartum preeclampsia:* After delivery

A less common classification divided the preeclampsia into early onset (delivery at <34 weeks of gestation) and late onset (delivery ≥34 weeks of gestation) preeclampsia, although it is not favored as it does not define the maternal and fetal prognosis.

The importance of onset of preeclampsia time is important not only for knowing the underlying etiology but also for the efficacy of various early preeclampsia testing strategies and for preeclampsia prophylaxis usage.[2,3]

DIAGNOSIS OF PREECLAMPSIA

As per the ISHPP, preeclampsia is diagnosed after 20 weeks of gestation with new-onset hypertension (systolic blood pressure ≥140 mm Hg and/or diastolic blood pressure ≥90 mm Hg in an average of two measurements) in a previously normotensive patient with any other signs or symptoms of preeclampsia which include:[4]

- Proteinuria (protein/creatinine ≥30 mg/mmol in a spot urine sample or >0.3 g/day)
- Acute kidney injury (AKI)
- Liver involvement (elevated transaminases)
- Neurological symptoms (eclampsia, altered mental status, blindness, stroke, clonus, severe headaches, and persistent visual scotomata)
- Hematological abnormalities (thrombocytopenia with platelet count below 150,000/μL, disseminated intravascular coagulation, and hemolysis)
- Cardiorespiratory complications (pulmonary edema, myocardial ischemia or infarction, oxygen saturation <90%, ≥50% inspired oxygen for >1 hour or intubation other than for cesarean section)
- Uteroplacental dysfunction (fetal growth retardation, angiogenic imbalance, and placental abruption).

These updated guidelines are significantly different from the 2001 guidelines which required the presence of proteinuria in addition to newly diagnosed hypertension beyond 20 weeks of gestation in a previously normotensive mother.[5,6] This update resulted in higher number of pregnancies being diagnosed with preeclampsia and better prognostication of the mothers and offsprings.[5]

CLINICAL FEATURES

The clinical presentation of preeclampsia includes several distinct features as following:

- *Hypertension:* Hypertension typically manifests earliest and serves as a primary indicator.
- *Epigastric and upper abdominal pain:* Severe cases often feature discomfort in the epigastric, upper abdominal, or retrosternal regions, particularly at night. This pain, sometimes radiating to other areas, can indicate the severe end of the disease spectrum and may indicate hepatic complications such as rupture. With nausea or vomiting when persistent and associated with fatty liver of pregnancy should be ruled out. Acute pancreatitis should also be ruled out as it is a rare complication of preeclampsia.
- *Headache:* Headaches may stem from vascular dysfunction or impaired autoregulation within the cerebral vasculature (vasospasm of the cerebral vasculature,

impaired cerebrovascular autoregulation, leading to areas of both vasoconstriction and vasodilation). Rarely posterior reversible leukoencephalopathy syndrome (PRESS) may be present.

- *Chest pain:* It may indicate cardiac disease (ischemia, acute spontaneous coronary artery dissection).
- *Visual symptoms:* Visual disturbances, also indicative of severe disease, may arise from retinal arteriolar spasm or cerebral edema. These can include blurred vision, cortical blindness, amaurosis fugax photopsia, scotomata, diplopia, or temporary blindness.
- *Mental status changes:* Confusion or altered behavior may occur from neurological involvement.
- *Pulmonary edema:* Severe cases may involve pulmonary edema, though this occurs in a minority of cases (<10%).
- *Oliguria:* Reduced urine output, attributed to intravascular space contraction and intrarenal vasospasm
- *Generalized edema:* While common in pregnancy, sudden and significant weight gain or facial swelling may suggest preeclampsia and require evaluation.
- *Placental abruption:* A serious complication, especially in severe preeclampsia cases, placental abruption can threaten both maternal and fetal well-being.
- *Uterine and umbilical artery Doppler:* Doppler studies may reveal increase in the uterine artery pulsatility index and uterine artery notching on Doppler.
- *Risk of maternal mortality:* Preeclampsia poses a heightened risk of severe obstetric or medical complications (such as eclampsia, stokes, pulmonary edema, AKI, liver rupture, and abruption) contributing to a notable proportion of maternal deaths globally.

SUSPECTED PREECLAMPSIA

In mothers with hypertension without definite presence of obvious preeclampsia symptoms or signs, ISHPP recommends the evaluation for angiogenic imbalance as a marker of uteroplacental insufficiency.[1] The National Institute for Health and Care Excellence (NICE) guidelines recommend the use of measurements of placental growth factor (PlGF) alone or in combination with measurement of soluble fms-like tyrosine kinase 1 protein (sFLT-1) to rule out suspected preeclampsia with 14 days of the measurement.[5] PlGF is a protein involved in the placental angiogenesis and elevated levels have been observed in the blood and the serum which peak at 26–30 weeks in a normal pregnancy. Failure of the PlGF levels to rise may indicate placental dysfunction and point toward early preeclampsia. Along with clinical judgment and other tests, PlGF levels may help to diagnose preeclampsia in the second and third trimester and aid in early diagnosis of this disorder[5,6] **(Box 1)**.

Soluble fms-like tyrosine kinase 1 is another placental released angiogenic factor which typically increases 5 weeks before the onset of preeclampsia.[4,7] The ratio of sFLT-1 to PlGF is, therefore, a helpful tool in confirming the diagnosis of preeclampsia. Typically, a ratio of sFLT-1 to PlGF of <38 can reliably rule of the diagnosis in mothers with suspected preeclampsia.[8]

Another less commonly studied placental angiogenic factor is maternal soluble serum endoglin which has a pattern-like sFLT-1 that leads to disturbed angiogenesis and vasoconstriction which causes most symptoms of preeclampsia. It may prove to be a good predictive marker for preeclampsia though is not widely available at present.[9]

BOX 1: Advantages of using PIGF-based testing.

- Along with clinical judgement, helps diagnosis of preeclampsia in the 2nd and 3rd trimester
- Reduces the time to clinical confirmation and may improve the maternal and fetal morbidity
- Faster and more accurate diagnosis with improved risk assessment for adverse outcomes
- Allows women in whom preeclampsia has been ruled out to return to standard community care as against remaining admitted in a hospital for observation
- Helps predict complications in pregnancies and chalk out a better management plan including the timing of delivery
- Aids in the prediction or confirmation of a diagnosis of preeclampsia, fetal growth restriction, stillbirth, and preterm birth (PIGF levels <50 pg/mL associated with stillbirths in women suspected with preeclampsia)

(PIGF: placental growth factor)

Uncommon presentations in preeclampsia include:

Early onset (<20 weeks): Most cases before 20 weeks gestation are linked with molar pregnancy or antiphospholipid syndrome (APS). Lupus nephritis, hereditary thrombotic thrombocytopenic purpura, and hemolytic-uremic syndrome may also present similarly.

Postpartum onset (>2 days): This is termed delayed-onset or late postpartum preeclampsia, occurring more than 2 days but less than 6 weeks post-birth.

Severe symptoms without hypertension: While rare, severe symptoms without hypertension can occur, notably in HELLP syndrome and sometimes in eclampsia.

Isolated hypertension: New-onset mild hypertension without other preeclampsia criteria or underlying hypertensive disease is termed gestational hypertension. Close monitoring is crucial as up to half may later meet full preeclampsia criteria.

PROGRESSION OF DISEASE

Every woman, irrespective of the time of onset of preeclampsia, is at a risk for rapid disease progression and worsening severity history of chronic hypertension with worsening of systolic blood pressures or elevation of serum creatinine level may predict progression of severity. Various multivariate predictive models have been devised to predict the progression of preeclampsia and adverse maternal outcomes well.

The fullPIERS model is one such predictive tool that can foresee adverse maternal outcomes and perinatal outcomes with reasonable accuracy (AUROC 0.88, 95% CI 0.84–0.92).[10] It considers assessment of maternal signs and symptoms apart from laboratory findings to generate a valid and reliable algorithm. The model predicts the increased risk of adverse outcomes up to 7 days prior to their onset and thus helps planning the timing of delivery and place of care for the mother and child. Apart from gestational age, this model also takes into consideration the presence of chest pain and dyspnea, oxygen saturation, platelet levels, serum creatinine, and liver enzymes.

Another commonly used predictive model is the PREP-S prediction model which predicts the risk time of adverse outcomes at various time periods and can be used up to 34 weeks of gestation. The factors used in this model include maternal age, gestational age at diagnosis, presence or absence of tendon reflexes, presence or absence of preexisting conditions (hypertension, renal disease, diabetes mellitus, autoimmune disease, and previous preeclampsia), and systolic blood pressure.[11]

An sFLT1 to PlGF ratio of ≤38 had a negative predictive value of 98.9% (95% CI 97.6–99.6%) and a ratio of >38 had a positive predictive value of 53.5% (95% CI 45.0–61.8%) for a composite of adverse maternal outcomes (including death, pulmonary edema, acute renal failure, cerebral hemorrhage, cerebral thrombosis, and disseminated intravascular coagulation) as seen in a study from Asia.[12]

SCREENING FOR PREECLAMPSIA

The fetal medicine foundation (FMF) competing risks model is an effective screening algorithm which has been validated worldwide. It uses maternal age, along with ethnicity, weight and height, medical and obstetric history, mean arterial blood pressure, maternal circulating PlGF levels at 11–13 weeks of gestation, and uterine artery pulsatility index on ultrasonography to estimate the individual risk of developing preeclampsia in the mother.[4] There are NICE guidelines also for screening the individual risk in mothers which are based on a variety of maternal characteristics such as age, previous history of preeclampsia, and medical history like presence of chronic hypertension, CKD, and diabetes[13] **(Box 2)**. FMF screening is particularly effective for preterm preeclampsia, identifying ~90% of women which may develop preeclampsia at <34 weeks of gestation and ~80% of women which may develop preeclampsia at <37 weeks of gestation.[14] The limitation of the FMF risk model is the difficulty in procuring a uterine artery Doppler of PlGF levels especially in the low and low-middle income countries. Assessing the patient based on the medical and obstetric history and maternal characteristics followed by procuring either the uterine doppler or the PlGF levels have been found to be equally effective in predicting the risk.[14]

BOX 2: Risk assessment and screening using the NICE criteria.

High-risk factors:
- Previous preeclampsia
- Chronic renal disease
- Chronic hypertension
- Diabetes mellitus
- SLE or APLA

Moderate-risk factors:
- First pregnancy
- Age ≥35 years
- Body mass index ≥30 kg/m^2
- Interpregnancy interval >10 years
- Family history of preeclampsia
- Black ethnicity
- Low socioeconomic status

(APLA: antiphospholipid antibodies; SLE: systemic lupus erythematosus)

PREVENTION

- Aspirin prophylaxis in those at risk from first trimester onward reduces the risk as shown by ASPRE trial (Aspirin for Evidence-based Preeclampsia Prevention),[15] CLASP trial,[16] the Italian Study of Aspirin in Pregnancy (ISAP),[17] and ASPIRIN trials.[18] Candidates for aspirin prophylaxis include diabetics, those with CKD, autoimmune disease (SLE and APLA), chronic hypertension, multifetal gestation, and those with PE in prior pregnancy. Also, those with two or more moderate risk factors, i.e., family history of preeclampsia in mother or sister, age ≥35 years, sociodemographic characteristics (black persons and lower income level), personal risk factors (e.g., previous pregnancy with low birth weight or small for gestational age newborn, previous adverse pregnancy outcome, e.g., stillbirth, interval >10 years between pregnancies) (Level A evidence). Low-dose aspirin (75 mg) should be initiated for preeclampsia prevention at ≥12 weeks of gestation, and ideally prior to 16 weeks of gestation but in case not initiated earlier, it can be initiated even up to 28 weeks.[18] Initiation of aspirin after the development of PE has no benefit and, in fact, may increase the complications.

- Antihypertensive therapy prevents severe HT and sequelae, and magnesium sulfate prevents seizures. In the 2022, Control of Mild Hypertension during Pregnancy (CHAP) Trial, a strategy of treating pregnant patients with blood pressures ≥140/90 mm Hg compared with a strategy of reserving treatment only for severe hypertension reduced the incidence of any preeclampsia, preeclampsia with severe features and preterm births.[19]
- The ARRIVE trial showed that low-risk nulliparas assigned to induction of labor at 39–40 weeks of gestation were less likely to develop a hypertensive disorder of pregnancy than those assigned to expectant management >40 weeks.[20,21]
- In populations where baseline dietary calcium intake is low, World Health Organization (WHO) recommends 1,500–2,000 mg elemental calcium supplementation per day for pregnant individuals to reduce the risk of preeclampsia.
- Other protective interventions include prepregnancy weight loss in obese females, exercise, statin and metformin therapy, and anticoagulation in those at high risk. Omeprazole, sulfasalazine, etc. interventions like vitamin C, D, or E and folic acid supplementation were not found to be effective. Similarly, fish oil and NO oxide donors like arginine did not have any benefit.

MANAGEMENT

While the American College of Obstetricians and Gynecologists (ACOG) suggests initiating therapy at higher blood pressure levels (≥160/≥110 mm Hg) with target goals of 120–160/80–110 mm Hg, other organizations like the International Society for the Study of Hypertension in Pregnancy (ISSHP) and the National Institute for Health and Care Excellence (NICE) advocate for a more aggressive stance, recommending treatment at lower thresholds (≥140/≥90 mm Hg).

Inpatient Management

Hospitalization is recommended for those with severe features or those who are nonadherent to monitoring. Even in a hospital, the management can be expectant and immediate delivery may not be required unless indications for imminent delivery are present.

Fetal and Maternal Assessment

An initial assessment is conducted to determine eligibility for expectant management. Maternal stabilization, continuous monitoring of BP and symptoms, and laboratory evaluations are performed.

Fetal ultrasound for estimated fetal weight is conducted, and continuous fetal monitoring is done until stability and eligibility for expectant management are confirmed.

The fullPIERS model is intended for use at any time in pregnancy and predicts adverse maternal outcomes in the next 48 hours. The fullPIERS calculator is available online and is based on gestational age, chest pain or dyspnea, oxygen saturation, creatinine, platelets, and aspartate aminotransaminase (AST) or alanine aminotransaminase (ALT).[10] The PREP-S prediction model is intended for use up to 34 weeks' gestation.[11]

Monitoring of inpatients undergoing expectant management of PE:

Maternal evaluation: Monitoring of blood pressure and symptoms of severe disease, as well as the use of antihypertensive medications to maintain blood pressure below 160/110. Laboratories are conducted at least weekly, with frequency adjusted as needed on an individual basis.

Fetal evaluation: Daily nonstress tests (NST), biophysical profile (BPP) tests twice a week, Doppler studies if indicated for fetal growth restriction (FGR), and ultrasound for growth every 2–4 weeks.

Management of Eclampsia

The management of eclampsia can be divided into two parts. The medical management of hypertension in preeclampsia and the medical and obstetric management of severe preeclampsia.

Women with preeclampsia should be assessed for adverse risk factors and clinical examination at each antenatal visit and offered hospital-based management in the presence of the following variables that affect maternal and fetal outcomes:[22,23]

- *Persistent systolic blood pressure of ≥160 mm Hg:*
  - Any maternal biochemical or hematological investigations that cause concern, like:
    - Rise in creatinine

    Or
    - Rise in alanine transaminase (over 70 IU/L, or twice upper limit of normal range)

    Or
    - *Thrombocytopenia:*
      - Signs of impending eclampsia
      - Signs of impending pulmonary edema
      - Suspected fetal compromise
      - Any other clinical signs that cause concern

Antihypertensive therapy offered should be based on the presenting blood pressure and clinical condition of the patient. While nonsevere hypertension can be treated with first-line agents like oral methyldopa, labetalol, and nifedipine, severe hypertension (SBP ≥160 mm Hg or DBP ≥110 mm Hg) should trigger the offer of inpatient care and monitored use of IV labetalol or hydralazine.[24]

While the use of magnesium sulfate to prevent recurrent seizures in patients with eclampsia is well established, it should also be given to women with severe hypertension and proteinuria or neurological signs and symptoms. The use of magnesium sulfate has been clearly shown to decrease the incidence and recurrence of eclampsia.[25]

Timing of the Delivery

Any woman with hypertensive disorders of pregnancy should be considered for termination of pregnancy if they present with the following risk factors:

- Abnormal neurological features (such as eclampsia, severe intractable headache, or repeated visual scotomata)
- Repeated episodes of severe hypertension despite maintenance treatment with three classes of antihypertensive agents
- Pulmonary edema
- Progressive thrombocytopenia or platelet count <50 × 10^9/L
- Transfusion of any blood product
- Abnormal and rising serum creatinine
- Abnormal and rising liver enzymes
- Hepatic dysfunction (INR >2 in absence of DIC or warfarin), hematoma, or rupture
- Abruption with evidence of maternal or fetal compromise
- Nonreassuring fetal status (including death)

Fetal gestational age deemed to be nonviable should also be an indication for termination of pregnancy unless access to a center with expertise in the care of very preterm babies is available. Initiation of delivery is recommended at a gestation age >37 weeks and expectant care including the administration of antenatal corticosteroids for gestational age from deemed viability to 34 weeks.[26] Studies looking at the gray area between 34 and 37 weeks suggest a trade-off between maternal safety outcomes and increased respiratory or neurodevelopmental complications for the baby.[26,27]

Postpartum Care

Blood pressure must be monitored postpartum in women who were on antenatal antihypertensives and the decision to continue medication or reduce and stop must be made based on recorded BP values. Medications may be reduced at BP <130/80 mm Hg. Patients must be reviewed at 3 months to ensure BP, urinalysis and laboratory abnormalities have normalized and advised regarding the risk of gestational hypertension and recurrent preeclampsia in subsequent pregnancies.[28]

CARDIOVASCULAR SYSTEM IN PREECLAMPSIA: LOOKING BEYOND A NEPHRON-CENTRIC VIEW

Despite decades of exhausting research, the only unifying theory explaining the pathophysiology of preeclampsia continues to be centered around the placental deficiency and the subsequent vascular reactivity cascade.[29,30] We need to think beyond this hypothesis given that it fails to explain many facts about most preeclampsia cases. It has been an established fact for a long time that preeclampsia has a long-term impact on the mother with regards to her cardiovascular health.[31,32] Preeclampsia is a major risk factor for major cardiovascular, renal, and neurovascular events in the future. As compared to a woman with a normal pregnancy, preeclamptic pregnancy increases the risk of a cardiovascular-related death in the future by as much as fivefold.[31] However, the emerging evidence now suggests that the impact on cardiovascular health is not only in the future but also profound in the immediate period.[32]

Thus, since the cardiovascular problems in these women are observed before, during, and after the index preeclamptic pregnancy, it would be reasonable to believe that the cardiovascular system is not only a victim of preeclampsia but may also play a role in the pathogenesis of preeclampsia.[33] The risk factors which have described in detail for preeclampsia are largely cardiovascular in nature **(Box 3)**.

Thus, it becomes imperative that these mothers are educated about the

BOX 3: Overlapping risk factors for preeclampsia and cardiovascular diseases.

Maternal factors:
- Advanced age
- Obesity
- Ethnicity (Blacks/Hispanics)

Hormonal factors:
- Polycystic ovarian syndrome
- Premature ovarian failure

Autoimmune factors:
- APLA syndrome
- SLE

Metabolic factors:
- Diabetes mellitus
- Abnormal serum lipid levels

Renal factors:
- Chronic kidney disease
- Previous episodes of acute kidney injury

Others factors:
- Chronic hypertension
- Kidney donation

(APLA: antiphospholipid antibodies; SLE: systemic lupus erythematosus)

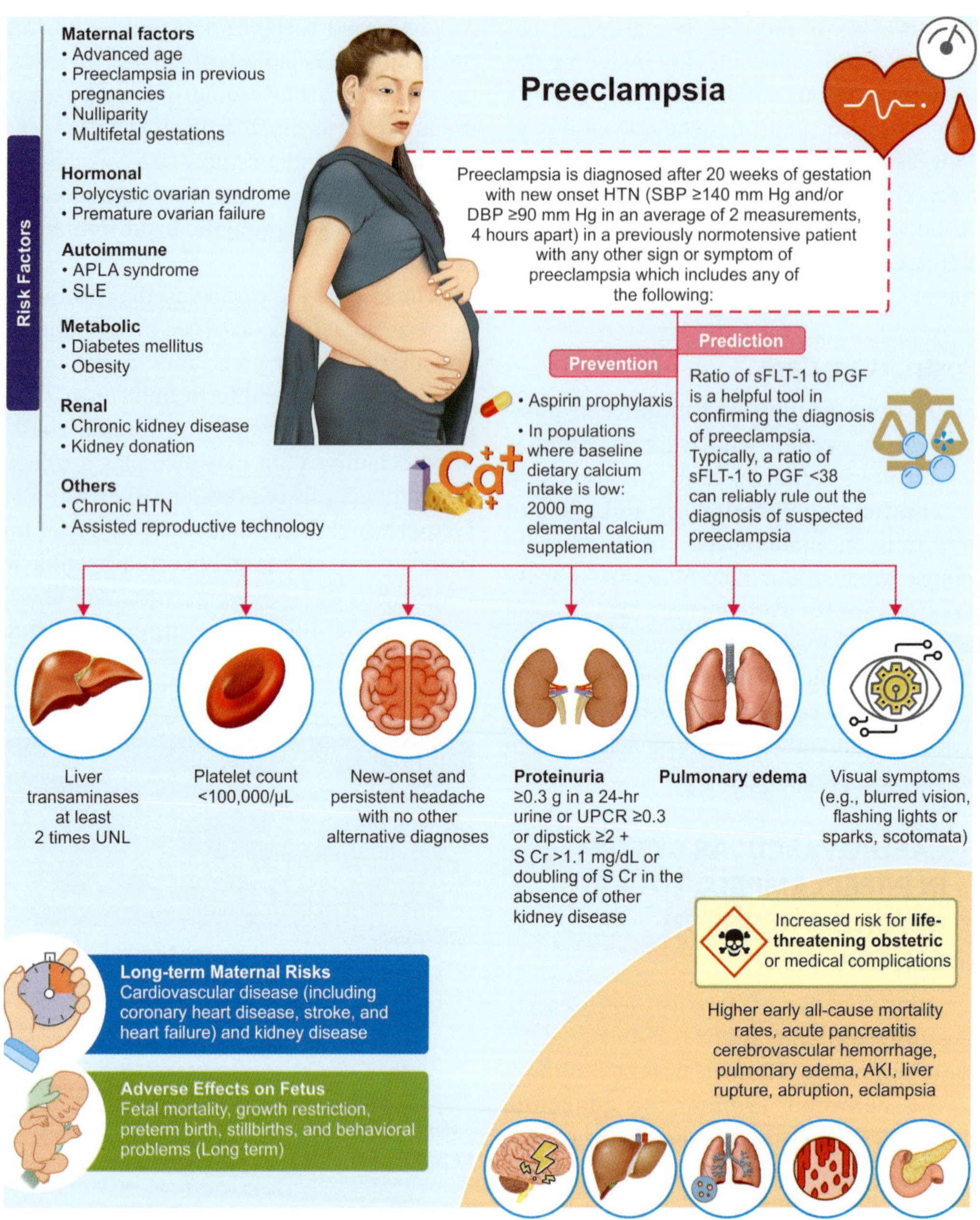

Fig. 1: Summary of the chapter. (DBP: diastolic blood pressure; HTN: hypertension; SBP: systolic blood pressure; Scr: serum creatinine; UNL: upper normal limit; UPCR: urine protein/creatinine ratio)

Courtesy: Dr Priti Meena

immediate- and long-term cardiovascular effects of preeclampsia and are counseled regarding risk mitigation that continues after delivery. Also, these mothers need to be followed up for screening and early diagnosis of cardiovascular diseases and hypertension even after delivery and in the long term. A strong focus on better postnatal cardiovascular assessment after preeclampsia is an absolute necessity so as not to waste a unique opportunity for a timely intervention in the disease trajectory and to improve the cardiovascular and cerebrovascular health outcomes of these women. **Figure 1** summarizes the key points in preeclampsia.

CONCLUSION

Preeclampsia continues to remain an enigmatic disorder having immediate and long-term health effects on the mother and the child. Despite significant strides having been made in the pathophysiology of the disorder as well as diagnosis and screening with risk assessment, there continue to be major gaps in our knowledge. Potential therapies and preventive methods which may effectively prevent preeclampsia and its immediate- and long-term adverse effects on the mother and child are areas of research which need to be pursued rigorously. The follow-up of these mothers needs to be continued in the long term to identify and treat the various long-term complications of preeclampsia.

REFERENCES

1. Magee LA, Brown MA, Hall DR, Gupte S, Hennessy A, Karumanchi SA, et al. The 2021 International Society for the Study of Hypertension in Pregnancy Classification, Diagnosis and Management Recommendations for international practice. Pregnancy Hypertens. 2022;27:148-69.
2. O'Gorman N, Wright D, Poon LC, Rolnik DL, Syngelaki A, de Alvarado M, et al. Multicenter screening for pre-eclampsia by maternal factors and biomarkers at 11–13 weeks' gestation. Ultrasound Obstet Gynecol. 2017;49:756.
3. Rolnik D, Wright D, Poon LC, O'Gorman N, Syngelaki A, de Paco Matallana C, et al. Aspirin versus placebo in pregnancies at high risk for preterm preeclampsia. N Engl J Med. 2017;377:613-22.
4. Dimitriadis E, Rolnik DL, Zhou W, Estrada-Gutierrez G, Koga K, Francisco RPV, et al. Pre-eclampsia. Nat Rev Dis Primers. 2023;9(1):8.
5. Webster K, Fishburn S, Maresh M, Findlay SC, Chappell LC. Diagnosis and management of hypertension in pregnancy: summary of updated NICE guidance. BMJ. 2019;366:l5119.
6. Duhig KE, Myers J, Seed PT, Sparkes J, Lowe J, Hunter RM, et al. Placental growth factor testing to assess women with suspected pre-eclampsia: a multicentre, pragmatic, stepped-wedge cluster-randomised controlled trial. Lancet. 2019;393:1807-18.
7. Verlohren S, Galindo A, Schlembach D, Zeisler H, Herraiz I, Moertl MG, et al. An automated method for the determination of the sFlt-1/PIGF ratio in the assessment of preeclampsia. Am J Obstet Gynecol. 2010;202:161.e1-161.e11.
8. Zeisler H, Llurba E, Chantraine F, Vatish M, Staff AC, Sennström M, et al. Predictive value of the sFlt-1:PlGF ratio in women with suspected preeclampsia. N Engl J Med. 2016;374:13-22.
9. Margioula-Siarkou G, Margioula-Siarkou C, Petousis S, Margaritis K, Alexandratou M, Dinas K, et al. Soluble endoglin concentration in maternal blood as a diagnostic biomarker of preeclampsia: a systematic review and meta-analysis. Eur J Obstet Gynecol Reprod Biol. 2021;258:366-81.
10. Von Dadelszen P, Payne B, Li J, Ansermino JM, Broughton Pipkin F, Côté AM, et al. Prediction of adverse maternal outcomes in pre-eclampsia: development and validation of the fullPIERS model. Lancet. 2011;377:219-27.
11. Thangaratinam S, Allotey J, Marlin N, Dodds J, Cheong-See F, von Dadelszen P, et al. PREP Collaborative Network. Prediction of complications in early-onset pre-eclampsia (PREP): development and external multinational validation of prognostic models. BMC Med. 2017;15(1):68.

12. Bian X, Biswas A, Huang X, Lee KJ, Li TK, Masuyama H, et al. Short-term prediction of adverse outcomes using the sFlt-1 (soluble fms-like tyrosine kinase-1)/PlGF (placental growth factor) ratio in Asian women with suspected preeclampsia. Hypertension. 2019;74:164-72.
13. O'Gorman N, Wright D, Syngelaki A, Akolekar R, Wright A, Poon LC, et al. Competing risks model in screening for preeclampsia by maternal factors and biomarkers at 11–13 weeks gestation. Am J Obstet Gynecol. 2016;214(1):103.e1-103.e12.
14. Wright D, Wright A, Nicolaides KH. The competing risk approach for prediction of preeclampsia. Am J Obstet Gynecol. 2020;223(1):12-23.e7.
15. Poon LC, Wright D, Rolnik DL, Syngelaki A, Delgado JL, Tsokaki T, et al. Aspirin for Evidence-Based Preeclampsia Prevention trial: effect of aspirin in prevention of preterm preeclampsia in subgroups of women according to their characteristics and medical and obstetrical history. Am J Obstet Gynecol. 2017;217(5):585.e1-e5.
16. CLASP Collaborative Group. CLASP: a randomised trial of low-dose aspirin for the prevention and treatment of pre-eclampsia among 9364 pregnant women. CLASP (Collaborative Low-dose Aspirin Study in Pregnancy) Collaborative Group. Lancet. 1994;343(8898):619-29.
17. Italian Study of Aspirin in Pregnancy. Low-dose aspirin in prevention and treatment of intrauterine growth retardation and pregnancy-induced hypertension. Italian study of aspirin in pregnancy. Lancet. 1993;341(8842):396-400.
18. Mendoza M, Bonacina E, Garcia-Manau P, López M, Caamiña S, Vives À, et al. Aspirin discontinuation at 24 to 28 weeks' gestation in pregnancies at high risk of preterm preeclampsia: a randomized clinical trial. JAMA. 2023;329(7):542-50.
19. Tita AT, Szychowski JM, Boggess K, Dugoff L, Sibai B, Lawrence K, et al.; Chronic Hypertension and Pregnancy (CHAP) Trial Consortium. Treatment for Mild Chronic Hypertension during Pregnancy. N Engl J Med. 2022;386(19):1781-92.
20. Grobman WA, Rice MM, Reddy UM, Tita ATN, Silver RM, Mallett G, et al; Eunice Kennedy Shriver National Institute of Child Health and Human Development Maternal–Fetal Medicine Units Network. Labor Induction versus Expectant Management in Low-Risk Nulliparous Women. N Engl J Med. 2018;379(6):513-23.
21. Hurrell A, Duhig K, Vandermolen B, Shennan AH. Recent advances in the diagnosis and management of pre-eclampsia. Fac Rev. 2020;9:10.
22. Chappell LC, Brocklehurst P, Green ME, Hunter R, Hardy P, Juszczak E, et al. Planned early delivery or expectant management for late preterm pre-eclampsia (PHOENIX): a randomised controlled trial. Lancet. 2019;394:1181-90.
23. Magee LA, von Dadelszen P, Rey E, Ross S, Asztalos E, Murphy KE, et al. Less-tight versus tight control of hypertension in pregnancy. N Engl J Med. 2015;372:407-17.
24. Garovic VD, Dechend R, Easterling T, Karumanchi SA, McMurtry Baird S, Magee LA, et al.; American Heart Association Council on Hypertension; Council on the Kidney in Cardiovascular Disease, Kidney in Heart Disease Science Committee; Council on Arteriosclerosis, Thrombosis and Vascular Biology; Council on Lifestyle and Cardiometabolic Health; Council on Peripheral Vascular Disease; and Stroke Council. Hypertension in Pregnancy: Diagnosis, Blood Pressure Goals, and Pharmacotherapy: A Scientific Statement From the American Heart Association. Hypertension. 2022;79(2):e21-e41.
25. Altman D, Carroli G, Duley L, Farrell B, Moodley J, Neilson J, et al. Do women with pre-eclampsia, and their babies, benefit from magnesium sulphate? The Magpie trial: a randomised placebo-controlled trial. Lancet. 2002;359:1877-90.
26. Broekhuijsen K, van Baaren GJ, van Pampus MG, Ganzevoort W, Sikkema JM, Woiski MD, et al. Immediate delivery versus

expectant monitoring for hypertensive disorders of pregnancy between 34 and 37 weeks of gestation (HYPITAT-II): an open-label, randomised controlled trial. Lancet. 2015;385:2492-501.

27. Cluver C, Novikova N, Koopmans CM, West HM. Planned early delivery versus expectant management for hypertensive disorders from 34 weeks gestation to term. Cochrane Database Syst Rev. 2017;1(1):CD009273.
28. Cairns AE, Pealing L, Duffy JMN, Roberts N, Tucker KL, Leeson P, et al. Postpartum management of hypertensive disorders of pregnancy: a systematic review. BMJ Open. 2017;7:e018696.
29. Thilaganathan B, Kalafat E. Cardiovascular system in preeclampsia and beyond. Hypertension. 2019;73(3):522-31.
30. Mongraw-Chaffin ML, Cirillo PM, Cohn BA. Preeclampsia and cardiovascular disease death: prospective evidence from the child health and development studies cohort. Hypertension. 2010;56:166-71.
31. Davis EF, Lazdam M, Lewandowski AJ, Worton SA, Kelly B, Kenworthy Y, et al. Cardiovascular risk factors in children and young adults born to preeclamptic pregnancies: a systematic review. Pediatrics. 2012;129:e1552-61.
32. Maher GM, O'Keeffe GW, Kearney PM, Kenny LC, Dinan TG, Mattsson M, et al. Association of hypertensive disorders of pregnancy with risk of neurodevelopmental disorders in offspring: a systematic review and meta-analysis. JAMA Psychiatry. 2018;75:809-19.
33. Behrens I, Basit S, Melbye M, Lykke JA, Wohlfahrt J, Bundgaard H, et al. Risk of post-pregnancy hypertension in women with a history of hypertensive disorders of pregnancy: nationwide cohort study. BMJ. 2017;358:j3078.

CHAPTER 6

Complement-Mediated Disorders of Pregnancy

Anuja Java, Shannon Lyons, Manuel Urra,
Corina Gabriela Teodosiu, Richard Burwick

HIGHLIGHTS

- Complement disorders in pregnancy often arise from a mismatch between complement activation and regulation.
- HELLP (hemolysis, elevated liver enzymes, and low platelet count) is definitively treated by delivery of fetus and placenta.
- Complement-mediated thrombotic microangiopathy (CM-TMA) in pregnancy is hard to differentiate from HELLP. Persistence of symptoms and laboratory abnormalities >72 hours after delivery is strongly suggestive of CM-TMA and should be treated with anti-complement therapy. Patients should undergo testing for complement genetic mutations and autoantibodies.
- Antiphospholipid syndrome (APS) is characterized by recurrent pregnancy loss and thrombotic events. In pregnancy, anticoagulation with low-molecular-weight heparin (LMWH) ± low-dose aspirin is indicated in patients with a history of former thrombotic event or fetal loss with + aPL antibody.

INTRODUCTION

Pregnancy is a time of significant change within the body. The complement system plays a significant role in the maternal–fetal relationship during pregnancy through multiple mechanisms. One mechanism represents a delicate balance between complement regulation which prevents complement-mediated damage to the trophoblast and placenta, and ongoing complement activation, which contributes to vascular remodeling of the spiral arteries and protection from infectious organisms. Complement-mediated disorders occur when this careful balance is upset, with pregnancy and the postpartum period being a high-risk time for such disorders to manifest. Three major types of complement-mediated disorders in pregnancy are hemolysis, elevated liver enzymes and low platelets (HELLP) syndrome often seen in conjunction with preeclampsia with severe features (PE-SF), thrombotic microangiopathy (TMA) associated with antiphospholipid syndrome (APS), and complement-mediated thrombotic microangiopathy (CM-TMA) or atypical hemolytic uremic syndrome (aHUS). It can be challenging to differentiate between these various etiologies given the clinical and laboratory similarities; however, timely diagnosis is key for appropriate management and to prevent end-stage kidney disease (ESKD) and other associated complications including myocardial ischemia, seizures, strokes, and even death.

This chapter will discuss expected complement changes in pregnancy as well as the above-mentioned complement disorders including their epidemiology, pathophysiology, clinical presentation, and various treatment strategies.

COMPLEMENT CHANGES IN PREGNANCY

There are expected changes to the complement system in pregnancy that maintain the balance between complement activation and regulation **(Fig. 1)**. Pregnancy represents an allogeneic-type mismatch between the fetus and the maternal immune system. Since the fetus encounters maternal immunocompetent cells during trophoblast invasion, healthy placentation depends on a collaboration between efficient trophoblast invasion and the mother's immune system. During trophoblast invasion, many immune cells infiltrate the decidua, allowing them to reach the endometrium and spiral arteries. In healthy pregnancies, nonrecognition of these trophoblasts by maternal immune cells promotes maternal–fetal tolerance. However, an overactive maternal immune system can negatively impact this process. It can activate trophoblast apoptosis significantly disrupting their migration and placental vascularization which can lead to placental ischemia and release of inflammatory mediators by the placenta. As the mother's blood circulates in the intervillous space, cellular debris containing placental/ trophoblast fragments will further activate the maternal complement system. Regulated complement activation will help clear these fragments from maternal circulation and decrease inflammation; however, improper clearance of such components, driven by an inadequately regulated complement system, may cause deposition of debris in tissues and vascular walls. This then leads to an overly exuberant inflammatory response, resulting in endothelial injury and placental dysfunction. Several studies have supported this theory by showing that pregnant

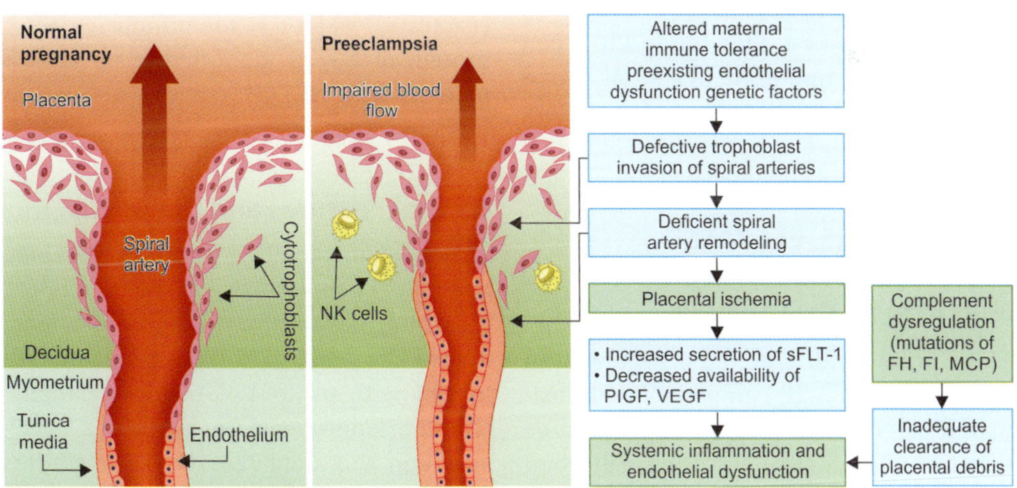

Fig. 1: Changes in vasculature of placenta in preeclampsia. (FH: factor H; FI: Factor I; MCP: membrane cofactor protein; NK cells: natural killer cells; PIGF: placental growth factor; sFLT- 1: soluble fms like tyrosine kinase-1; VEGF: vascular endothelial growth factor)

women have higher levels of complement components including MBL (mannose-binding lectin), C3, C3a, C4, C4d, and SC5b-9 compared to nonpregnant women. Under normal conditions of pregnancy, this augmented complement activation is kept in check by increased expression of complement regulatory proteins including CD55, CD46, and CD59 which promote the inactivation of anaphylatoxins and breakdown of the membrane attack complex (MAC).[1]

Complement activation can also occur as a result of imbalance in the production between antiangiogenic [soluble fms-like tyrosine kinase-1 (sFlt-1)] and proangiogenic factors [vascular endothelial growth factor (VEGF) and placental growth factor (PlGF)] by placenta. In vitro studies have shown that VEGF induces complement Factor H synthesis by endothelial cells and protects the endothelium through modulation of local complement proteins. sFLT-1 is an endogenous inhibitor of VEGF and can thereby promote aberrant complement activation and complement-mediated placental damage through VEGF inhibition at the maternal–fetal interface. Increased secretion of sFLT-1 that binds PlGF can also result in impaired placental blood flow, oxygenation, and poor spiral artery remodeling further contributing to placental inflammation and endothelial dysfunction.[2]

HEMOLYSIS, ELEVATED LIVER ENZYMES, AND LOW PLATELET SYNDROME

The HELLP syndrome, often occurring in the context of PE-SF, can occur in approximately 0.5–1% of all pregnancies with more than two-thirds of cases occurring in the third trimester, with some cases occurring in the immediate postpartum period.[3] It is also the most common cause of TMA in pregnancy and is often difficult to differentiate from CM-TMA. The maternal mortality rate of HELLP syndrome is estimated at 1.1% and perinatal death rate reported at 7–34% of cases.[4,5]

Etiology/Pathophysiology

The exact pathophysiologic mechanism for the development of HELLP is not fully understood. It is generally accepted that abnormal placentation plays a significant role in its development. As discussed above, under normal conditions, there should be a balance between complement activation by fetal antigens and complement regulation by complement regulatory proteins and when this balance is upset, HELLP can develop in certain cases. This has been supported by reports in the literature demonstrating an increase in markers of complement activation (C5a and C5b-9) in PE/HELLP. Additionally, it has been shown that C5b-9 deposition on endothelial cells was increased following exposure to plasma from women with PE/HELLP syndrome.[6] A dysregulated complement system can also occur due to genetic mutations in complement proteins (Factor H, Factor I, membrane cofactor protein or C3) as identified in up to 45% patients with HELLP (range 5–45% across numerous studies).[7]

Clinical Features and Diagnosis

Presenting maternal symptoms may include abdominal pain localized to the right upper quadrant, nausea, vomiting, and fatigue. Acute kidney injury (AKI) has been reported in 10% with up to 40% of those patients requiring kidney replacement therapy (KRT), although this data reflects older studies which may not have sufficiently evaluated for aHUS.[8,9] In general, severe kidney injury is generally uncommon in HELLP and aHUS/CM-TMA should be considered in the differential in these cases.

The diagnosis of HELLP is made by the presence of elevated lactate dehydrogenase (LDH) with a level >600 IU/L, transaminases [aspartate aminotransferase (AST) or alanine aminotransferase (ALT)] greater than twice the upper limit of normal, and thrombocytopenia with platelet count <100k/μL. Additional testing is recommended to confirm that LDH elevation in HELLP is due to microangiopathic hemolysis (e.g., haptoglobin, peripheral smear). HELLP is often associated with PE-SF which is defined as BP >160/110 mm Hg on more than two occasions, and the presence of one of the following clinical or laboratory findings: thrombocytopenia with platelet count <100k/μL, abnormal liver function tests with transaminase levels twice the upper limit of normal or persistent right upper quadrant pain, AKI, intractable headache, pulmonary edema, or visual disturbances. A recent study conducted in hospitalized patients between 23 and 35 weeks of gestation showed that serum sFLT-1:PlGF ratio ≥40 was a marker of disease severity and predictive of severe PE and adverse outcomes.[10]

TREATMENT AND PROGNOSIS

Definitive treatment of HELLP syndrome centers around delivery of the fetus and placenta regardless of gestational age and should begin to resolve within 3–4 days of delivery **(Table 1)**. Persistence of severe thrombocytopenia (<30,000/μL) or AKI in the postpartum period beyond 72 hours should prompt consideration of an alternate diagnosis, such as thrombotic thrombocytopenic purpura (TTP) or CM-TMA. TTP can be ruled out by checking an ADAMTS13 activity level. If there is a delay in the turnaround time for this diagnostic test, empiric treatment with plasmapheresis should be initiated while awaiting results, especially if profound thrombocytopenia or neurologic symptoms are present. HELLP can potentially be differentiated from CM-TMA by the combination of serum creatinine and LDH discussed in the CM-TMA section of this chapter. Individuals who experience HELLP syndrome are at

TABLE 1: Complement-mediated disorders in pregnancy.

	HELLP	*CM-TMA*	*APS*
Diagnosis	• LDH >600 IU/L • AST, ALT ≥2 times the upper limit of normal • Platelet count <150k/μL	• Genetic testing for variants in complement proteins • Anti-FH antibody titers	• aPL antibody titers (LA, anticardiolipin IgG/IgM, anti-beta-2 glycoprotein I)
Treatment	• Delivery of fetus and placenta	• C5 inhibitors (eculizumab) • *If complement inhibitors are not available:* plasma exchange	• *Previous thrombotic event:* LMWH + LDA • *History of pregnancy morbidity without previous thrombotic event:* LMWH or LDA • *Previous pregnancy losses despite appropriate anticoagulation:* IVIG

(aPL: antiphospholipid; APS: antiphospholipid syndrome; CM-TMA: complement-mediated thrombotic microangiopathy; HELLP: hemolysis, elevated liver enzymes, and low platelet count syndrome; IVIG: intravenous immunoglobulin; LA: lupus anticoagulant; LDA: low-dose aspirin; LDH: lactate dehydrogenase; LMWH: low-molecular-weight heparin) an increased risk for development of preeclampsia and HELLP during subsequent pregnancies and for the development of chronic hypertension, seizures, stroke, cardiovascular disease, pulmonary edema, ESKD, and depression. Fetal complications can include intrauterine growth restriction (IUGR) and prematurity.

COMPLEMENT-MEDIATED TMA

Complement-mediated TMA is a potential complication of both pregnancy and postpartum period. Pregnancy-related CM-TMA is reported to occur in 1 in 25,000 pregnancies accounting for 7% of all TMA cases with 79% of these presenting in the postpartum period.[11,12] Morbidity is also high in CM-TMA with 81% of patients requiring dialysis and 46% progressing to ESKD.[13]

Etiology/Pathophysiology

Thrombotic microangiopathy is a well-described syndrome characterized by microangiopathic hemolytic anemia (hemoglobin level <10 g/dL, serum LDH level >1.5 upper limit of normal, undetectable serum haptoglobin, negative direct erythrocyte antiglobulin test, and presence of schistocytes on peripheral smear), thrombocytopenia (platelet count <150 × 10^9/L), and end organ damage with a predilection for the renal, cardiac, and nervous systems. The clinical manifestations occur due to endothelial injury and microthrombi formation in small blood vessels, leading to ischemic organ injury.

Complement-mediated TMA results from an overactivation of the alternative pathway (AP) of complement **(Fig. 2)**. The AP has the capacity to deposit on a pathogen without need for prior exposure. This innate immune self-amplifying defense mechanism leads to generation of small amount of autoactivated C3 continuously generated in blood at 1–2%/hour called tick-over.[14] If it deposits on healthy self-tissue or ticks over in the fluid phase, host regulatory proteins immediately inactivate it. However, if it is deposited on a microbe, activated C3

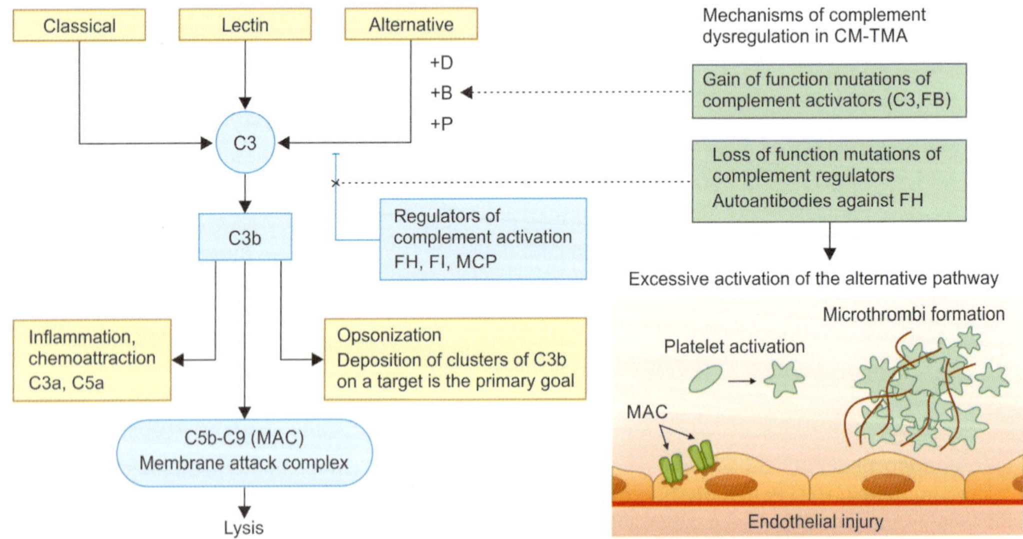

Fig. 2: Overactivation of the alternative complement pathway leading to endothelial injury.

can be rapidly amplified by engaging two proteases, Factor B and Factor D, along with a stabilizing protein, properdin (P), to create the powerful AP C3 convertase. Contained within the AP is an efficient feedback or amplification loop for the generation of large amounts of C3b to opsonize a pathogen. As previously discussed, the complement system requires strict control to avoid damage to self. Inhibition of complement activation is mediated by host regulators in the plasma as well as on cells. In CM-TMA, an excessive degree of AP activation takes place in the setting of dysfunctional control, leading to microthrombi, especially in the glomeruli of the vulnerable kidney.[14]

The most common etiology of a dysregulated complement system in CM-TMA is a heterozygous, loss-of-function mutation in a regulator of the AP such as in Factor H (FH), Factor I (FI), or membrane cofactor protein (MCP, CD46) that leads to haploinsufficiency as identified in 60–70% patients.[14] In these cases, the protein is generally (1) not synthesized, (2) synthesized but not secreted, or (3) secreted in normal amounts but is dysfunctional. Less frequently, a gain-of-function mutation in a complement activator (C3, Factor B) is identified. Acquired deficiencies in the form of autoantibodies against FH also occur in ~5–10% of patients.[15] A genetic defect, namely a homozygous deletion in CFHR1 and CFHR3 (complement FH-related 1 and 3), may predispose to the development of FH autoantibodies. Disease penetrance is ~50%, suggesting that an environmental trigger is necessary in most cases. Pregnancy is considered one of the major triggers for CM-TMA.

Clinical Features and Diagnosis

Presenting symptoms vary widely and consist of nausea, vomiting, abdominal pain, headache, altered mental status, and hypertension. Renal impairment is almost always seen with CM-TMA. Markedly elevated creatinine and LDH strongly suggest pregnancy-associated CM-TMA and can be used to differentiate from HELLP in the postpartum period. A serum creatinine of ≥1.9 mg/dL or an LDH ≥1832 U/L or a serum creatinine ≥1.9 mg/dL + LDH ≥600 U/L is reported to be >95% specific for a diagnosis of CM-TMA.[16]

A kidney biopsy (when feasible) can be performed to confirm the diagnosis of TMA. Biopsy can also be useful to evaluate the extent of organ damage and to rule out other etiologies of kidney failure. Pathologically, TMA is characterized on light microscopy by the presence of fibrin thrombi within the glomeruli. However, in some biopsies, overt thrombosis is not seen. Nonthrombotic features include endothelial swelling and mesangiolysis (in active lesions), double contours of the glomerular basement membrane (in chronic lesions), as well as accumulation of fluffy material in the subendothelium. Intramural fibrin deposition, myxoid intimal thickening, and concentric myointimal proliferation (onion skinning) may occur in arteries and arterioles.

Evaluation for underlying genetic variants in complement proteins should be conducted in all patients. The clinically validated next-generation sequencing-based complement, multiplex ligation-dependent probe amplification (MLPA) and coagulation disease panel, currently consists of 15 genes (*ADAMTS13, C3, CD46, CFB, CFH, CFHR1, CFHR2, CFHR3, CFHR4, CFHR5, CFI, DGKE, THBD, MMACHC*, and *PLG*). If identified, interpretation of variants may require additional functional assays, biomarker testing, or need for recombinant protein production followed by structure–function assessment of the variants. Genetic and functional testing can take up to 4–6 weeks, therefore are not used to make a diagnosis of CM-TMA but are important to determine risk of relapse and recurrence of disease as well as to establish duration of treatment.

Treatment and Prognosis

Prior to the approval of C5 inhibitors, treatment with plasma exchange and plasma infusion was the mainstay for the management of CM-TMA although overall efficacy was poor **(Table 1)**. The rationale behind this treatment is to reduce the quantity of a mutant protein by plasmapheresis and then deliver functionally normal protein by plasma infusion. Plasma therapies remain the initial treatment of choice when complement inhibitors are not available.

Eculizumab is a humanized monoclonal antibody to C5 which blocks activation of the terminal pathway and prevents MAC formation. Multiple studies and case reports have shown relative efficacy and safety of eculizumab in pregnancy.[17,18] When used during pregnancy, eculizumab has been detected at low concentrations in umbilical cord blood, suggesting that it crosses the placenta at low levels; however, it does not seem to alter the complement system activity of the fetus. It is also considered safe with lactation and has not been detected in breast milk samples of women receiving eculizumab.[18]

A newer longer acting C5 inhibitor, ravulizumab, is also approved for CM-TMA. Ravulizumab has been engineered from eculizumab by changing four amino acids which preserves the binding of ravulizumab to C5 in serum but allows it to dissociate from C5 in the acidified endosome (pH 6.0).[19] These alterations also result in an increased efficiency of ravulizumab recycling via neonatal Fc receptor and increased affinity of ravulizumab for this receptor by more than 10 times compared to eculizumab. This leads to an increased half-life of ~52 days compared to ~11 days for eculizumab but also, higher uptake into the fetal circulation and breastmilk. Due to this, its use is not recommended in pregnancy or lactation, but its use in postpartum CM-TMA has been reported with complete response in 87.5% of patients by 31 days and discontinuation of dialysis by 21 days.[19]

The predominant concern with using any anticomplement therapy is a life-threatening infection with *Neisseria meningitidis*. Meningococcal vaccination must be administered to everyone undergoing treatment with C5 inhibitor. This vaccine is considered safe to administer with pregnancy and lactation. In addition, if C5 inhibitor must be given urgently, appropriate prophylactic antibiotics should be used for at least 14 days following the first dose of meningococcal vaccine.

Several other drugs for CM-TMA are also in development or undergoing clinical trials. These novel complement inhibitors include crovalimab (anti-C5), nomacopan (anti-C5), pegcetacoplan (anti-C3), iptacopan (anti-factor B), and narsoplimab [mannose-binding lectin-associated serine protease 2 (MASP-2)]. Prospective, randomized controlled trials are required to investigate the utility of these therapies in CM-TMA and particularly their efficacy and safety in pregnancy-associated CM-TMA.

Maternal complications of pregnancy-associated CM-TMA include increased risk of preterm delivery, disseminated intravascular coagulation (DIC), ESKD, stroke, and even death. Babies born to mothers with CM-TMA are often small-for-gestational age and have low birth weight with increased risk for fetal morbidity and mortality.[11] When diagnosed and treated promptly with C5 inhibition, outcomes of pregnancy-associated CM-TMA are considerably improved with decreased progression to ESKD, less time on dialysis, and successful remission of disease.[17,18]

ANTIPHOSPHOLIPID SYNDROME

Antiphospholipid syndrome is a systemic autoimmune disorder characterized by development of antiphospholipid antibodies (aPLAb) which include lupus anticoagulant (LA), anticardiolipin antibodies (aCLAb), and anti-beta2 glycoprotein I (anti-beta2GPIAb). The estimated prevalence of APS ranges from 17 to 50 patients per 1,000,000.[20,21] It is estimated that aPLAbs are associated with 50,000 pregnancy losses, 110,000 strokes, 100,000 myocardial infarctions, and 30,000 deep vein thromboses (DVT) every year in the US.[22] APS can occur as a primary condition in ~50% patients or in the setting of systemic lupus erythematosus (SLE) or another systemic autoimmune disease.[23]

Etiology/Pathophysiology

Antiphospholipid antibodies can lead to thrombosis by inhibition of the anticoagulant cascade and fibrinolytic activity and enhancing platelet aggregation as well as complement activation **(Fig. 3)**. The current model of aPLAb-mediated thrombosis, however, is better defined by a "two-hit" hypothesis since thrombosis alone is often not sufficient to explain the placental damage

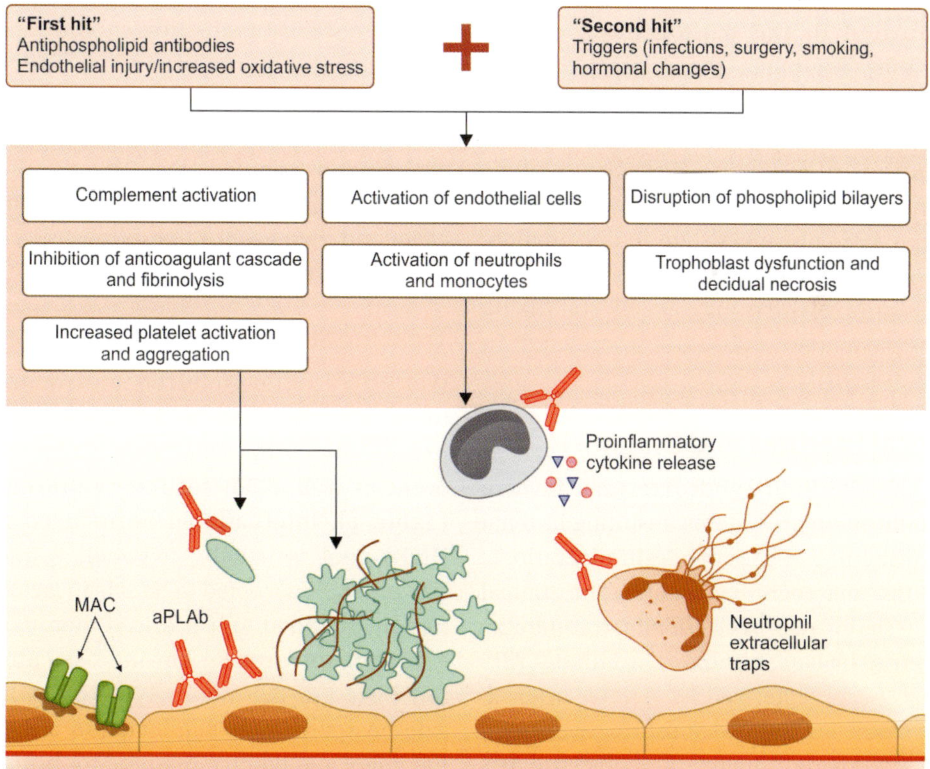

Fig. 3: "Two-hit" hypothesis in antiphospholipid antibody syndrome.

observed in APS. Patients with positive aPL antibodies (first hit) often need an additional inciting agent or trigger (second hit) to manifest disease. Triggers can include infection, sepsis, surgery, smoking or commonly, hormonal changes during pregnancy. Together, these mechanisms result in a proinflammatory state involving activation of neutrophils and monocytes, disruption of the phospholipid bilayer, and complement activation.[24] Animal models have demonstrated that inflammatory processes involving complement activation contribute most to poor obstetric outcomes by promoting coagulation and cellular injury. Additionally, the interaction of aPLAb with the disrupted phospholipid bilayer can lead to trophoblast dysfunction and decidual necrosis. Neutrophil extracellular traps (NETs) have also been implicated in the pathogenesis of APS and may aggravate thrombosis through activation of the coagulation cascade and inhibition of anticoagulant factors. Antiphospholipid antibodies themselves promote NET formation. Moreover, NETs formed in APS appear resistant to degradation. Anti-NET antibodies (particularly immunoglobulin M), which may act by stabilizing NETs, are also markedly increased in patients with APS.

Clinical Features and Diagnosis

Antiphospholipid syndrome may involve virtually all organ systems, resulting in renal impairment, TMA, stroke, skin ulcerations, seizures, and cognitive decline. The clinical manifestations can be classified as thrombotic, obstetric, or catastrophic. Thrombotic APS is mainly characterized by venous, arterial, and small vessel thrombotic events in different organs. A hallmark of obstetric APS is pregnancy complications, which include preeclampsia, recurrent early pregnancy loss, fetal death, or premature birth due to IUGR. LA positivity has been shown in several prospective studies to be a strong predictor of poor pregnancy outcomes.[25] Patients who carry all three autoantibodies (triple aPL positivity) are reported to have significantly worse pregnancy outcomes with increased risk of fetal loss. Approximately 1% of patients with APS may develop catastrophic APS (CAPS) which is a severe and life-threatening form characterized by microvascular and macrovascular thrombosis that develop simultaneously or over a short period of time leading to multiorgan failure and a significantly increased risk of mortality.[24]

Diagnosis should be suspected when patients present with thrombotic events and adverse pregnancy outcomes especially in the setting of recurrent miscarriages and/or SLE. Laboratory evaluation should include complete blood count, renal function panel, coagulation profile, urinalysis and urine protein evaluation, antinuclear Ab, anti-double-stranded DNA Ab, and aPLAb. aPL antibodies are usually obtained at time of event and then again 12 or more weeks later to confirm the diagnosis.

Treatment and Prognosis

Warfarin is the preferred anticoagulant for nonpregnant or postpartum patients presenting with their first thrombotic event as well as for secondary prevention **(Table 1)**. International normalized ratio (INR) goal is usually between 2 and 3. It is generally accepted to be safe in lactation. Aspirin is added to warfarin if there is also a history of arterial thrombosis and at low dose (75–325 mg daily) is considered safe postpartum during lactation although the infant should be monitored for bruising/bleeding.

In pregnancy, low-molecular-weight heparin (LMWH) is used in place of warfarin due to its known teratogenicity. If there is a history of former thrombotic event, expert opinion recommends LMWH along with low-dose aspirin due to the prothrombotic nature of pregnancy. In patients with no prior history of thrombosis but with laboratory criteria for aPL and ≥1 fetal loss at ≥10 weeks of gestation or ≥3 unexplained consecutive, spontaneous pregnancy losses at <10 weeks of gestation, treatment also consists of low-dose aspirin and prophylactic LMWH. If a patient has positive aPL antibodies and ≥1 preterm delivery before 34 weeks of gestation or other findings consistent with placental insufficiency without prior thrombotic event, patient is treated with low-dose aspirin or LMWH alone. Intravenous immunoglobulin (IVIG) is reserved for those with a history of pregnancy losses despite appropriate anticoagulation. The management of CAPS is similar, and patients are treated with anticoagulation, highdose solumedrol, and plasma exchange or IVIG. If refractory to treatment, a trial of rituximab or eculizumab can be considered.

Statins upregulate endothelial nitric oxide synthase and may be protective in APS. While statins are no longer considered contraindicated in pregnancy, their use in APS during pregnancy is still not recommended.[26] Hydroxychloroquine can also be considered for those with APS secondary to SLE. Direct oral anticoagulants (DOACs) are not used since they have been associated with increased risk of thrombotic events and strokes in several studies.[27]

Long-term outcomes for pregnant patients with APS can vary, however, the overall rate of live birth is lower (~73%) compared to the general US population (~90%).[28,29] The most common obstetric complication is recurrent miscarriage which occurs in about 1% of the general population as compared to 10–15% of women with APS.[30,31] High-titer aCLAb and prior fetal loss carry an 80% risk of future pregnancy loss.[1] After pregnancy, women with APS remain at higher risk of venous thromboembolism and ischemic cerebrovascular disease. Children born to mothers with APS may also have higher rates of learning disabilities although these studies have been small and conclusive evidence of this association remains to be seen.

CONCLUSION

Diagnosing and differentiating between various complement disorders in pregnancy can be challenging given several overlapping features between the three most common etiologies. A thorough clinical history, laboratory data, and careful attention to presenting features can serve to clarify the diagnosis in many cases **(Table 1)**. Prompt treatment is necessary to avoid significant morbidity and mortality as well as the potential long-term complications for both the mother and infant.

REFERENCES

1. Lockshin MD, Qamar T, Druzin ML, Goei S. Antibody to cardiolipin, lupus anticoagulant, and fetal death. J Rheumatol. 1987;14(2):259-62.
2. Yonekura Collier AR, Zsengeller Z, Pernicone E, Salahuddin S, Khankin EV, Karumanchi SA. Placental sFLT-1 is associated with complement activation and syncytiotrophoblast damage in pre-eclampsia. Hypertens Pregnancy. 2019; 38(3):193-9.
3. Kirkpatrick CA. The HELLP syndrome. Acta Clin Belg. 2010;65(2):91-7.
4. Sibai BM, Ramadan MK, Usta I, Salama M, Mercer BM, Friedman SA. Maternal morbidity and mortality in 442 pregnancies

with hemolysis, elevated liver enzymes, and low platelets (HELLP syndrome). Am J Obstet Gynecol. 1993;169(4):1000-6.
5. van Lieshout L, Koek GH, Spaanderman MA, van Runnard Heimel PJ. Placenta derived factors involved in the pathogenesis of the liver in the syndrome of haemolysis, elevated liver enzymes and low platelets (HELLP): A review. Pregnancy Hypertens. 2019;18: 42-8.
6. Palomo M, Blasco M, Molina P, Lozano M, Praga M, Torramade-Moix S, et al. Complement activation and thrombotic microangiopathies. Clin J Am Soc Nephrol. 2019;14(12):1719-32.
7. Burwick RM, Feinberg BB. Complement activation and regulation in preeclampsia and hemolysis, elevated liver enzymes, and low platelet count syndrome. Am J Obstet Gynecol. 2022;226(2S):S1059-S1070.
8. Fang JT, Chen YC, Huang CC. Unusual presentation of mesangial proliferative glomerulonephritis in HELLP syndrome associated with acute renal failure. Ren Fail. 2000;22(5):641-6.
9. Gupta A, Ferguson J, Rahman M, Weber-Shrikant E, Venuto R. Acute oliguric renal failure in HELLP syndrome: case report and review of literature. Ren Fail. 2012;34(5):653-6.
10. Thadhani R, Lemoine E, Rana S, Costantine MM, Calsavara VF, Boggess K, et al. Circulating angiogenic factor levels in hypertensive disorders of pregnancy. NEJM Evidence. 2022;1(12):EVIDoa2200161.
11. Fakhouri F, Roumenina L, Provot F, Sallée M, Caillard S, Couzi L, et al. Pregnancy-associated hemolytic uremic syndrome revisited in the era of complement gene mutations. J Am Soc Nephrol. 2010;21(5):859-67.
12. Asif A, Nayer A, Haas CS. Atypical hemolytic uremic syndrome in the setting of complement-amplifying conditions: case reports and a review of the evidence for treatment with eculizumab. J Nephrol. 2017;30(3):347-62.
13. Fremeaux-Bacchi V, Fakhouri F, Garnier A, Bienaimé F, Dragon-Durey MA, Ngo S, et al. Genetics and outcome of atypical hemolytic uremic syndrome: a nationwide French series comparing children and adults. Clin J Am Soc Nephrol. 2013;8(4):554-62.
14. Liszewski MK, Java A, Schramm EC, Atkinson JP. Complement dysregulation and disease: Insights from contemporary genetics. Annu Rev Pathol. 2017;12:25-52.
15. Sinha A, Gulati A, Saini S, Blanc C, Gupta A, Gurjar BS, et al. Prompt plasma exchanges and immunosuppressive treatment improves the outcomes of anti-factor H autoantibody-associated hemolytic uremic syndrome in children. Kidney Int. 2014;85(5): 1151-60.
16. Burwick RM, Moyle K, Java A, Gupta M. Differentiating hemolysis, elevated liver enzymes, and low platelet count syndrome and atypical hemolytic uremic syndrome in the postpartum period. Hypertension. 2021;78(3):760-8.
17. Fakhouri F, Scully M, Provôt F, Blasco M, Coppo P, Noris M, et al. Management of thrombotic microangiopathy in pregnancy and postpartum: report from an international working group. Blood. 2020;136(19): 2103-17.
18. Kelly RJ, Höchsmann B, Szer J, Kulasekararaj A, de Guibert S, Röth A, et al. Eculizumab in pregnant patients with paroxysmal nocturnal hemoglobinuria. N Engl J Med. 2015;373(11):1032-9.
19. Gackler A, Schönermarck U, Dobronravov V, La Manna G, Denker A, Liu P, et al. Efficacy and safety of the long-acting C5 inhibitor ravulizumab in patients with atypical hemolytic uremic syndrome triggered by pregnancy: a subgroup analysis. BMC Nephrol. 2021;22(1):5.
20. Radin M, Sciascia S, Bazzan M, Bertero T, Carignola R, Montabone E, et al. Antiphospholipid Syndrome Is Still a Rare Disease-Estimated Prevalence in the Piedmont and Aosta Valley Regions of Northwest Italy: Comment on the Article by Duarte-Garcia et al. Arthritis Rheumatol. 2020;72(10):1774-6.
21. Duarte-Garcia A, Crowson CS, Warrington KJ, Matteson EL. Reply. Arthritis Rheumatol. 2020;72(10):1776.

22. Andreoli L, Chighizola CB, Banzato A, Pons-Estel GJ, Ramire de Jesus G, Erkan D. Estimated frequency of antiphospholipid antibodies in patients with pregnancy morbidity, stroke, myocardial infarction, and deep vein thrombosis: a critical review of the literature. Arthritis Care Res (Hoboken). 2013;65(11):1869-73.
23. Cervera R, Serrano R, Pons-Estel GJ, Ceberio-Hualde L, Shoenfeld Y, de Ramón E, et al. Morbidity and mortality in the antiphospholipid syndrome during a 10-year period: a multicentre prospective study of 1000 patients. Ann Rheum Dis. 2015;74(6):1011-8.
24. Giannakopoulos B, Krilis SA. The pathogenesis of the antiphospholipid syndrome. N Engl J Med. 2013;368(11):1033-44.
25. Yelnik CM, Laskin CA, Porter TF, Branch DW, Buyon JP, Guerra MM, et al. Lupus anticoagulant is the main predictor of adverse pregnancy outcomes in aPL-positive patients: validation of PROMISSE study results. Lupus Sci Med. 2016;3(1):e000131.
26. Laufs U, La Fata V, Plutzky J, Liao JK. Upregulation of endothelial nitric oxide synthase by HMG CoA reductase inhibitors. Circulation. 1998;97(12):1129-35.
27. Woller SC, Stevens SM, Kaplan D, Wang TF, Branch DW, Groat D, et al. Apixaban compared with warfarin to prevent thrombosis in thrombotic antiphospholipid syndrome: a randomized trial. Blood Adv. 2022;6(6):1661-70.
28. Chen HY, Shih JC, Tsai MH, Chung CH. Long-term survival and renal outcomes of thrombotic microangiopathy in pregnancy: A retrospective cohort study. Int J Gynaecol Obstet. 2023;163(3):940-7.
29. Boklage CE. Survival probability of human conceptions from fertilization to term. Int J Fertil. 1990;35(2):75, 79-80, 81-94.
30. Rai RS, Regan L, Clifford K, Pickering W, Dave M, Mackie I, et al. Antiphospholipid antibodies and beta 2-glycoprotein-I in 500 women with recurrent miscarriage: results of a comprehensive screening approach. Hum Reprod. 1995;10(8):2001-5.
31. Stirrat GM. Recurrent miscarriage. Lancet. 1990;336(8716):673-5.

CHAPTER 7

Acute Kidney Injury in Pregnancy

Arpita Ray Chaudhury (Lahiri)

HIGHLIGHTS

- Acute kidney injury in pregnancy (Pr-AKI) is poorly defined as physiologic changes in pregnancy that lead to a significant increase in glomerular filtration rate (GFR) and 50% fall of creatinine, making it unsuitable to fit in standard AKI definition criteria by RIFLE (risk, injury, failure, loss, end-stage kidney disease), Acute Kidney Injury Network (AKIN), and Kidney Disease: Improving Global Outcomes (KDIGO), and a baseline creatinine is often not available.
- Pr-AKI has decreased globally because of improved obstetric care and better health care access; however, in developing countries, puerperal sepsis, hemorrhages, and severe preeclampsia remain a cause of poor maternal and fetal outcome. In developed world, pregnancy at a higher age exposes the mother to AKI due to many comorbidities like hypertension, diabetes, obesity, and chronic kidney disease.
- The thrombotic microangiopathies-associated causes of Pr-AKI, atypical hemolytic uremic syndrome (aHUS), thrombotic thrombocytopenic purpura (TTP), and antiphospholipid antibody (APLA)-related syndrome are rare but difficult to differentiate from relatively common causes like preeclampsia, HELLP (hemolysis, elevated liver enzymes, low platelet count) syndrome, or lupus nephritis flare in pregnancy. The clinical clue-based high suspicion index and differential-based battery of tests may be able to clinch the right diagnosis early. Early goal-directed therapy may improve both fetal and maternal outcome.
- Puerperal infections and hemorrhage may initiate a cascade of multifactorial AKI and may remain one of the most important preventable causes of PR-AKI. An interdisciplinary collaborative approach for sepsis prevention and early diagnosis is necessary to improve outcome.
- Management of Pr-AKI includes treatment of underlying cause, preserving kidney function, and providing supportive care for those who need dialysis and intensive care unit (ICU) support.

INTRODUCTION

Compared to acute kidney injury (AKI) in general population, obstetric AKI or AKI patients in pregnancy (Pr-AKI) are particularly prone to facing adverse outcomes, both short and long term.[1] It demands more attention as it accounts for risk of two lives and is largely preventable. Short-term outcome is a rise in maternal and fetal mortality and morbidity in resource-limited setting of the developing world. Severe AKI in pregnancy often leads to bilateral cortical necrosis and either progresses to immediate dialysis-dependent end-stage renal disease (ESRD) or gradually progresses to chronic kidney disease (CKD). The main reason lies in limited access to obstetric care and inadequate sepsis-prevention measures. Long-term consequences include progression to CKD and increased cardiovascular risk in surviving patients and high healthcare resource utilization. In an Indian scenario, many studies have highlighted that puerperal sepsis is the main reason of increased maternal mortality, which is a highly preventable cause. Increased awareness and early diagnosis with well-adopted preventive measures may change the scenario in countries with high Pr-AKI prevalence, like India, Bangladesh, or Pakistan.

EPIDEMIOLOGY

Currently in India, majority of Pr-AKI occurs in the postpartum period or late third trimester. The postabortion sepsis of early pregnancy has decreased from 9–10% in 1980–1990 to 1.5–2% in 2014.[2] PIH remains important cause if the whole spectrum of AKI (both dialysis requiring and non requiring) is taken in account, because most of the AKI due to PIH is nondialysis requiring and resolves once the baby is delivered. However, when severe AKI or dialysis-requiring AKI is considered, puerperal sepsis and postpartum hemorrhage (PPH) remain main contributors along with currently rising diagnosis of pregnancy-related thrombotic microangiopathy (P-TMA). It is important to understand that Pr-AKI is often multifactorial, and difficult or delayed access to right health care often worsens the prognosis. In India, there are encouraging reports of declining incidence of Pr-AKI,[2,3] particularly due to decline of septic abortion and improved antenatal care (ANC) access, but postpartum sepsis still remains an important cause of mortality, and P-TMA [atypical hemolytic uremic syndrome (aHUS)/ thrombotic thrombocytopenic purpura (TTP)] is increasingly being diagnosed as a cause of poor renal and maternal outcome of Pr-AKI.

Although a more sinister problem of low- to middle-income countries (LMIC), Pr-AKI is still considered as a global problem and two recent reports from Canada and US had shown a recent rise of AKI (an increase in the incidence of Pr-AKI from 2.4 per 10,000 deliveries in 1999–2001 to 6.3 per 10,000 deliveries in 2010–2011 in the US and 1.66 per 10,000 deliveries in 2003–2004 to 2.68 per 10,000 deliveries in 2009–2010) due to increasing incidence of preeclampsia pregnancy occurring in the setting of older maternal age and higher comorbidities (CKD, hypertensive disorders, diabetes, and obesity) along with higher detection of AKI. The studies also registered a higher incidence in native Americans and blacks where education is limited, thus compromising timely access to obstetric care, echoing a similar crisis in developing nations.[4,5]

DEFINITION AND DIAGNOSIS OF ACUTE KIDNEY INJURY IN PREGNANCY

Acute kidney injury in general population has well-validated diagnostic criteria evolving over time (2004–2007) by RIFLE (risk, injury, failure, loss, end-stage kidney disease) criteria,[6,7] Acute Kidney Injury Network (AKIN) criteria,[8] and Kidney Disease: Improving Global Outcomes (KDIGO) staging,[9] but these are not validated in pregnant population because of the unique physiological changes occurring during pregnancy.[10]

Pregnancy-related increase in blood volume and cardiac output with decline in systemic vascular resistance results in hyperfiltration, which gives rise to increased effective plasma renal flow; consequently, glomerular filtration rate (GFR) increases by 40–60%, with a decrease in creatinine value during pregnancy, usually 0.4–0.6 mg/dL, which confounds the detection of creatinine-based diagnosis of AKI in obstetric population. In an Indian study reporting 253 pregnant individuals with AKI, Pr-AKI was diagnosed based on sudden increase of >1 mg/dL in serum creatinine, oliguria/anuria >12 hours, and/or the need for dialysis.[2] A similar definition was picked up in other studies.[3,11] A creatinine prior to pregnancy is not available most of the time. In a clinically relevant condition, e.g., new-onset hypertension in pregnancy with low platelets, an increase of even smaller magnitude than that accepted in AKIN (0.3 mg/dL change accepted as stage 1) criteria, like 0.2 mg/dL, may be considered a significant pointer toward AKI [HELLP (hemolysis, elevated liver enzymes, low platelet count) or aHUS in the third trimester and postpartum] and may set up an alarm for a close follow-up with serial creatinine and relevant serologies. Renal ultrasounds that are performed to rule out postrenal causes of AKI or an underlying kidney disease may show hydronephrosis, which may be physiologic rather than pathologic. Serum complements estimation is important for diagnosing autoimmune diseases such as lupus nephritis (flare or first appearance) but may lose significance as serum complements are higher in pregnancy because of increased synthesis by the liver. Proteinuria also increases in pregnancy likely because of hyperfiltration, and higher normal has been set to 300 mg/day; therefore, the preeclampsia diagnosis includes urine protein–creatinine ratio (UPCR) >0.3 as a diagnostic criterion. It might be a reflection of tubular proteinuria too, as some studies have shown a rise in urinary retinol-binding protein (RBP) in pregnancy. Hence, albuminuria has not been the criterion for diagnosis. Increased UPCR in absence of hypertension which may be seen in 15% of normal pregnancy may mandate a close follow-up in a selective clinical scenario because pregnancy may be complicated by nephrotic syndrome as well. Kidney biopsy in pregnancy in early trimester may be of help to resolve a doubt between preeclampsia and nephrotic syndrome and may ask for a change in therapy. Late-trimester biopsy-related complications are more; people preferably may wait till the postdelivery period for biopsy.[12]

Many studies have arbitrarily considered a diagnosis of AKI when creatinine exceeds 1 mg/dL. Also, routine creatinine monitoring is not practiced as standard of care in pregnancy. All these together make early detection of AKI in pregnancy challenging and mandate a good clinical differential and blood biochemistry evaluation as soon as AKI is diagnosed in pregnancy.

ETIOLOGY OF ACUTE KIDNEY INJURY IN PREGNANCY

Causes of AKI in pregnancy may be unique to the causes related to pregnancy when an otherwise healthy woman suffers from hyperemesis gravidarum, septic abortion, puerperal sepsis, aHUS, HELLP syndrome, or preeclampsia or else it may be categorized as per causes similar in general population (prerenal, renal, and postrenal).

For *prerenal causes*, a hemodynamic compromise with volume depletion starts in the setting of hyperemesis gravidarum, septic abortion, pyelonephritis or postpartum sepsis, and antepartum or postpartum hemorrhage. There is a reversible reduction in GFR; left untreated, it leads to ischemic acute tubular injury [acute tubular necrosis (ATN)]. Usually, ATN is more common and reversible and renal function comes back in 7–21 days but in association with pregnancy, it has a predilection to progress to irreversible acute cortical necrosis (ACN) in most severe cases. Relatively rare causes of prerenal AKI include amniotic fluid embolism, acute fatty liver of pregnancy (AFLP), and chorioamnionitis.

Acute cortical necrosis is a pathologic diagnosis resulting from compromised vascular supply to kidney in a setting of severe hypotension with septic shock or obstetric hemorrhage or from intravascular thromboses in the interlobular and afferent arterioles diffusely involving the cortex while sparing the medulla. Often, it leads to dialysis-dependent CKD. Why ACN is fairly common in pregnancy-related AKI probably finds explanation in the fact that pregnancy is a hypercoagulable state with increased levels of coagulation factors with suppressed fibrinolysis and with any additional trigger, a series of complex and self-enhancing cascades are activated, like coagulation cascade, renin–angiotensin and complement pathways. Disseminated intravascular coagulation (DIC) may be the end result of such complex interactions, and renal recovery becomes unlikely.[13] The incidence of pregnancy-associated ACN, like overall pregnancy-related AKI, however, is decreasing. An Indian study showed a decrease in the incidence from 4.7% to 0.5% between the years 1984 and 2005.[14] While legalization of abortion has decreased the incidence of septic abortion, other causes like pregnancy-related TMA are increasingly diagnosed and both TMA and puerperal sepsis are coming up as potential causes of ACN in the postpartum period.[2,3]

Pregnancy-related *intrarenal* causes include the spectrum of diseases under hypertensive disorders in pregnancy like preeclampsia, AFLP, and HELLP syndrome. Other conditions which may be precipitated and worsened by pregnancy include pyelonephritis, sepsis, lupus nephritis, and TTP/complement-mediated aHUS. Whatever may be the initiating insult, a fullblown Pr-AKI is often multifactorial and AKI requiring dialysis often has a poor outcome leading to death or progression to dialysis-dependent CKD.[2,3]

Among *postrenal causes*, obstructive uropathy is a rare cause of Pr-AKI. The physiologic right-sided hydronephrosis occurs in up to 90% of pregnancies due to the compression of the ureter at the pelvic brim by the growing uterus, and progesterone induced smooth muscle relaxation, unless complicated by pyelonephritis this hydronephrosis causes neither decrease in urine output nor decline in GFR. Bilateral hydronephrosis, on the other hand, due to bilateral renal calculi, gravid uterus, especially with multiple gestations, polyhydramnios, and large fibroids can cause Pr-AKI. Post-delivery obstructive voiding symptoms have been reported after emergency cesarean delivery, following prolonged operation time, and postoperative analgesia that requires bladder catheterization. Iatrogenic injuries to the bladder and ureters from the cesarean section remain to be an uncommon cause for Pr-AKI. Postsurgical AKI when occurs due to breach in aseptic precaution, may result in grave consequences.

Causes of AKI in pregnancy are shown in **Figures 1 and 2**.

CLINICAL APPROACH TO PR-AKI

Medical History and Physical Examination

Whenever a Pr-AKI patient is seen in ward or emergency, both pregnancy-specific and pregnancy-unrelated AKI causes should be kept in mind. Medical history may reveal prior autoimmune diseases, like lupus nephritis, coexistent hypertension, and/or diabetes which are important, and history of nephrotoxic drugs like nonsteroidal

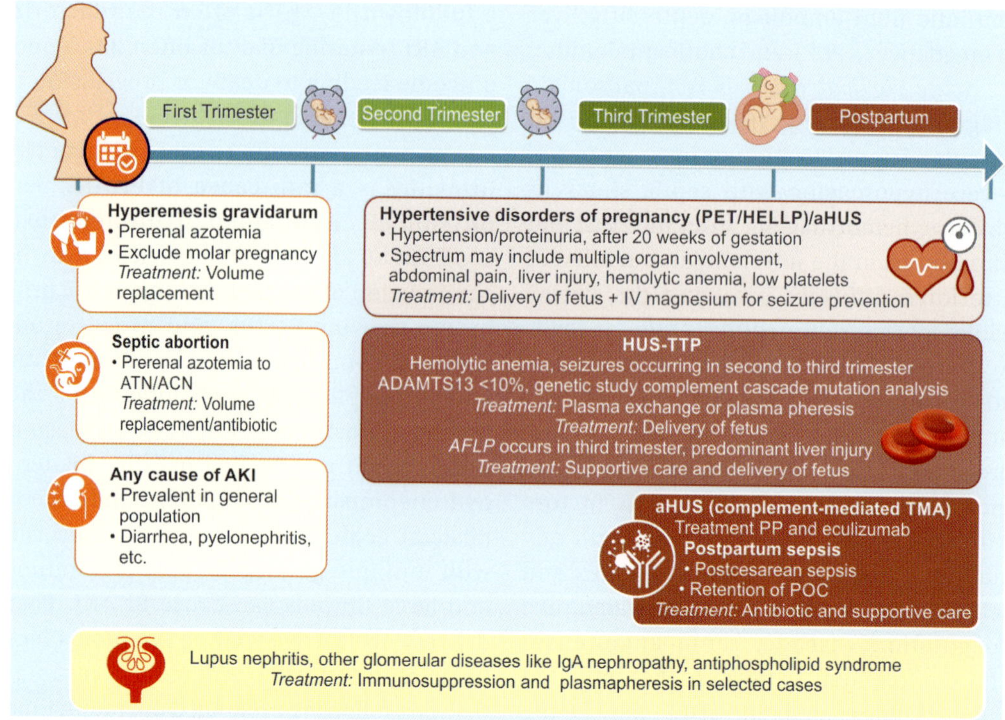

Fig. 1: Main causes of pregnancy-related AKI corresponding to timing during pregnancy with key diagnostic features. (ACN: acute cortical necrosis; AFLP: acute fatty liver of pregnancy; aHUS: atypical hemolytic uremic syndrome; AKI: acute kidney injury; APS: antiphospholipid antibody syndrome; ATN: acute tubular necrosis; HELLP: hemolysis, elevated liver enzymes, low platelets; PET: preeclamptic toxemia; POC: product of conception; TMA: thrombotic microangiopathy; TTP: thrombotic thrombocytopenic purpura)

Courtesy: Dr Priti Meena

anti-inflammatory drugs (NSAIDs) as post-lower uterine cesarean section analgesia may worsen the outcome of a resolving preeclampsia. The onset of preeclampsia is usually after 20 weeks; new-onset hypertension before 20 weeks may raise the probability of molar pregnancy, preexisting undiagnosed CKD, and inflammatory conditions like antiphospholipid antibody (APLA) syndrome (APS). Prior history of a similar episode or family history may be found in preeclampsia, congenital, or recurrent TTP.

Physical examination may detect volume depletion, dehydration, signs of other organ involvement in multisystem diseases or systemic vasculitis appearing in pregnancy, signs of enlarged tender liver in AFLP, heart failure with pregnancy and heart or kidney disease, signs of volume overload, severe anemia, and jaundice in Pr-TMA diseases.

Investigations

Urine examination may provide important information; proteinuria alone in a setting of new onset hypertension is most likely due to preeclampsia; but if associated with hematuria should bring in other glomerular diseases like lupus nephritis, systemic vasculitis and IgA nephropathy under differential diagnosis. A direct Coombs positive anemia, low C3, ANA, and anti-dsDNA positivity may

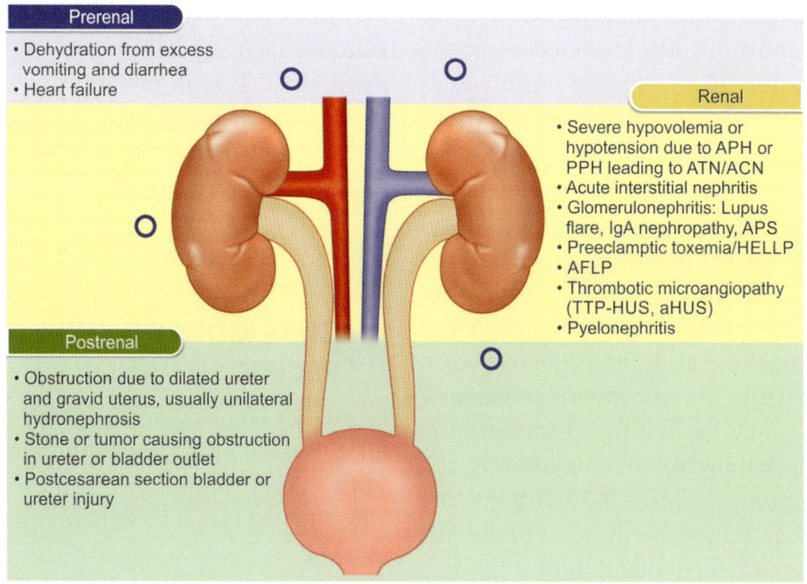

Fig. 2: Causes of AKI in pregnancy. (ACN: acute cortical necrosis; AFLP: acute fatty liver of pregnancy; aHUS: atypical hemolytic uremic syndrome; AKI: acute kidney injury; APH: antepartum hemorrhage; APS: antiphospholipid antibody syndrome; ATN: acute tubular necrosis; HELLP: hemolysis, elevated liver enzymes, low platelets; PET: preeclamptic toxemia; PPH: postpartum hemorrhage; TMA: thrombotic microangiopathy; TTP: thrombotic thrombocytopenic purpura)

Courtesy: Dr Priti Meena

confirm the diagnosis of lupus but other glomerular disease exclusion by renal biopsy. Baseline urine and blood biochemistry along with imaging is able to pick up diagnosis. The investigations done are:

- Dipstick urinalysis and microscopic analysis of sediment.
- Quantitation of protein excretion by either 24-hour urine collection or by protein-to-creatinine ratio.
- Urine culture
- Hemoglobin level and platelet count with peripheral blood smear to evaluate for microangiopathic hemolysis and thrombocytopenia.
- Total, direct, and indirect bilirubin concentration, haptoglobin, and lactate dehydrogenase (LDH) to evaluate for hemolysis.
- Serum aspartate aminotransferase (AST) and/or alanine aminotransferase (ALT) to assess liver injury in infection-associated and HELLP syndrome.
- *In specific cases:* Evaluation of the complement levels, autoantibodies of specific association like ANA, anti-ds DNA, ANA profile, perinuclear anti-neutrophil cytoplasmic antibody (p-ANCA) and cytoplasmic ANCA (c-ANCA), ADAMTS13, and antibody to ADAMTS13.
- *Imaging:* USG abdomen and thorax. The need of limited radiation exposure may be a challenge to establish diagnosis. Transvaginal ultrasonography, MRI, and low-dose CT remain the alternatives if needed.

TIMING OF ACUTE KIDNEY INJURY

The timing of AKI during pregnancy may serve as an important clue for making a differential diagnosis and plan relevant investigations. After significant decline in septic abortion, AKI that occurs in the first trimester in developing countries is mostly prerenal and may include any cause occurring in general population. First-onset lupus or flare of lupus nephritis may occur, and hyperemesis may be another pregnancy-specific cause. Any hypertensive disorder in early pregnancy should raise the suspicion of undiagnosed pre-existing hypertension and CKD and needs exclusion of molar or twin pregnancy. Urine microscopy and proteinuria evaluation may be helpful to identify the underlying kidney disease or identify the need for biopsy which may change the management of the patient. Most of the AKI occurring in the second and third trimesters are due to hypertensive complications such as preeclampsia/HELLP and TTP/HUS, where genetic predisposition also plays a role. Abruption placentae, severe hemorrhage, or DIC also decreased in frequency in India due to improved access to obstetric care. AFLP with AKI occurring in the third trimester may contribute to increased maternal mortality and morbidity. This relatively rare disease stands as an important differential with preeclamptic toxemia (PET)/HELLP. Atypical HUS, however, generally occurs late in the third trimester or postpartum after delivery and clinically stands as a differential of HELLP syndrome or puerperal sepsis. Pregnancy-related TTP may present in the early third trimester, earlier in timing than aHUS, and neurologic symptoms may be more prominent than renal involvement. Diagnosis of aHUS in the postpartum period often requires a high degree of suspicion, as AKI in this situation becomes multifactorial. Evaluation of intravascular hemolysis (anemia, thrombocytopenia, high LDH, low haptoglobin, and schistocytes in peripheral blood smear) may clinch the diagnosis early. Many of these diseases exhibit overlapping features, such as preeclampsia/HELLP, lupus nephritis, TTP/HUS, and AFLP.

Timing of recovery is also important. PE/HELLP/AFLP often tends to resolve following delivery, while Pr-aHUS does not.

Figure 3 shows signs and symptoms of overlapping syndromes of AKI.

ACUTE KIDNEY INJURY IN SPECIFIC SITUATIONS

Pregnancy is considered as a high-risk period for the development of different kinds of TMA. Three major syndromes including TTP, PE/HELLP, and aHUS may account for Pr-TMA

During pregnancy, immune tolerance toward the semiallogeneic fetus is necessary for the physiologic progression of gestation and the postpartum period is associated with the recovery of a pregestational immunocompetent state, where autoantibody-mediated diseases [e.g., acquired TTP, lupus nephritis, APLA syndrome, aHUS, complement mediated TMA (c-TMA)] may make their first or relapsing appearance.

The diagnostic challenge and therapeutic dilemma lie in their overlapping clinical features and at least sometimes, coexistence of more than one pathogenic mechanism. Each disorder terminates in the final event of endothelial damage and fibrin thrombi formation in the microcirculation. Both fragmented RBCs and platelet aggregates interfere with blood supply and cause ischemic injury to the target organs (kidney, brain, gastrointestinal tract, or liver). As the treatment differs, early diagnosis of the main pathologic mechanism may be crucial to intervene and improve fetal and maternal outcome.

Box 1 shows characteristics of TMA.

	PET/HELLP	TTP-HUS	aHUS	AFLP	APS	Lupus flare
Timing in pregnancy	>20 weeks	Higher in second trimester	Higher in postpartum	Last trimester	All gestational ages	All gestational ages
Blood pressure	3+	0–3+	2+	0–2+	0–3+	0–3+
Neurological involvement	0-3+	2+ to 3+	0–1+	0	0–3+	0–3+
Fever	0	1+ to 3+	0	1+ to 3+	2+	2+
Schistocytes in PBS >2%	0–2+	3+	2+	0–1+	2+	0
Thrombocytopenia	0–3+	2+ to 3+	3+	1+ to 3+	1+ to 2+	1+ to 2+
ADAMTS13 level	0–1+	3+	1+	0	0	0
Elevated liver enzymes	0–3+	0–1+	0–1+	2+ to 3+	0–1+	0
Proteinuria	0–1+	0–1+	0–1+	1+	0–1+	1+ to 3+
Treatment	Delivery of fetus	Plasmapheresis	Plasmapheresis and eculizumab	Delivery of fetus	Aspirin + anticoagulation	Immunosuppression

Fig. 3: Signs and symptoms of overlapping syndromes of acute kidney injury. (ADAMTS13: alpha disintegrin and metalloprotease with a thrombospondin type 1 motif member 13; AFLP: acute fatty liver of pregnancy; aHUS: atypical hemolytic uremic syndrome; APS: antiphospholipid antibody syndrome; HELLP: hemolysis, elevated liver enzymes, low platelets; PBS: peripheral blood smear; PET: preeclamptic toxemia; TTP: thrombotic thrombocytopenic purpura)

Notes: Ratings: 0 = Unlikely or not present, 1+ = Mild or low likelihood, 2+ = Moderate likelihood, 3+ = High likelihood.

BOX 1: Characteristics of thrombotic microangiopathy (TMA).

TMA is defined by a pathological pattern, endothelial cell swelling, detachment from the basement membrane, thrombi in the microcirculation, and, in the kidney, "double contour" aspects of the glomerular basement membrane and a dissolution or attenuation of the mesangial matrix (mesangiolysis); it is however usually diagnosed based on a clinicopathological triad:

- Peripheral thrombocytopenia (platelet count $<100 \times 10^9$/L)
- Mechanical hemolytic anemia (hemoglobin <10 g/dL, LDH >upper limit of normal, undetectable haptoglobin, schistocytes on blood smear)
- Organ injury

(LDH: lactate dehydrogenase)

Thrombotic Thrombocytopenic Purpura (Box 2)

Thrombotic thrombocytopenic purpura is a rare hematologic condition that is caused by a severe deficiency of the von Willebrand factor (vWF)-cleaving protease ADAMTS13, resulting in excess of highly adhesive unusually large vWF multimers, which causes inappropriate platelet clumping in the microvasculature under high shear stress conditions, leading to severe thrombocytopenia and occlusive microangiopathy. The classical description of TTP consists of the pentad of microangiopathic hemolytic anemia (MAHA), thrombocytopenia, fever, and renal and neurological dysfunction, though this pentad is present in only 40% of cases. TTP is classified as

BOX 2: Characteristics of thrombotic thrombocytopenic purpura (TTP), hemolytic uremic syndrome (HUS) and catastrophic antiphospholipid syndrome (CAPS).

TTP:
- TMA with mainly hematological, neurological, and potentially cardiac involvement
- Usually associated with a complete hereditary or immune deficiency in ADAMTS13 plasma activity

HUS:
- TMA with mainly renal involvement and potentially neurological and cardiac involvement
- May be linked to various types of endothelial cell injury
- Atypical HUS is caused by a dysregulation of the complement alternative pathway
- HUS can include extrarenal manifestations and TTP may be associated with significant renal disease; it may prove difficult to distinguish the two entities on clinical grounds alone

CAPS:
CAPS is defined by the occurrence of fulminant multiorgan damage (brain, kidney, lung, skin, etc.) resulting from extensive small-vessel thrombosis in the setting of persistent antiphospholipid antibodies (lupus anticoagulant, anticardiolipin, and anti-beta 2GPI antibodies); it is usually associated with thrombocytopenia and mechanical hemolytic anemia

immune-mediated TTP (iTTP) if the patient is positive for anti-ADAMTS13 autoantibodies and as congenital TTP (cTTP) if *ADAMTS13* gene abnormalities are detected. Along with the clinical picture of predominant neurological abnormalities, convulsions being the most common, renal insufficiency, nonspecific systemic symptoms, biochemical tests supporting anemia, thrombocytopenia, high LDH with direct Coombs test being negative, and ADAMTS13 (a vWF-cleaving protease) activity <10%, a diagnosis of TTP is considered. If antibody to ADAMTS13 is positive, a diagnosis of iTTP is established and a negative antibody test with low activity is diagnostic of cTTP or hereditary TTP. The maternal and fetal outcome is worse if cTTP occurs early in pregnancy or is associated with superimposed preeclampsia. If not diagnosed early and left untreated, end-organ damage and death may ensue. In the case of hereditary TTP, there is decreased production of ADAMTS13 from a genetic mutation, a syndrome known as Upshaw-Schulman syndrome (USS). In many patients of cTTP the disease may appear during pregnancy for the first time, as thrombophilia state of pregnancy acts as a second hit of thrombophilic state of pregnancy with high VWF and relatively low ADAMTS13 to manifest the disease and has a higher risk of appearing recurrently in pregnancy. Similarly, acquired TTP, occurring in adolescents and adults, may first appear in pregnancy. Physiologic gestation is characterized by a hypercoagulable state which is highest by the end of the third trimester to minimize bleeding complication during delivery. In normal pregnancy, VWF increases progressively toward the end of pregnancy and the protease is consumed, so ADAMTS13 decreases from the second trimester to the term up to an extent of 25–30% of the normal. These physiological changes of pregnancy may explain why for every congenitally deficient patient, the protease may go below 5–10% to trigger an acute episode.

The disease is a known mimicker of preeclampsia, and often the two entities can coexist within the same patient as initial and recurrent TTP presents most often in the second trimester (55.5%) after 1–2 days of signs/symptoms. One large study identified TTP with preeclampsia (n = 28) which exhibits two to four times higher AST values and lower total LDH to AST ratios =13:1, compared with TTP without preeclampsia (LDH to AST ratio = 29:1). Maternal mortality is higher with initial TTP (26% vs. 10.7%), especially with concurrent preeclampsia (44.4% vs. 21.8%; p <0.02).[15] Another UK TTP Registry[16] also confirmed. Prognosis was worse when TTP appeared in the 2nd or 3rd trimester than postpartum presentation. Although maternal mortality with TTP has substantially declined after utilization of plasma therapy, if there is delay of diagnosis and clinical picture of initial TTP gets confounded by preeclampsia/HELLP syndrome, there may be significant maternal-perinatal threat. Awareness of possibilities, right interpretation of clinical history, and availability of rapid laboratory testing to quickly diagnose TTP and HELLP syndrome/preeclampsia are desperately needed to improve care. Two scores have been developed—French and plasmic scores— but both are out of pregnancy setting, because of delayed or unavailable ADAMTS13 in low resource setting. Creatinine >2 mg/dL and platelets >30,000/μL are likely to exclude the diagnosis of TTP.

Treatment involves either replacement of the deficient ADAMTS13 with plasma infusion or removal of antibody or inhibitor, if present, by therapeutic plasma exchange (TPE) together with immune suppression in autoimmune (acquired) TTP with steroids and other immunosuppressants. Platelet therapy is only indicated to manage severe bleeding complication. Decision for expedited delivery depends on gestational age, fetal maturity, and clinical condition of the mother. The question remains whether to allow pregnancy the next time, as recurrence is 92% for cTTP and 42–45% for acquired TTP in subsequent pregnancy. The decision should be taken by family with risks explained and availability of higher center care and need to continue immunosuppression in acquired TTP. Use of heparin or low-dose aspirin is not practiced universally.[17]

Preeclampsia/HELLP Syndrome (Box 3)

Preeclampsia defined by new-onset hypertension and proteinuria after 20 weeks of

BOX 3: Clinical features of preeclampsia/eclampsia (PE/E) and HELLP (hemolysis, elevated liver enzymes and low platelet count) syndrome.

- PE is defined as gestational hypertension (systolic blood pressure ≥140 mm Hg and/or diastolic blood pressure ≥90 mm Hg) accompanied by ≥1 of the following new-onset conditions at ≥20 weeks' gestation:[4]
  - Proteinuria
  - Acute kidney injury (serum creatinine ≥90 μmol/L)
  - Alanine or aspartate aminotransferase >40 IU/L ± right upper quadrant or epigastric abdominal pain
- Eclampsia, in addition to the criteria defining PE, is characterized by altered mental status, blindness, stroke, clonus, severe headaches, and persistent visual scotomata
- Platelet count <100 g/L, disseminated intravascular coagulation, hemolysis
- Fetal growth restriction, abnormal umbilical artery Doppler waveform analysis, or stillbirth
- HELLP syndrome is considered part of PE/E (the most severe part of the spectrum of PE/E)
- PE/E and HELLP syndrome are associated with an imbalance between angiogenic (placental growth factor) and antiangiogenic (soluble Flt1) factors
- To date, PE/E and HELLP syndrome have not been linked to acquired or hereditary severe (<20%) deficiency in ADAMTS13 activity nor to a hereditary complement dysregulation

pregnancy is a relatively common condition, affecting 3–7% of pregnancies; when severe, it becomes an important contributor to maternal and fetal morbidity and mortality, not only in developing but also in the developed world. It has a long-term increased risk of cardiovascular diseases and premature death. Risk factors for preeclampsia include a previous history of preeclampsia, primiparity, obesity, maternal preexisting diabetes, hypertension, family history of preeclampsia, and multiple pregnancies. Early onset and presence of severe features are associated with poor outcome of both mother and baby. Proteinuria is not absolutely essential to diagnose preeclampsia; new-onset hypertension with proteinuria UPCR >0.3 and other laboratory markers like thrombocytopenia and altered liver function test (LFT) with typical symptoms being involved may define preeclampsia.[18]

Preeclampsia manifests with hypertension and proteinuria, and if hypertension is treated adequately AKI is unlikely. The patient recovers completely with delivery of the baby, sometimes the delivery may need to be expedited even with a preterm baby and compromised fetal outcome. AKI occurs only in 1% cases. But when associated with severe features, the pathophysiology of HELLP syndrome appears full blown and AKI incidence increases up to 7–15% of cases. Timing of onset of preeclampsia and association of severe features may be a challenge for diagnosis and therapy decision, as TTP/aHUS, AFLP, and lupus nephritis may come as important differentials. Clinical clues and simple investigations can help to formulate a working diagnosis.

The pathology of preeclampsia starts at the level of placenta. The placenta is attached to the maternal decidua by anchoring villi. During normal placentation, cytotrophoblasts cross these placental–maternal bridges and invade the maternal decidua and adjacent spiral arteries. They penetrate the walls of the arteries and replace part of the maternal endothelium, stimulating remodeling of the arterial wall such that the smooth muscle is thinned out and the artery dilates facilitating placental perfusion. Also, immune NK cells and macrophages in placenta facilitate deep invasion of cytotrophoblasts in the myometrial segments. In poor placentation syndrome, failure of remodeling of spiral artery leads to placental hypoperfusion and resultant fetal growth restriction and consequent ischemia and endothelial dysfunction. The maternal constitution and susceptibility often added to the placental syndrome and endothelial dysfunction lead to a more severe systemic circulatory inflammation response. The key player remains the soluble receptor for vascular endothelial growth factor (VEGF)-1, also known as sFlt-1 (soluble fms-like tyrosine kinase 1). It binds with the VEGFs and placental growth factor (PlGF), leading to severe placental hypoxia. It is also secreted by trophoblasts into the maternal circulation, and this antiangiogenic factor excess can explain many clinicopathological conditions of preeclampsia like glomerular endotheliosis, proteinuria and hypertension, liver function abnormalities, and coagulopathy. The systemic inflammatory response generated by excess sFlt-1 triggers platelets' activation, the release of vasoconstrictors, and impaired vascular relaxation in mother as well. This imbalance between angiogenic (decreased VEGF and PlGF) and increased antiangiogenic factors like sflt-1 may serve as advanced biochemical markers that may help in discriminating between preeclampsia and chronic hypertension, CKD, lupus nephritis, and ESRD patients on dialysis.[19-24]

Patients with HELLP syndrome who do not improve in terms of platelet recovery and increased liver enzymes within 48 hours of delivery are likely to need plasma exchange and develop dialysis-dependent AKI with progression to worse outcome.[25]

Acute Fatty Liver of Pregnancy

Acute fatty liver of pregnancy is a rare entity which occurs in ~1 in 20,000 deliveries. The maternal liver is exposed to excess fetal fatty acids produced due to deficiency of long-chain 3-hydroxyl coenzyme A dehydrogenase (LCHAD), which cross the placenta and are hepatotoxic to the mother. Women usually present in the third trimester with fatigue, nausea, vomiting, jaundice, and abdominal pain with ascites; hypoglycemia and lactic acidosis are not uncommon. AKI is not universal but may occur in 50–75% patients and in most cases, are nondialysis requiring. More conspicuous is the liver involvement, i.e., altered transaminases, high bilirubin, hyperammonemia, leukocytosis, thrombocytopenia, and coagulopathy with hypofibrinogenemia and in 50% cases with AKI it may be associated with proteinuria.

Therefore, the differential diagnoses mainly considered are HELLP syndrome and preeclampsia with severe features.[26] There is lot of clinical overlap among these three. Hypertension is present in essentially 100% of patients with preeclampsia, 85% of patients with HELLP, and up to about 50% of patients with AFLP. More severe liver involvement with AKI and features of multiorgan involvement like AKI and acute respiratory distress syndrome (ARDS) with liver failure usually indicate AFLP. Diagnosis usually does not need a liver biopsy. Ultrasound of abdomen may show fatty liver, hepatomegaly. Clinical clues and blood biochemistry often establish the correct diagnosis or may clinch the correct diagnosis; however, the treatments are usually the same for all three, i.e., expedited delivery and supportive care.[27]

Pregnancy-related Atypical HUS

Pregnancy-specific aHUS (p-aHUS), which is reported mostly in the postpartum period (80%) in different pregnancy AKI cohorts, or in third trimester of pregnancy in some cases, is a rare and severe form of TMA associated with poor renal prognosis as well as high maternal death rate. Initially, it was classified under secondary TMA (like autoimmune disease, drug, infection- or malignancy-associated TMA). But increasing evidence of complement gene abnormality associations in multiple aHUS cohorts like French, Spanish, and several others,[28-30] suggested that p-aHUS should be considered complement-mediated primary TMA, though 40% of the global aHUS registry[30] did not show any genetic mutation or autoantibody when tested for more than five complement genes, *C3, CFH, B, I*, *CD46* (membrane cofactor protein), and thrombomodulin. 98% of them had their initial TMA in the first pregnancy and 2nd pregnancy was not reported in 98% of them, suggesting poor renal recovery or and/or compromised survival of the patient particularly in the preeculizumab era. The recently published global registry analysis challenged many previous concepts. It showed that the demographic data, clinical features, genetic association, and treatment response to plasma exchange or plasmapheresis or eculizumab are comparable in p-aHUS and non-p-aHUS in women of child-bearing age. 43% of the p-aHUS group had pathogenic variants in complement genes or anti-complement factor H (CFH) antibodies. Women who develop p-aHUS fare poorly with two-third to three-fourth of them developing ESRD in the pre-eculizumab era, which is still true for India. With regard to the treatment of aHUS in pregnancy, the mainstay of therapy, similar to nonpregnant patients, is plasmapheresis and treatment with eculizumab, a humanized monoclonal anti-C5 antibody that selectively targets and inhibits the terminal portion of the complement cascade. The efficacy of eculizumab is proved in four prospective clinical trials and has been supported by additional data from registries and other real-world patient studies. Another terminal complement C5 inhibitor ravulizumab, along with eculizumab, has been approved as targeted treatments for patients with aHUS. Eculizumab seems to be relatively safe during pregnancy based on data indicating that it does not impair complement function in newborns.[31]

Antiphospholipid Antibody Syndrome

Antiphospholipid antibody syndrome is an autoimmune thrombophilic complication, in which antiphospholipid antibodies in the blood target the phospholipid-binding proteins. It is characterized by recurrent arterial and venous thromboses and multiple pregnancy complications like recurrent miscarriage, preterm delivery, oligohydramnios, prematurity, intrauterine growth restriction, fetal distress, fetal or neonatal thrombosis, and preeclampsia/eclampsia. HELLP syndrome, arterial or venous thrombosis, and placental insufficiency are the most severe APS-related complications for pregnant women. Antiphospholipid antibodies promote activation of endothelial cells, monocytes, and platelets, causing an overproduction of tissue factor and thromboxane A2. Complement activation might have a central pathogenetic role. These factors, associated with the typical changes in the hemostatic system during normal pregnancy, result in a hypercoagulable state. This is responsible of thrombosis that is presumed to provoke many of the pregnancy complications associated with APS. The mainstay of management is anticoagulation, in a background of lupus with aPLA positive patients, with history of thrombosis, or obstetric APS defined as more than three pregnancy losses and late first-trimester fetal loss. Anticoagulation of choice is either aspirin or unfractionated heparin. Warfarin cannot be used as it has the potential hemorrhagic risk and teratogenicity.

Immunosuppression is reserved for those who, in addition to APS, have active systemic lupus erythematosus (SLE). Women with a history of APS and arterial thrombotic events should be advised against pregnancy due to high risks for not only pregnancy loss, but also stroke and maternal morbidity and mortality.[32]

Lupus Nephritis

Lupus nephritis, a multisystem autoimmune disease, if diagnosed prior to pregnancy, needs a preconception planning, as any flare of lupus during pregnancy may be associated with adverse outcomes like miscarriage, preeclampsia, intrauterine growth restriction, and preterm delivery. Recent studies report much better maternal and fetal outcome; counseling is therefore not against conception. Fecundity is not diminished in lupus unless creatinine is high and APS is present. Some drugs need to be discontinued like mycophenolate mofetil that is used frequently for remission maintenance (increasing evidence of teratogenicity) and antiproteinuric angiotensin receptor blockers in patients of lupus nephritis planning pregnancy. Conception should be avoided within 6 months of lupus flare and

9 months of lupus nephritis flare. The risk for flare increases if hydroxychloroquine (HCQS) is discontinued or conception comes in <6 months of last lupus flare. The patient may continue on steroids and azathioprine and HCQS when planning conception and should ideally be in proteinuric as well as disease remission state. Any flare may be confused with preeclampsia, as pedal edema and hypertension are common to both and systemic involvement like anemia, thrombocytopenia, and headache may mimic severe eclampsia. The risk of preeclampsia ranges from 11% to 35%, although most reports show that the risk is closer to 30% compared with a risk of approximately 5% in the general population.[33] Urine examination may reveal RBCs which may be a pointer towards presence of other glomerular diseases. Low complement levels, ANA and anti ds-DNA positivity may establish the diagnosis of lupus nephritis. Renal biopsy may be done to ensure class-specific treatment but is avoided in late pregnancy.[34] It is difficult to distinguish between preeclampsia and lupus at the onset, and some studies had shown that an imbalance of angiogenic factors like sFlt-1 and PlGF between 16 and 19 weeks in pregnancy may predict an adverse pregnancy outcome (including preeclampsia). The adverse pregnancy risk is highest with the lowest quartile of PIGF (<70.3 pg/mL) and highest quartile of sFlt-1 (>1,872 pg/mL). This distinction is critical because lupus nephritis is managed with immunosuppression, whereas delivery, even remote from term, is indicated for severe and superimposed preeclampsia.[35]

Treatment

Usually mycophenolate mofetil, cyclophosphamide, and rituximab-based common induction therapy is avoided. An active flare should be treated with IV methylprednisolone followed by oral prednisolone taper and azathioprine. If needed, tacrolimus may be used. HCQS should be continued; it is safe in pregnancy and has shown efficacy in decreasing the risk of anti-RO positive mothers by at least 50% and congenital heart block in neonates.

Acute Kidney Injury with Infections in Pregnancy

Many physiologic changes in the female genital tract may predispose a pregnant lady to antepartum urinary tract infections and pyelonephritis. The World Health Organization (WHO) defined puerperal sepsis as an infection of the genital tract occurring at any time between the rupture of membranes or labor and the 42nd day postpartum, in which two or more of the following are present: Pelvic pain, fever, abnormal vaginal discharge, and delay in the reduction of the size of the uterus. The WHO also recognizes the term puerperal infections, inclusive of both genital and nongenital infections, and the recent epidemiology shows that puerperal infection-related maternal death rate is still high in the obstetric population in the developing countries. Along with that, an increased chance of instrumental and operative trauma and obstetric complications like premature rupture of membranes, abruptio placentae, complicated abortions, and intrauterine fetal death makes this population an easy target for multiple hospital-acquired polymicrobial infections. The common clinical pointers to sepsis, i.e., tachycardia, tachypnea, and hypotension, may be attributed to blood loss, and sepsis diagnosis is often delayed.

Infections of urinary tract(UTI) are not uncommon during pregnancy, post abortion and puerperium also may have association with increased incidence of UTI. Asymptomatic bacteriuria needs active treatment in this population. It occurs in about 2–7% of pregnant women and is associated with an increased risk of low birth weight, preterm delivery, urinary tract infection, and pyelonephritis; the most common organism recovered is *Escherichia coli*. It is important to ensure eradication by a repeat culture a week or two later as 30% of pregnant women may fail to clear the infection and may progress to pyelonephritis, which needs hospital admission and aggressive treatment with IV antibiotics. Inadequately treated, 20% of these patients may develop complications such as septic shock or ARDS.[36]

Cesarean section, particularly in low resource setting, has been identified as a common factor for puerperal infection, particularly when further associated with prolonged rupture of membrane, wound hematoma, and surgical misfortune. Septic abortion has come down drastically in most countries, but still, termination of pregnancy may be associated with postabortive sepsis due to unhygienic practice, lack of antibiotic stewardship in peripheral units, and retained products of conception. Untreated pelvic and endometrial infection may later turn up with septic shock to ICUs.[37]

Treatment

Aggressive management of septic shock will require multidisciplinary care in ICU, appropriate IV antibiotics, hemodynamic or ventilatory support, and may become dialysis requiring. It is important to mention that obstetric AKI requiring dialysis has poorer prognosis. Multiple Indian studies have shown dialysis dependence in 16–20% patients, cause of Pr-AKI, anemia, and hypoalbuminemia remaining important predictors.[38]

Obstructive Uropathy

Obstructive uropathy is not common in pregnancy. It can be a rare cause of AKI. The complex physiological and mechanical changes of pregnancy alter the risk of stone formation due to presence of physiological hydronephrosis in almost 90% pregnancies. The hydronephrosis favors stasis and infection as well as longer contact time between lithogenic factors. The stasis and infection, along with hypercalciuria in pregnancy and increased pH in the urinary tract, may lead to calcium phosphate stone formation. The presentation is usually with abdominal pain, nausea, and vomiting. Fever may be present if complicated with infection. USG remains the first diagnostic modality. Alternatives remain transvaginal ultrasonography, MRKUB, and low-dose CT. Good pain protocol, kidney with normal anatomy, and stone size <1 cm are usually managed conservatively. Anatomically complex kidney, along with presence of infection with stone size >2 cm, may demand surgical intervention. Depending on the clinical condition of the mother, nephrostomy or definitive surgery may be planned. Conditions like bilateral renal calculi and gravid uterus, especially with multiple gestations, polyhydramnios, and large fibroids, may cause bilateral hydroureteronephrosis which can cause Pr-AKI.[39] Postpartum voiding dysfunctions are reported following C-section and emergency surgery. Iatrogenic injuries to bladder and uterus are rare, but remain an uncommon cause of AKI.[40]

CONCLUSION

The changing epidemiology of Pr-AKI demands new introspection into the challenges and adoption of preventive measures. Maternal sepsis is a cause of unacceptably high maternal mortality where improved access to hygienic obstetric care with enforced practice of universal precaution and availability of high-end antibiotics in public sector hospitals remain an unmet need. Eculizumab has come up as a very effective intervention in TMAs but still not available at a comfortable price so as to meet the need of obstetric population. The promise of use of angiogenic factors in both diagnosis and treatment may be an area of new hope in this area.

REFERENCES

1. Liu Y, Ma X, Zheng J, Liu X, Yan T. Pregnancy outcomes in patients with acute kidney injury during pregnancy: a systematic review and meta-analysis. BMC Pregnancy Childbirth. 2017;17(1):235.
2. Prakash J, Pant P, Prakash S, Sivasankar M, Vohra R, Doley PK, et al Changing picture of acute kidney injury in pregnancy: Study of 259 cases over a period of 33 years. Indian J Nephrol. 2016;26(4):262-7.
3. Saini S, Chaudhury AR, Divyaveer S, Maurya P, Sircar D. The Changing Face of Pregnancy-Related Acute Kidney Injury from Eastern Part of India: A Hospital-Based, Prospective, Observational Study. Saudi J Kidney Dis Transplant. 2020;31(2):493-502.
4. Rao S, Jim B. Acute Kidney Injury in Pregnancy: The Changing Landscape for the 21st Century. Kidney Int Rep. 2018;3(2):247-57.
5. Mehrabadi A, Dahhou M, Joseph KS, Kramer MS. Investigation of a Rise in Obstetric Acute Renal Failure in the United States, 1999–2011. Obstet Gynecol. 2016;127(5):899-906.
6. Mehrabadi A, Liu S, Bartholomew S, Hutcheon JA, Magee MA, Kramer MS, et al. Hypertensive disorders of pregnancy and the recent increase in obstetric acute renal failure in Canada: population based retrospective cohort study. BMJ. 2014;349:g4731.
7. Bellomo R, Ronco C, Kellum JA, Mehta RL, Palevsky P. Acute renal failure - definition, outcome measures, animal models, fluid therapy and information technology needs: the Second International Consensus Conference of the Acute Dialysis Quality Initiative (ADQI) Group. Crit Care. 2004;8(4):R204-12.
8. Mehta RL, Kellum JA, Shah SV, Molitoris BA, Ronco C, Warnock DG, et al. Acute Kidney Injury Network: report of an initiative to improve outcomes in acute kidney injury. Crit Care. 2007;11(2):R31.
9. Lin CY, Chen YC. Acute kidney injury classification: AKIN and RIFLE criteria in critical patients. World J Crit Care Med. 2012;1(2):40-5.
10. Machado MN, Nakazone MA, Maia LN. Acute kidney injury based on KDIGO (Kidney Disease Improving Global Outcomes) criteria in patients with elevated baseline serum creatinine undergoing cardiac surgery. Rev Bras Cir Cardiovasc. 2014;29(3):299-307.
11. Davison JM, Dunlop W. Renal hemodynamics and tubular function normal human pregnancy. Kidney Int. 1980;18(2):152-61.
12. Piccoli GB, Daidola G, Attini R, Parisi S, Fassio F, Naretto C, et al. Kidney biopsy in pregnancy: evidence for counselling? A systematic narrative review. BJOG. 2013;120(4):412-27.
13. Matlin RA, Gary NE. Acute cortical necrosis. Case report and review of the literature. Am J Med. 1974;56(1):110-8.
14. Prakash J, Vohra R, Wani IA, Murthy AS, Srivastva PK, Tripathi K, et al. Decreasing incidence of renal cortical necrosis in patients with acute renal failure in developing countries: a single-centre experience of 22 years from Eastern India. Nephrol Dial Transplant. 2007;22(4):1213-7.
15. Martin JN, Jr, Bailey AP, Rehberg JF, Owens MT, Keiser SD, May WL. Thrombotic thrombocytopenic purpura in 166 pregnancies: 1955-2006. Am J Obstet Gynecol. 2008;199(2):98-104.
16. Scully M, Yarranton H, Liesner R, Cavenagh J, Hunt B, Benjamin S, et al. Regional UK TTP registry: correlation with laboratory ADAMTS 13 analysis and clinical features. Br J Haematol. 2008;142(5):819-26.
17. Fyfe-Brown A, Clarke G, Nerenberg K, Chandra S, Jain V. Management of pregnancy-associated thrombotic thrombocytopenia purpura. AJP Rep. 2013;3(1):45-50.
18. American College of Obstetricians and Gynecologists; Task Force on Hypertension in Pregnancy: Hypertension in pregnancy. Report

of the American College of Obstetricians and Gynecologists' Task Force on Hypertension in Pregnancy. Obstet Gynecol. 2013;122:1122-31.

19. Sibai B, Dekker G, Kupferminc M. Preeclampsia. Lancet. 2005;365:785-99.
20. Staff AC, Dechend R, Pijnenborg R. Learning from the placenta: acute atherosis and vascular remodeling in preeclampsia-novel aspects for atherosclerosis and future cardiovascular health. Hypertension. 2010;56: 102634.
21. Redman CW, Sargent IL. Latest advances in understanding preeclampsia. Science. 2005;308:1592-4.
22. Gul A, Aslan H, Cebeci A, Polat I, Ulusoy S, Ceylan Y. Maternal and fetal outcomes in HELLP syndrome complicated with acute renal failure. Ren Fail. 2004;26:557-9.
23. Sibai BM, Ramadan MK, Usta I, Salama M, Mercer BM, Friedman SA. Maternal morbidity and mortality in 442 pregnancies with hemolysis, elevated liver enzymes, and low platelets (HELLP syndrome). Am J Obstet Gynecol. 1993;169:1000-6.
24. Philipps EA, Thadhani R, Benzing T, Ananth Karumanchi S. Preeclampsia: pathogenesis, novel diagnostics and therapies. Nat Rev Nephrol. 2019;15:275-89.
25. Simetka O, Klat J, Gumulec J, Dolezalkova E, Salounova D, Kacerovsky M. Early identification of women with HELLP syndrome who need plasma exchange after delivery. Transfus Apher Sci. 2015;52(1):54-9.
26. Casey LC, Fontana RJ, Aday A, Nelson DB, Rule JA, Gottfried M, et al. Acute Liver Failure (ALF) in Pregnancy: How Much Is Pregnancy Related? Hepatology (Baltimore, Md.). 2020;72(4):1366-77.
27. Nelson DB, Yost NP, Cunningham FG. Acute fatty liver of pregnancy: clinical outcomes and expected duration of recovery. Am J Obstet Gynecol. 2013;209(5):456.e1-7.
28. Fakhouri F, Roumenina L, Provot F, Sallée M, Caillard S, Couzi L, et al. Pregnancy-associated hemolytic uremic syndrome revisited in the era of complement gene mutations. J Am Soc Nephrol JASN. 2010; 21(5):859-67.
29. Bruel A, Kavanagh D, Noris M, Delmas Y, Wong EKS, Bresin E, et al. Hemolytic uremic syndrome in pregnancy and postpartum. Clin J Am Soc Nephrol. 2017;12(8):1237-47.
30. Fakhouri F, Scully M, Ardissino G, Al-Dakkak I, Miller B, Rondeau E. Pregnancy-triggered atypical hemolytic uremic syndrome (aHUS): a Global aHUS Registry analysis. J Nephrol. 2021;34:1581-90.
31. Rondeau E, Cataland SR, Al-Dakkak I, Miller B, Webb NJA, Landau D. Eculizumab safety: five-year experience from the global atypical hemolytic uremic syndrome registry. Kidney Int Rep. 2019;4(11):1568-76.
32. Di Prima FA, Valenti O, Hyseni E, Giorgio E, Faraci M, Renda E, et al. Antiphospholipid syndrome during pregnancy: the state of the art. J Prenat Med. 2011;5(2):41-53.
33. Stanhope TJ, White WM, Moder KG, Smyth A, Garovic VD. Obstetric nephrology: lupus and lupus nephritis in pregnancy. Clin J Am Soc Nephrol. 2012;7(12):2089-99.
34. Lightstone L, Hladunewich MA. Lupus Nephritis and Pregnancy: Concerns and Management. Semin Nephrol. 2017;37(4): 347-53.
35. Kim MY, Buyon JP, Guerra MM, Rana S, Zhang D, Laskin CA, et al. Angiogenic factor imbalance early in pregnancy predicts adverse outcomes in patients with lupus and antiphospholipid antibodies: results of the PROMISSE study. Am J Obstet Gynecol. 2016;214(1):108.e1-108.e14.
36. Burlinson CEG, Sirounis D, Walley KR, Chau A. Sepsis in pregnancy and the puerperium. Int J Obstet Anesth. 2018;36:96-107.
37. Nicolle LE, Gupta K, Bradley SF, Colgan R, DeMuri GP, Drekonja D, et al. Clinical Practice Guideline for the Management of Asymptomatic Bacteriuria: 2019 Update by the Infectious Diseases Society of America. Clin Infect Dis. 2019;68(10):e83-e110.
38. Buddeberg BS, Aveling W. Puerperal sepsis in the 21st century: progress, new challenges and the situation worldwide. Postgrad Med J. 2015;91(1080):572-8.
39. Semins MJ, Matlaga BR. Kidney stones during pregnancy. Nat Rev Urol. 2014;11(3):163-8.
40. Liang CC, Wu MP, Chang YL, Chueh HY, Chao AS, Chang SD. Voiding dysfunction in women following cesarean delivery. Taiwan J Obstet Gynecol. 2015;54(6):678-81.

CHAPTER 8

Acute Fatty Liver of Pregnancy

Rajesh Jhorawat, Vinant Bhargava

HIGHLIGHTS

- Acute fatty liver of pregnancy (AFLP) is a rare complication, occurring in about 5 cases per 100,000 pregnancies, typically manifesting in late pregnancy.
- It poses risks for both maternal and fetal health and is characterized by acute liver dysfunction caused by fatty infiltration of liver tissue, leading to potential complications such as coagulopathy, electrolyte imbalance, and multiorgan failure.
- Defects related to the metabolism of fatty acids, particularly long-chain 3-hydroxyacyl-CoA dehydrogenase (LCHAD) deficiency, can lead to the accumulation of fatty acids in hepatocytes, resulting in cellular damage.
- LCHAD deficiency is implicated in approximately 20% of AFLP.
- Delivery of the fetus, along with supportive care for the mother, constitutes the primary treatment approach for AFLP.

INTRODUCTION

Acute fatty liver of pregnancy (AFLP) is an uncommon yet potentially life-threatening medical condition marked by hepatic failure. It usually manifests in the third trimester or early postpartum period, and there is a risk of advancing to acute liver failure, leading to mortality and necessitating liver transplantation.[1,2] Sheehan described it as an "acute yellow atrophy of the liver" in 1940 and related it to chloroform, a commonly used anesthetic agent at that time. However, Burroughs et al. later provided a meticulous pathologic description of these women as having widespread microvesicular fatty infiltration of swollen hepatocytes with minimal necrosis and cholestasis. These women also had moderate-to-severe renal insufficiency and many had profound coagulopathic changes.[3] The documented occurrence ranges from 1 in 7,000 to 1 in 20,000 pregnancies, reflecting variations in study populations.[2] AFLP exhibits certain clinical and laboratory characteristics akin to other obstetric complications like HELLP (Hemolysis, Elevated Liver enzymes, and Low Platelet count) syndrome. Management of this severe clinical condition requires prompt recognition with close clinical surveillance and delivery.[2,3]

PATHOGENESIS

In a normal pregnancy, the fetal-placental unit metabolizes free fatty acids to support fetal growth and development. Placental enzymes facilitate the breakdown of triglycerides into free fatty acids, subsequently transferring them to the fetus.[2] These autosomal recessive fatty acid oxidation (FAO) defects are potentially fatal and now are being increasingly diagnosed, not limited to AFLP, but also extending to the HELLP (hemolysis, elevated liver enzymes, and low platelets) syndrome, preeclampsia and placental infarction.[2,4] When such defects exist in the FAO pathway of the fetal–placental unit, the products—intermediate fatty acid metabolites—accumulate and enter the maternal circulation. Maternal liver disease, particularly acute fatty liver, has been associated with pregnancies in which the fetus is affected with long-chain 3-hydroxyacyl-CoA dehydrogenase (LCHAD) deficiency.[4,5] However, several authors have demonstrated that short- and medium-chain defects can also be implicated in maternal liver disease during pregnancy.[6,7] The accumulation of fatty acids and metabolites in the maternal compartment is driven by two processes. Firstly, the fetal–placental unit experiences a homozygous or compound heterozygous mutation, resulting in an enzyme defect. Secondly, a heterozygous mother exhibits a reduced ability to carry out FAO in late pregnancy, leading to an inability to efficiently clear accumulated fatty acid metabolites transferred from the deficient fetal–placental unit.[2,8] Given this association, it is recommended to test for fatty oxidation disorders in the infant when maternal acute fatty liver is present. Prenatal diagnosis should be contemplated, especially in cases where the mother has previously had an affected child, making her an obligate heterozygote. Molecular analysis of fetal DNA, obtained through chorionic villus sampling (CVS) or amniocentesis, is feasible if the disease-causing mutation is known. In cases where the mutation is unidentified, biochemical analysis can be conducted by assessing FAO enzymatic activity in CVS or amniocyte cultures.[5,9]

RISK FACTORS

Important risk factors associated with AFLP are as follows:

- Fetal FAO disorders
- Multifetal gestations
- Male fetus
- Previous episode of AFLP
- Nulliparity
- Low body mass index (BMI) (<20 kg/m^2)

While the majority of cases typically present in the third trimester, there have been reported occurrences in the second trimester.[2,10-12]

CLINICAL PRESENTATIONS

Most women diagnosed with AFLP are in the third trimester of pregnancy, and the mean gestational age is 35–36 weeks, with a range of 28–40 weeks and a few isolated cases reported in 26 weeks of gestation to immediately postpartum periods.[1,2,13] The manifestations of AFLP range from minimal clinical findings and laboratory derangements to overt liver failure with hepatic encephalopathy. Patients often present with nonspecific symptoms such as headache, anorexia, nausea, vomiting, fatigue, and pain in abdomen. On physical examination, the patient is usually febrile and had jaundice, which is very common and eventually occurs in more than 70% of patients with AFLP as the condition progresses. In severe cases, the patient can present with multisystem involvement, including acute renal failure, encephalopathy, gastrointestinal bleeding, pancreatitis, and coagulopathy. The symptoms and signs of AFLP are highlighted in **Table 1**.

Other clinical conditions can also present with similar clinical presentation in the third trimester like jaundice (intrahepatic cholestasis of pregnancy, preeclampsia/eclampsia, HELLP syndrome, Dubin-Johnson syndrome), upper abdominal

TABLE 1: Common symptoms and signs of AFLP.[1]

Symptoms and signs	*Frequency (%)*
Nausea and vomiting	50–60
Abdominal pain	50–60
CNS (delirium, seizure, or coma)	60–80
Pyrexia	50
Tachycardia	50
Jaundice	>70
Oliguria	40–60
Acute renal failure	>60
GI bleed	20–60
DIC	55

(AFLP: acute fatty liver of pregnancy; CNS: central nervous system; DIC: disseminated intravascular coagulation; GI: gastrointestinal)

pain (preeclampsia/eclampsia, HELLP syndrome, acute hepatic rupture, Budd-Chiari syndrome); nausea and vomiting (preeclampsia/eclampsia, HELLP syndrome), and thrombocytopenia (preeclampsia/eclampsia, HELLP syndrome).[13]

LABORATORY FINDING AND DIAGNOSTIC CRITERIA

To interpret the array of laboratory tests employed in diagnosing AFLP, it is crucial to comprehend the normal physiological changes during pregnancy and the corresponding alterations in laboratory values. The term "normal values," as indicated by an electronic medical record (EMR), often rely on reference ranges derived from males and/or nonpregnant females, which can significantly deviate from what is considered normal for pregnant patients.[2,14] In AFLP cases, all patients exhibit elevated aminotransferases (aspartate aminotransferase or alanine aminotransferase), typically ranging from 5 to 10 times the upper limit of normal. Additional frequently encountered laboratory findings are outlined in **Table 2**.

TABLE 2: Laboratory findings in AFLP.[1,2]

Hematological parameters:	
• Hemoglobin	Normal
• Hematocrit	Normal
• WBCs	Raised (mild)
• Platelets	Normal/decrease (mild)
Liver parameters:	
• Aspartate aminotransferase	Raised (moderately)
• Alanine aminotransferase	Raised (moderately)
• Gamma-glutamyltransferase	Raised (mild)
• Alkaline phosphatase	Raised (moderately)
• Lactate dehydrogenase	Normal/decrease (mild)
• Bilirubin, total	Raised (moderately)
• Bilirubin, direct	Raised (moderately)
• Ammonia	Raised (mild)
• Glucose	Decreased (moderately)
• Cholesterol	Decreased (mild)
• Triglycerides	Decreased (mild)
Coagulation parameters:	
• International normalized ratio	Raised (moderately)
• Partial thromboplastin time	Raised (mild)
• Fibrinogen	Decreased (moderately)
• Fibrin split products	Present (+)
• Antithrombin III	Decreased (moderately)
Renal parameters:	
• Uric acid	Raised (moderately)
• Blood urea nitrogen	Raised (mild)
• Creatinine	Raised (moderately)

(AFLP: acute fatty liver of pregnancy)

Typically, the diagnosis of AFLP is confirmed using the Swansea criteria **(Table 3)**. To establish the diagnosis, six of the specified criteria must be satisfied.[15] These criteria are well validated and proven to be effective.

Applying the Swansea criteria to a cohort of 24 patients with suspected pregnancy-related liver disease who underwent biopsy, the presence of six or more abnormal variables

TABLE 3: Swansea criteria for diagnosis of AFLP.[2,15] Six features from below are required for the diagnosis.

Clinical features	• Nausea and vomiting • Abdomen pain • Encephalopathy • Polyuria and polydipsia
Laboratory features	• Bilirubin >0.8 mg/dL • Hypoglycemia <72 mg/dL • WBC >11 × 10^9/L • AST or ALT >41 IU/L • AKI or Serum creatinine >1.7 mg/dL • Coagulopathy or PT >14 seconds • Ammonia >47 µg/L • Urate >340 µg/L
Ultrasonographic features	Ascites or echogenic liver
Histological features	Microvascular steatosis on liver biopsy

(AFLP: acute fatty liver of pregnancy; AKI: acute kidney injury; ALT: alanine aminotransferase; AST: aspartate aminotransferase; PT: prothrombin time; WBC: white blood cell)

demonstrated a positive predictive value of 85% and a negative predictive value of 100% for detecting microvesicular steatosis.[16]

DIFFERENTIAL DIAGNOSIS

Pregnant women who present with abnormal liver enzymes should have an extensive workup that includes viral and autoimmune serology testing, coagulation studies, and consideration of imaging to determine the etiology of liver dysfunction. The differential diagnosis of acute liver failure in pregnancy can be divided into two broad categories:[17]

1. *Pregnancy related*:
   - Hyperemesis gravidarum
   - Benign jaundice of pregnancy
   - Intrahepatic cholestasis of pregnancy
   - Preeclampsia
   - HELLP syndrome
   - AFLP
2. *Nonpregnancy related*:
   - Drug-induced hepatitis
   - Acute viral hepatitis
   - Alcoholic hepatitis
   - Toxins
   - Trauma
   - Wilson's disease
   - Budd–Chiari syndrome

A detailed history including medical comorbidities, presenting signs and symptoms, physical examination, and investigational studies helps to differentiate between these etiologies.

TREATMENT

Prompt fetal delivery and supportive resuscitation form the cornerstone of therapy. As per the American College of Gastroenterology, expectant treatment is not appropriate and prompt delivery is strongly recommended.[10]

Treatment Algorithm

- Maternal supportive care and stabilization are to be initiated first
- Correction of electrolytes, fluid replacement (if required)
- Management of hypoglycemia
- Management of coagulopathy
- Monitoring of:
  - Maternal parameters
  - Fetal evaluation

The route of delivery is dependent upon fetal or maternal decompensation and/or presence of contraindications to vaginal birth. Vaginal delivery and labor induction may be done in the absence of contraindication to vaginal delivery. Platelet transfusion may be necessary in case of cesarean delivery. As per guidelines, a platelet count of >40,000–50,000 should be maintained.[10] Magnesium sulfate is given for pregnancies <32 weeks to prevent neonatal cerebral palsy.

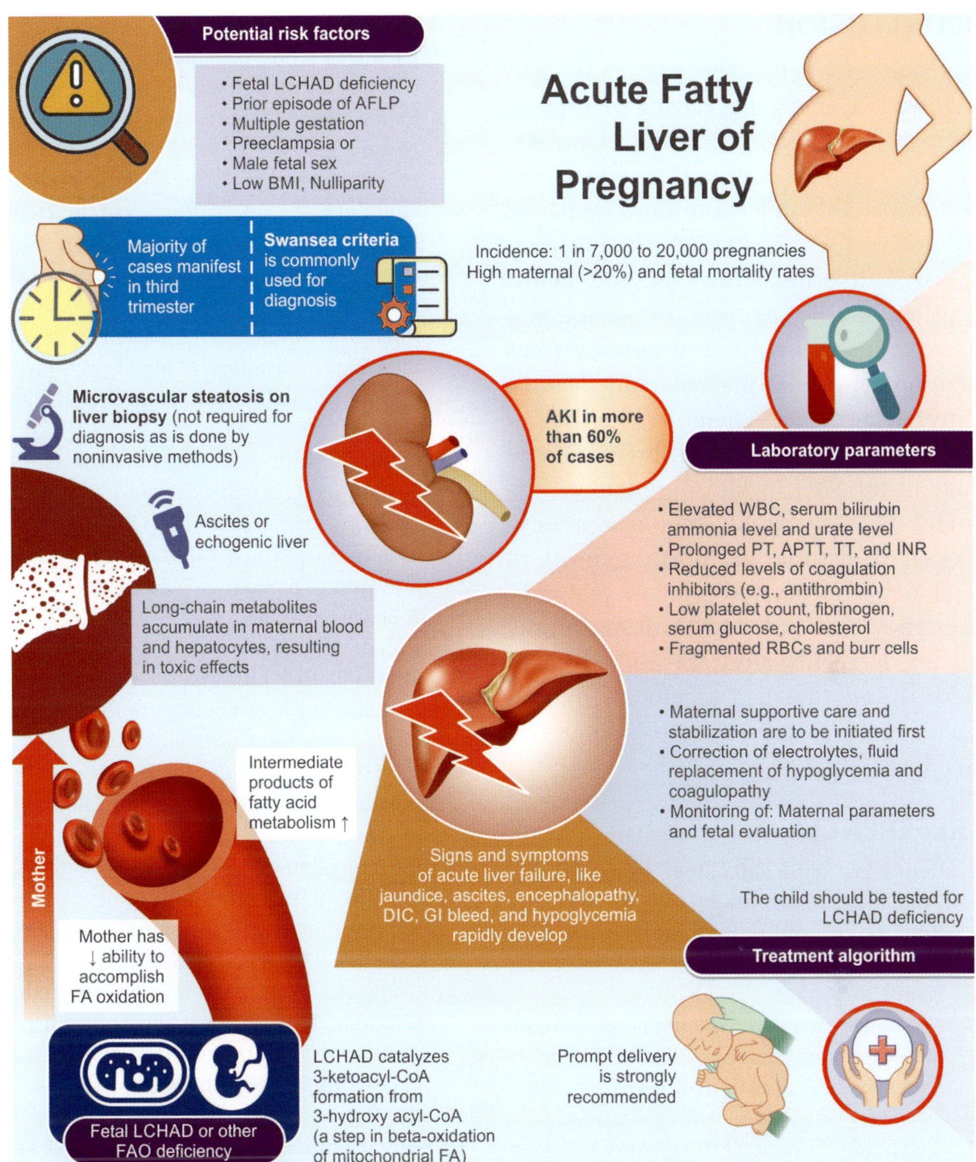

Fig. 1: Acute fatty liver of pregnancy (AFLP). (BMI: body mass index; DIC: disseminated intravascular coagulation; FA: fatty acid; FAO: fatty acid oxidation; HELLP: hemolysis, elevated liver enzymes, and low platelets; LCHAD: long-chain 3-hydroxyacyl-CoA dehydrogenase; PT: prothrombin time; RBCs: red blood cells; TT: thrombin time; WBC: white blood cell count)

Courtesy: Dr Priti Meena

Post delivery, monitoring of renal functions, hypoglycemia, and signs of bleeding has to be done. If hepatic dysfunction persists beyond delivery, liver transplantation may prove to be life-saving. The child should be tested for LCHAD deficiency apart from close monitoring for hypoglycemia and fatty liver.[5]

CONCLUSION

Acute fatty liver of pregnancy is a potentially fatal obstetric emergency having widespread microvesicular fatty infiltration of swollen hepatocytes with minimal necrosis and cholestasis. FAO defects in new-borns are responsible for this rare fatal autosomal-recessive disorder. However, the manifestation of this disorder necessitates a homozygous or compound heterozygous mutation in the fetal–placental unit, leading to an enzyme defect. A heterozygous mother with such a mutation exhibits reduced capacity for FAO in late pregnancy. It is crucial to distinguish this pregnancy-associated disorder from other forms of pregnancy-associated liver failure and non-pregnancy-associated disorders. Timely delivery is highly advised, and in cases where the mother has previously had an affected child, prenatal diagnosis should be considered.

REFERENCES

1. Reddy A. Acute fatty liver of pregnancy. Princ Crit Care Obstet. 2016;2(1):57-64.
2. Roux O, Durand F, Bernuau J. Acute fatty liver of pregnancy. Obstet Gynecol. 2021; 138(2):307.
3. Nelson DB, Yost NP, Cunningham FG. Acute fatty liver of pregnancy: Clinical outcomes and expected duration of recovery. Am J Obstet Gynecol. 2013;209(5):456.e1-6.e7.
4. Shekhawat P, Bennett MJ, Sadovsky Y, Nelson DM, Rakheja D, Strauss AW. Human placenta metabolizes fatty acids: Implications for fetal fatty acid oxidation disorders and maternal liver diseases. Am J Physiol Endocrinol Metab. 2003;284(6):1098-105.
5. Chetty S, Norton ME. Obstetric care in women with genetic disorders. Best Pract Res Clin Obstet Gynaecol. 2017;42(2017):86-99.
6. Browning MF, Levy HL, Wilkins-Haug LE, Larson C, Shih VE. Fetal fatty acid oxidation defects and maternal liver disease in pregnancy. Obstet Gynecol. 2006;107(1):115-20.
7. Nelson J, Lewis B, Walters B. The HELLP syndrome associated with fetal medium-chain acyl-CoA dehydrogenase deficiency. J Inherit Metab Dis. 2000;23(5):518-9.
8. Nelson DB, Schell R. Acute fatty liver of pregnancy. Contemp Ob Gyn. 2021;66(6):18-22.
9. Rinaldo P, Studinski AL, Matern D. Prenatal diagnosis of disorders of fatty acid transport and mitochondrial oxidation. Prenat Diagn. 2001;21(1):52-4.
10. Tran TT, Ahn J, Reau NS. ACG clinical guideline: Liver disease and pregnancy. Am J Gastroenterol. 2016;111(2):176-94.
11. Nelson DB, Byrne JJ, Cunningham FG. Acute fatty liver of pregnancy. Clin Obstet Gynecol. 2020;63(1):152-64.
12. Knight M, Nelson-Piercy C, Kurinczuk JJ, Spark P, Brocklehurst P. A prospective national study of acute fatty liver of pregnancy in the UK. Gut. 2008;57(7):951-6.
13. Ko HH, Yoshida E. Acute fatty liver of pregnancy. Can J Gastroenterol. 2006; 20(1): 25-30.
14. Abbassi-Ghanavati M, Greer LG, Cunningham FG. Pregnancy and laboratory studies: A reference table for clinicians. Obstet Gynecol. 2009;114(6):1326-31.
15. Ch'ng CL, Morgan M, Hainsworth I, Kingham JGC. Prospective study of liver dysfunction in pregnancy in Southwest Wales. Gut. 2002;51(6):876-80.
16. Goel A, Ramakrishna B, Zachariah U, Ramachandran J, Eapen CE, Kurian G, et al. How accurate are the Swansea criteria to diagnose acute fatty liver of pregnancy in predicting hepatic microvesicular steatosis? Gut. 2011;60(1):138-9.
17. Palmer J, Borhart J. What Is Acute Fatty Liver of Pregnancy? Gastrointest Emergencies Evidence-Based Answers to Key Clin Quest. 2019;130(3):375-6.

CHAPTER 9

Changing Spectrum of Pregnancy-related Acute Kidney Injury in India

Arunkumar S, Dipankar Bhowmik

HIGHLIGHTS

- Pregnancy-related acute kidney injury (PrAKI) is a global public health issue that significantly affects fetomaternal outcomes.
- The overall incidence of PrAKI has reduced with developments in healthcare in both developing and developed countries. However, there has been a recent increase in developed countries due to hypertensive and thrombotic disorders.
- India has witnessed a significant decline in PrAKI incidence over the last few decades largely due to decline in the rates of septic abortion and better healthcare facilities to manage pregnancy-related complications such as hemorrhage.
- Government programs including Janani Suraksha Yojana (JSY) and Pradhan Mantri Surakshit Matritva Abhiyan (PMSMA) aim to improve maternal health by providing financial incentives and they have had a positive impact, particularly in rural areas.
- The diagnosis of PrAKI can be challenging in part due to the lack of uniform diagnostic criteria and the multitude of causes that can cause AKI in pregnancy.
- The long-term impact of PrAKI in increasing the risk for chronic hypertension, chronic kidney disease, and cardiovascular disease mandates appropriate attention and close follow-up.

INTRODUCTION

Pregnancy-related acute kidney injury (PrAKI) is associated with considerable maternal morbidity and mortality and risk of fetal loss regardless of the cause of kidney injury. Though there are multiple causes of kidney injury, hypertensive disorders and thrombotic disorders are the most common causes in developed countries. In resource-limited settings, pregnancy-related hemorrhage and infective complications play a major role in the etiopathogenesis of PrAKI historically. The etiological spectrum for PrAKI has changed over the years with a significant decline in sepsis-associated causes even in these settings. The kidneys undergo significant anatomic and hemodynamic changes during pregnancy which affect practically all aspects of kidney function.[1] The important changes in renal physiology during pregnancy are described in detail in **Chapter 1**. In patients with preexisting kidney diseases, these changes are attenuated to various degrees. A thorough understanding of these physiologic processes is needed to identify the pathophysiological processes that can occur during pregnancy.

The diverse symptomatology combined with overlapping signs and laboratory investigations make the diagnosis of PrAKI a challenge. This is further accentuated by the lack of uniform diagnostic criteria for AKI in pregnancy. In addition to the immediate impact on fetal and maternal health, long-term risk of chronic kidney disease (CKD) and adverse fetal outcomes of preterm births and low birth weights necessitate timely diagnosis and management of obstetric AKI.

EPIDEMIOLOGY

The causes and incidence of PrAKI vary according to the geographical location. The overall landscape of obstetric AKI has changed across the world.[2] In developing countries, reduction in the incidence of PrAKI is mostly driven by reductions in septic abortions, puerperal sepsis, and hemorrhagic complications with better healthcare facilities to manage the obstetric complications. The improvements in antenatal care combined with the legalization of abortion have reduced the incidence of obstetric AKI from 22% of all causes of AKI in the 1970s to around 5–6% in the present era **(Table 1)**.[3] In contrast to the developing countries, high resource settings where marked socioeconomic development has occurred witness almost an elimination in pregnancy-associated AKI.

The incidence of PrAKI in developed countries like the United States and Canada dropped to less than 1 in 10,000 pregnancies by 2010.[12] In the United States, there was an increase in the reported incidence from 2003 to 2011 due to a change in the coding pattern of AKI. With regards to developing countries like India, the incidence of PrAKI has reduced but the proportion of severe cases is around 30% (of total cases of PrAKI).[13] Previously, AKI was more prevalent among younger women in rural areas, but it is now increasingly observed in older, urban women with preexisting medical comorbidities. A recent meta-analysis of 31 studies found that the pooled incidence of PrAKI was 2.0% worldwide, highlighting improvements in perinatal care.[14] However, the study also revealed that only 49.3% of women received antenatal care, underscoring the crucial role of antenatal care in preventing pregnancy-related complications.

The Indian AKI registry, a pilot project by the Indian Society of Nephrology, included all cases of community-acquired AKI from various centers across India between

TABLE 1: Relative frequency of acute kidney injury (AKI) in different settings across decades.

Study	*Sample (n)*	*Medical (%)*	*Surgical (%)*	*Obstetric (%) (PrAKI)*
Sitprija and Benyajati[4]	162	61	15	24
Chugh et al.[5]	325	67	22	11
Shah et al. (1985)[27]	816	56	32	21
Muthusethupathi and Shivakumar[6]	187	85	9	6
Ramachandran (1994)[28]	317	79	15	6
Jayakumar et al.[7]	1,112	88	9	3
Kaul et al.[8]	240	78	8	14
ISN 0by25 study[9]	4,018	92	7	1
AIIMS-ND (2014–17)	476	84	10	6
Goswami et al.[10]	286	77.2	9	13.9
ISN-AKI registry[11]	3,711	86.7	7.3	6.1

(AIIMS-ND: All India Institute of Medical Sciences, New Delhi; PrAKI: pregnancy-related acute kidney injury)

2016 and 2019. In this registry, the overall incidence of obstetric AKI was found to be 6.1%, indicating a reduction in incidence over the years.[11] In a vast country like India, regional variations in healthcare availability are likely. In a long-term study by Jai Prakash et al. from eastern India, the incidence of PrAKI, which was 12.8% from 1983 to 1995, decreased only slightly to 11.8% from 1992 to 2008.[15] However, developments over the past 15 years are expected to reduce this number more significantly. Government programs such as Janani Suraksha Yojana (JSY) and Pradhan Mantri Surakshit Matritva Abhiyan (PMSMA) have improved antenatal care, leading to better perinatal care over the last two decades. A follow-up study from the same center revealed a PrAKI incidence of 4.68% in the latest period (2003–2014) of analysis.[16] This is in line with data from across India and other developing countries.

Causes of Pregnancy-related Acute Kidney Injury

The clue to the etiology of PrAKI lies in the timing. The causes can be categorized, similar to those in the general population, into prerenal, renal, and postrenal or according to the stage of pregnancy (trimester-wise or postpartum).[17] See **Chapter 7** for details.

The risk factors for PrAKI are advanced maternal age, diabetes, hypertension, multiple pregnancy due to assisted reproductive techniques, and preexisting renal disease.[18] The causes of PrAKI have evolved over the years, with a notable decrease in postabortal AKI cases following the legalization of abortion.

Historically, septic abortion and postpartum hemorrhage were the primary causes of PRAKI. The legalization of abortion in India (1971) and the subsequent availability of safe abortion services have drastically decreased septic abortion rates. Also, better management of labor and delivery, including improved blood transfusion practices, has minimized the risks and complications of postpartum hemorrhage. This decline in traditional causes has been accompanied by a rise in other factors contributing to AKI. Hypertensive disorders of pregnancy, particularly preeclampsia and eclampsia, have emerged as a major concern. A rise in maternal age, increased prevalence of chronic diseases like diabetes and obesity, and potential changes in diagnostic practices are responsible for the change in causes of PrAKI.

In the study by Prakash et al., the relative fraction of patients of postabortal AKI reduced from 61.5% (1982–91) to 31.8% (2003–14). In the same period, puerperal sepsis increased from 9% (1982–91) to 26.4% (2003–14).[16] A systematic review of 7 studies with 477 PrAKI patients also reported sepsis (41.9%) to be the most important cause followed by hemorrhage (22.1%) and hypertensive disorders of pregnancy (20.9%).[19] Additionally, most studies showed that PrAKI occurs most often in the postpartum period in 60–80% of all cases.[19,20] Understanding the evolving causes and time frame of PrAKI is crucial for designing preventative strategies and management protocols.

OUTCOMES OF PREGNANCY-RELATED ACUTE KIDNEY INJURY

Pregnancy-related AKI is associated with considerable fetal morbidity and mortality. In spite of the declining incidence, the fetomaternal complications of PrAKI are serious and have long-lasting impact. Studies from India have shown that the perinatal mortality is around 20–45% in such cases.[16] The mortality rate is still approximately 5.8%

TABLE 2: Indian studies on pregnancy-related acute kidney injury (PrAKI).

Study	*Study design*	*Sample size*	*PrAKI incidence (%)*	*RRT requirement*	*Renal recovery (%)*	*Maternal mortality (%)*	*Fetal outcomes (%)*
Gopalakrishnan et al.[20]	Prospective	130	7.8	73.8	CR: 56 PR: 35 ESRD: 1	7.7	PD: 54
Prakash et al.[15]	Prospective	132	2.7	–	CR: 89.4 PR: 4.6 ESRD: 2	6	PD: 23.5
Krishna et al.[21]	Retrospective	98	–	100	CR: 75 PR: 12 ESRD: 13	18.4	PD: 16.3 Preterm: 9.2
Saini et al.[22]	Prospective	81	–	15	CR: 39 PR: 33 ESRD: 16	25	PD: 23
Chowdhary et al.[23]	Retrospective	107	3.2	68.2	CR : 88.2 PR : 7 ESRD : 4.7	20.5	PD: 14
Sharma et al.[24]	Prospective	26	25	–	CR : 53.8 PR : 23.1 ESRD : 7.7	15.4	PD: 6.9 SB: 7.7
Sahay et al.[25]	Retrospective	395	8.1	73.4	CR: 76 PR: 15.7 ESRD: 8.3	5	IUD:10.5 PD: 9
AIIMS-ND data (2014–17)	Prospective	30	8	60	CR: 73.4 PR: 16.6 ESRD: 10	16.6	–

(AIIMS-ND: All India Institute of Medical Sciences, New Delhi; CR: complete recovery; ESRD: end-stage renal disease; IUD: intrauterine death; PD: perinatal death; PR: partial recovery; RRT: renal replacement therapy; SB: stillbirth)

from recent studies from India. The various Indian studies on PrAKI outcomes are summarized in **Table 2**.

A recent meta-analysis also reported a 25.4% risk of stillbirth/abortion and 18.6% rate of intrauterine death with PrAKI.[14] Though 37.2% patients required renal replacement therapy (RRT) during hospitalization, only 8.5% remained dialysis dependent on follow-up.

There is paucity of data on the long-term outcome of fetuses exposed to PrAKI. Long-term outcomes with focus on renal recovery are limited. Severe AKI requiring RRT has a higher risk for CKD and progression to end-stage renal disease (ESRD). In a recent meta-analysis, 2.4% of PrAKI-affected patients progressed to ESRD.[26] This highlights the need for close monitoring of patients with PrAKI after hospital discharge.

CONCLUSION

Pregnancy-related AKI is an important cause of maternal and fetal morbidity and mortality. Though the overall incidence has decreased in India and in most other parts of the world, there are cases of AKI requiring dialysis which have adverse long-term outcomes including risk of ESRD. The spectrum of PrAKI in India has changed significantly over the years, reflecting changes in socioeconomic conditions and improvements in healthcare infrastructure. While significant progress has been made, challenges remain, particularly in rural and underserved areas. Addressing these challenges requires a comprehensive approach, including improving healthcare infrastructure, enhancing training for healthcare providers, and increasing public awareness about the importance of peripartum care. Regular surveillance and timely management of AKI will help improve overall patient outcomes. Future research should focus on refining diagnostic criteria for AKI, enhancing preventive or surveillance options, and improving treatment modalities.

REFERENCES

1. Beers K, Patel N. Kidney Physiology in Pregnancy. Adv Chronic Kidney Dis. 2020;27(6):449-54.
2. Rao S, Jim B. Acute Kidney Injury in Pregnancy: The Changing Landscape for the 21st Century. Kidney Int Rep. 2018; 3(2):247-57.
3. Prakash J, Prakash S, Ganiger VC. Changing epidemiology of acute kidney injury in pregnancy: A journey of four decades from a developing country. Saudi J Kidney Dis Transpl. 2019;30(5):1118-30.
4. Sitprija V, Benyajati C. Tropical diseases and acute renal failure. Ann Acad Med Singapore. 1975;4(Suppl 4):112-4.
5. Chugh KS, Singhal PC, Nath IV, Tewari SC, Muthusethupathy MA, Viswanathan S, et al. Spectrum of acute renal failure in North India. J Assoc Physicians India. 1978;26(3): 147-54.
6. Muthusethupathi MA, Shivakumar S. Acute renal failure in south India. Our experience with 187 patients. J Assoc Physicians India. 1987;35(7):504-7.
7. Jayakumar M, Prabahar MR, Fernando EM, Manorajan R, Venkatraman R, Balaraman V. Epidemiologic trend changes in acute renal failure—a tertiary center experience from South India. Ren Fail. 2006;28(5):405-10.
8. Kaul A, Sharma RK, Tripathi R, Suresh KJ, Bhatt S, Prasad N. Spectrum of community-acquired acute kidney injury in India: a retrospective study. Saudi J Kidney Dis Transpl. 2012;23(3):619-28.
9. Feehally J. The ISN 0by25 Global Snapshot Study. Ann Nutr Metab. 2016;68(Suppl 2):29-31.
10. Goswami S, Raju BM, Purohit A, Pahwa N. Clinical Spectrum of Community-Acquired Acute Kidney Injury: A Prospective Study from Central India. Saudi J Kidney Dis Transpl. 2020;31(1):224-34.
11. Prasad N, Jaiswal A, Meyyappan J, Gopalakrishnan N, Chaudhary AR, Fernando E, et al. Community-acquired acute kidney injury in India: data from ISN-acute kidney injury registry. Lancet Reg Health Southeast Asia. 2024;21:100359.
12. Mehrabadi A, Liu S, Bartholomew S, Hutcheon JA, Magee LA, Kramer MS, et al. Hypertensive disorders of pregnancy and the recent increase in obstetric acute renal failure in Canada: population based retrospective cohort study. BMJ. 2014;349:g4731.
13. Mahesh E, Puri S, Varma V, Madhyastha PR, Bande S, Gurudev KC. Pregnancy-related acute kidney injury: An analysis of 165 cases. Indian J Nephrol. 2017;27(2):113-7.
14. Trakarnvanich T, Ngamvichchukorn T, Susantitaphong P. Incidence of acute kidney injury during pregnancy and its prognostic value for adverse clinical outcomes: A systematic review and meta-analysis. Medicine. 2022;101(30):e29563.
15. Prakash J, Singh TB, Ghosh B, Malhotra V, Rathore SS, Vohra R, et al. Changing epidemiology of community-acquired acute kidney injury in developing countries: analysis of 2405 cases in 26 years from eastern India. Clin Kidney J. 2013;6(2):150-5.

16. Prakash J, Pant P, Prakash S, Sivasankar M, Vohra R, Doley PK, et al. Changing picture of acute kidney injury in pregnancy: Study of 259 cases over a period of 33 years. Indian J Nephrol. 2016;26(4):262-7.
17. Scurt FG, Morgenroth R, Bose K, Mertens PR, Chatzikyrkou C. Pr-AKI: Acute Kidney Injury in Pregnancy: Etiology, Diagnostic Workup, Management. Geburtshilfe Frauenheilkd. 2022;82(3):297-316.
18. Taber-Hight E, Shah S. Acute kidney injury in pregnancy. Adv Chronic Kidney Dis. 2020;27(6):455-60.
19. Gautam M, Saxena S, Saran S, Ahmed A, Pandey A, Mishra P, et al. Etiology of Pregnancy-related Acute Kidney Injury among Obstetric Patients in India: A Systematic Review. Indian J Crit Care Med. 2022;26(10):1141-51.
20. Gopalakrishnan N, Dhanapriya J, Muthukumar P, Sakthirajan R, Dineshkumar T, Thirumurugan S, et al. Acute kidney injury in pregnancy—a single center experience. Ren Fail. 2015;37(9):1476-80.
21. Krishna A, Singh R, Prasad N, Gupta A, Bhadauria D, Kaul A, et al. Maternal, fetal and renal outcomes of pregnancy-associated acute kidney injury requiring dialysis. Indian J Nephrol. 2015;25(2):77-81.
22. Saini S, Chaudhury AR, Divyaveer S, Maurya P, Sircar D, Dasgupta S, et al. The changing face of pregnancy-related acute kidney injury from eastern part of India: A hospital-based, prospective, observational study. Saudi J Kidney Dis Transpl. 2020;31(2):493-502.
23. Chowdhary PK, Tibrewal A, Kale SA. Postpartum Acute Kidney Injury in Tertiary Care Center: Single-Center Experience from Central India. Saudi J Kidney Dis Transpl. 2021;32(4):1111-7.
24. Sharma M, Mazumder MA, Alam S, Deka N, Shehwar D, Mahanta PJ, et al. Characteristics, maternal and neonatal outcomes of acute kidney injury in preeclampsia: A prospective, single-center study. Clin Nephrol. 2021; 96(5):263-9.
25. Sahay M, Priyashree, Dogra L, Ismal K, Vali S. Pregnancy-related Acute Kidney Injury in Public Hospital in South India: Changing Trends. J Assoc Physicians India. 2022;70(8):11-2.
26. Liu Y, Ma X, Zheng J, Liu X, Yan T. Pregnancy outcomes in patients with acute kidney injury during pregnancy: a systematic review and meta-analysis. BMC Pregnancy Childbirth. 2017;17(1):235.
27. Shah PP, Trivedi HL, Sharma RK, Shah PR, Joshi MN. Acute renal failure, experience of 816 patients in the tropics. Presented at the XVth Annual Conference of the Indian Society of Nephrology.
28. Ramachandran S. in Asian Nephrology (ed. Chugh KS) 378–383 (Oxford University Press, New Delhi, 1994).

CHAPTER 10

Glomerular Disease in Pregnancy

Priti Meena

HIGHLIGHTS

- Improvements in medical care and fertility technology have expanded the possibility of pregnancy for women with glomerular diseases.
- Prepregnancy counseling offers a unique opportunity to assess the diagnosis, disease activity, medications, and potential fetal impacts.
- The best pregnancy outcomes occur when the disease is in remission, with preserved renal function and absence of proteinuria or hypertension.
- Each type of glomerulonephritis requires specific considerations during pregnancy.
- Renal biopsy should only be pursued if essential to modify management and extend pregnancy with a viable fetus.

INTRODUCTION

The presence of glomerular diseases (GDs) in pregnancy creates a complex and intricate medical landscape, presenting formidable challenges to both patients and nephrologists alike. This chapter highlights the critical importance of preconception planning as an essential strategy for optimizing maternal and fetal outcomes in the context of GDs. This planning involves a multifaceted approach, involving comprehensive stratification, treatment optimization, and comorbidity assessment, which collectively empower nephrologists to engage in well-informed decision-making processes alongside their patients. Recognizing the multifaceted nature of this field, a multidisciplinary approach is imperative to meet the intricate healthcare needs of pregnant individuals with GDs.

This chapter discusses the difficult issues of diagnosing GDs and the importance of preconception counseling. Additionally, we discuss prenatal and postnatal care and how glomerular disorders affect each stage of pregnancy. This chapter also sheds light on the management and prognosis of glomerular disorders and the prudent use of immunosuppressives.

EPIDEMIOLOGY

Due to variations in reporting and the range of study groups and types of studies, precise statistics on the prevalence and type of GDs in pregnancy are limited. The most common GD found by kidney biopsies during pregnancy or postpartum is focal segmental glomerulosclerosis (FSGS), which is followed by IgA nephropathy (IgAN) and lupus nephritis (LN).[1] However, IgAN was the most commonly reported GN in a recently published systematic review on pregnancy and glomerular illness.[2] GDs accounted for

35–56% of end-stage kidney disease (ESKD) cases among women who started dialysis before or after pregnancy, as well as those who received a kidney transplant, according to the Australian and New Zealand Dialysis and Transplantation Registry.[3]

DIAGNOSTIC CHALLENGES

In the pregnant state, glomerular filtration rate (GFR) estimation equations based on serum creatinine are unreliable. Among the frequently employed methods, measuring 24-hour urinary creatinine clearance has been deemed the standard of care, despite the fact that (scheduled) timed urine collection is challenging in pregnancy due to urinary stasis. Nonetheless, serum creatinine levels of >0.75 mg/dL during pregnancy indicate renal impairment.[4] The urine protein–creatinine ratio (UPCR) and urine albumin–creatinine ratio (UACR) have been validated in the assessment of proteinuria in pregnancies with preeclampsia, but data in GN patients is limited. Proteinuria during pregnancy is commonly defined as >300 mg/24 hours or a spot UPCR of >0.3 (dipstick 1+). Proteinuria is usually not associated with maternal and fetal (adverse) outcomes in preeclampsia, although it is in pregnant women with GDs.[5] Increase in proteinuria does not always imply worsening of GD during pregnancy. Other than glomerular reasons, hematuria in pregnancy might arise as a result of uterine distension, increased vascularity, venous pressures, and, rarely, nutcracker syndrome. The presence of acanthocytes and red blood cell (RBC) casts in urine may be a strong indicator of glomerular inflammation. Isolated microhematuria does not appear to suggest deteriorating GN in IgAN, but it does in LN, as microhematuria is part of the lupus flare description and implies active glomerular inflammation.[6] The complement system is integrally engaged in the maintenance of normal placentation, and studies have shown that C3 and C4 levels rise, particularly in the second and third trimesters, but C5b-9 (the terminal component) remains largely unaltered.[7] Antineutrophil cytoplasmic antibody (ANCA) titers have only limited predictive value in pregnant women with ANCA-associated vasculitis. In the case of other GDs, such as MN, data on the use of anti-PLA2R (phospholipase A2 receptor) autoantibodies in the routine follow-up of these pregnancies is limited.[8]

Typically, the differentiation between preeclampsia and pregnancy-associated relapse of GN can be effectively made by the presence of active urine sediments, acanthocyturia, and cellular casts in conjunction with hypocomplementemia; occasionally, the laboratory results may be equivocal. Studies have clarified the role of the ratio of placental growth factor (PlGF) to soluble fms-like tyrosine kinase 1 (sFlt-1), which is significantly increased in preeclampsia but not in lupus or chronic kidney disease (CKD) pregnancy. In other circumstances, the differentiation may be very difficult due to the absence of particular markers. **Chapter 11** describes how to distinguish between LN flare and preeclampsia. The utility of kidney biopsy has been explained in **Chapter 12**.

DE NOVO GLOMERULAR DISEASES

De novo GDs is considered a potential diagnosis when pregnant individuals, who do not have a documented history of GD, present with abnormalities such as proteinuria and/or hematuria, while maintaining normal kidney function. Additionally, de novo GD may be suspected if pregnant individuals experience subacute or acute kidney injury (AKI) accompanied by proteinuria or nephrotic syndrome. If the presence of proteinuria is identified prior to the 20th week of gestation, it is probable that GD was already established prior to the commencement of the pregnancy. After a duration of 20 weeks, the primary differential diagnosis encompasses isolated proteinuria, preeclampsia, and other GDs. While the available evidence on the occurrence of de novo GDs during pregnancy is limited, there have been reported instances of de novo minimal change disease (MCD), focal segmental glomerular sclerosis (FSGS), antiglomerular basement membrane (anti-GBM) disease, and vasculitis.[8-10] There is a limited number of case reports documenting instances of de novo membranous nephropathy, wherein the presence of positive anti-M-type PLA2R antibodies has been observed. Although the transplacental transfer of PLA2R antibodies has been documented, neonates did not exhibit proteinuria at birth or during later follow-up examinations. Additionally, it has been observed that PLA2R antibodies are capable of being transmitted from the mother to the fetus during pregnancy, as well as being present in breast milk.[10]

PREPREGNANCY AND ANTENATAL CARE

Patients with GD should receive antenatal care (ANC) before pregnancy. It should include pregnancy planning, risk stratification, kidney disease treatment optimization, and comorbidity evaluation to improve maternal and fetal outcomes. A multidisciplinary team must address complex demands. After setting expectations, planning should address fertility and pregnancy timing. Keeping fertility is the goal. Avoid alkylating agents like cyclophosphamide (CYC) if the patient desires to conceive.

To determine pregnancy timing, evaluate GD activity, proteinuria, and hypertension. To pragmatically assess GD activity, serum creatinine, proteinuria, and baseline-specific antibody levels should be tested. Contraception is recommended until the pregnancy is safe. Guidelines recommend targeting preconception blood pressure of <140/90 mm Hg [European Society of Cardiology/International Society of Hypertension (ESC/ISH) class IA].[11] It is strongly advised to refrain from using renin–angiotensin–aldosterone (RAAS) blockers during pregnancy because of the established hazards associated with their exposure during the second and third trimesters. There exists a paucity of data about the potential risk of congenital abnormalities linked to exposure during the initial trimester of pregnancy. Their association with a congenital malformation on exposure in the first trimester is questionable.[12] Nevertheless, Kidney Disease: Improving Global Outcomes (KDIGO) recommends optimizing BP readings before conception with alternate antihypertensives.[13]

According to KDIGO guidelines, sodium–glucose cotransporter-2 inhibitors (SGLT-2i) are now the first-line nephroprotective treatment for IgAN class 1A without preconception considerations.[13] No well-controlled trials on pregnant women and SGLT2 inhibitors exist.

It is recommended to discontinue CYC and mycophenolate mofetil (MMF) before conception (3 months for CYC, 6 weeks for MMF) to replace them with nonteratogenic alternatives while maintaining GD stability.[14] Also, it has been advocated to use two contraceptives (typically barrier and hormonal) when switching to safer choices.

Antenatal care should focus on proteinuria, GN disease activity, and blood pressure control. Monitoring and frequency of visits should be tailored depending on GN type, activity, CKD stage, comorbidities, and psychosocial setting. Every woman with CKD or GN should have her prenatal plan reviewed based on maternal and fetal progress. GN flares or relapses, maternal comorbidities, fetal abnormalities, and preeclampsia should be monitored closely. All women with preeclampsia risk, including GDs, should start low-dose aspirin (100–150 mg) before 12–14 weeks of gestation. Controlling blood pressure to <140/90 mm Hg in women with persistent hypertension can reduce severe episodes without harming fetal health.[15,16] In the setting of an increased risk of venous thromboembolism such as antiphospholipid antibody (APLA) syndrome, consider low-molecular-weight heparin anticoagulation.[17]

In severe nephrotic syndrome and edema, diuretics may be required yet overdiuresis reduces blood pressure, placental perfusion, and amniotic fluid volume.[17]

Nutritional assessment helps address hematinic, vitamin, and other nutritional deficits, and proper protein and micronutrient intake should be ensured.

TREATMENT

A pregnant patient with biopsy-proven GDs who relapses with nephrotic range proteinuria in the third trimester or close to term can be treated conservatively with moderate salt restriction, antiedema measures, and antihypertensives. Steroids have been successfully used in the treatment of MCD and FSGS in newly diagnosed patients and relapses during the first and second trimesters. Calcineurin inhibitors (tacrolimus and cyclosporine) can be used in steroid-resistant instances and membranous glomerulonephritis (MGN); however, they increase gestational hypertension and diabetes risk.[14] Due to its unknown teratogenic risk, rituximab is avoided at least a year before the anticipated pregnancy.[18]

Antineutrophil cytoplasmic antibody-associated vasculitis is uncommon in reproductive-age women, and high-dose steroids may not be adequate in patients with organ- and life-threatening disease activity. Rituximab and CYC have been used in some cases of early and late pregnancy in published literature, respectively, as well as plasma exchange.[8,19] The management of IgAN during pregnancy primarily centers around managing hypertension and renal insufficiency. In general, it is not advisable to use immunosuppressive medications during pregnancies for IgAN with the exception of steroids which may be used to manage proteinuria and rapidly declining kidney function. Management of LN is described in the **Chapter 11**. and atypical hemolytic uremic syndrome (aHUS) in **Chapter 6**.

Table 1 shows maternal and fetal complications of various immunosuppressive drugs.

DELIVERY AND POSTPARTUM CARE

Regular discussion about the ideal delivery time should balance the benefits of extended gestational age against the danger of maternal–fetal complications if gestation is continued after fetal viability. Continuous monitoring of renal parameters, blood pressure, and serological markers to assess maternal health and ultrasound growth, amniotic fluid volume, Doppler, and cardiotocography to monitor fetal growth is crucial.

Women should be followed for postpartum hypertension, disease flare, and renal function decline. In proteinuric women, RAAS blockage must be restored.

TABLE 1: Maternal and fetal complications of various immunosuppressive drugs.

Immunosuppressive drug	*Category*	*Fetal and maternal complications*
Glucocorticoids	C	• *Maternal:* Increases lower urinary tract infections, gestational diabetes, gestational hypertension • Earlier associated with cleft palate (not proven), transient adrenal insufficiency, thymic hypoplasia
Calcineurin inhibitors (cyclosporine, tacrolimus)	C	• *Fetal:* Reversible nephrotoxicity and hyperkalemia in the newborn have been reported • *Maternal:* Worsening of gestational hypertension and diabetes (in prone patients)
Azathioprine	C Active metabolite, 6-mercaptopurine does not cross placenta	• *Fetal:* Transient lymphopenia • *Maternal:* Gastrointestinal side effects, bone marrow suppression including cytopenias, increased risk of infections
Mycophenolate mofetil (MMF)	D	• *MMF embryopathy:* Ear, mouth, fingers, ocular organ malformation (EMFO tetrad) (risk of malformations 20%) • *Maternal:* Gastrointestinal side effects, bone marrow suppression, infections
Cyclophosphamide	D	• Congenital malformations, suppressed bone marrow function, neuronal defects reported
Hydroxychloroquine	C	No increase in congenital malformations in fetus noted
Rituximab	C	• Increased preterm deliveries, nonspecific malformation syndromes (causation unclear) • Depletion of fetal/infant B lymphocytes and increased risk for neonatal infection
Eculizumab	C	Limited data, safe in case series

Quinapril and enalapril can be taken by breastfeeding women. Breastfeeding is rarely contraindicated in most women.[20]

The impact of pregnancy on GDs and the reciprocal impact of GDs on pregnancy can be detrimental. There are also potential ramifications for fetal well-being. The most significant predictors of potential complications, such as maternal kidney disease progression, maternal or fetal death, preterm, small-for-gestational-age baby, or admission to the neonatal intensive care unit, include CKD stage, preexisting hypertension, and proteinuria.[21] There exists a substantial body of published data pertaining to LN and IgAN, whereas the available data regarding other GDs is very sparse.

Furthermore, there is a scarcity of data regarding long-term follow-up after pregnancy.

According to a study on pregnancy outcomes in 48 GD patients, preeclampsia accounted for 33% of complications, urine protein doubled in 39%, and serum creatinine ≥50% in 27%. Perinatal mortality was 13%, and 48% of newborns were preterm. GD subtypes did not differ significantly, while FSGS had the highest renal function reduction.[22]

The Cure Glomerulonephropathy project showed that a history of complicated pregnancy was associated with greater eGFR decline in the years following glomerulonephropathy (GN) diagnosis. Specifically, those with MN exhibited the lowest likelihood of reporting complications. Conversely, individuals with FSGS reported the highest incidence of complications.[23]

Notwithstanding these obstacles, the prospects for women with GDs who desire to conceive are favorable. Through meticulous strategizing and effective monitoring, the majority of women have the capability to successfully give birth to offspring of sound health. Nevertheless, it is imperative to adopt a pragmatic approach toward the potential hazards and collaborate closely with a healthcare team in order to formulate a tailored strategy that aligns with the specific requirements of each individual. There exists considerable potential for substantial advancements in the domains of personalized risk assessment, extended post-treatment monitoring, and timely detection of underlying pathologies. The establishment of collaborative research endeavors including nephrologists, obstetricians, and other healthcare providers is imperative in order to facilitate advancements in the area and enhance results for young women afflicted with glomerular disorders who desire to get pregnant.

CONCLUSION

Managing glomerular diseases during pregnancy presents significant challenges. Pregnancy can exacerbate GDs, and GDs can adversely affect pregnancy outcomes, with potential ramifications for fetal well-being. Key predictors of complications include chronic kidney disease stage, preexisting hypertension, and proteinuria. While substantial research exists on lupus nephritis (LN) and IgA nephropathy (IgAN), data on other GDs are limited. Potential complications include the progression of maternal kidney disease, maternal or fetal death, preterm birth, small-for-gestational-age infants, and neonatal intensive care unit admissions.

REFERENCES

1. Day C, Hewins P, Hildebrand S, Sheikh L, Taylor G, Kilby M, et al. The role of renal biopsy in women with kidney disease identified in pregnancy. Nephrol Dial Transplant. 2007;23(1):201–6.
2. De Castro I, Easterling TR, Bansal N, Jefferson JA. Nephrotic syndrome in pregnancy poses risks with both maternal and fetal complications. Kidney Int. 2017;91(6): 1464-72.
3. Wyld ML, Clayton PA, Kennedy SE, Alexander SI, Chadban SJ. Pregnancy outcomes for kidney transplant recipients with transplantation as a child. JAMA Pediatr. 2015;169(2):e143626.
4. Gao M, Vilayur E, Ferreira D, Nanra R, Hawkins J. Estimating the glomerular filtration rate in pregnancy: The evaluation of the Nanra and CKD-EPI serum creatinine-based equations. Obstet Med. 2021;14(1):31-4.
5. Fishel Bartal M, Lindheimer MD, Sibai BM. Proteinuria during pregnancy: definition, pathophysiology, methodology, and clinical significance. Am J Obstet Gynecol. 2022; 226(2):S819-34.
6. Brown MA, Holt JL, Mangos GJ, Murray N, Curtis J, Homer C. Microscopic hematuria in pregnancy: relevance to pregnancy outcome. Am J Kidney Dis. 2005;45(4):667-73.
7. Girardi G, Lingo JJ, Fleming SD, Regal JF. Essential role of complement in pregnancy: from implantation to parturition and beyond. Front Immunol. 2020;11:1681.
8. Singh P, Dhooria A, Rathi M, Agarwal R, Sharma K, Dhir V, et al. Successful treatment outcomes in pregnant patients with

ANCA -associated vasculitides: a systematic review of literature. Int J Rheum Dis. 2018;21(9):1734-40.

9. Uchino E, Takada D, Mogami H, Matsubara T, Tsukamoto T, Yanagita M. Membranous nephropathy associated with pregnancy: an anti-phospholipase A2 receptor antibody-positive case report. CEN Case Rep. 2018;7(1):101-6.
10. Saleem M, Iftikhar H. (2023). Anti-phospholipase A2 Receptor Antibody-Negative Membranous Nephropathy in Pregnancy. Cureus. [online] Available from: https://www.cureus.com/articles/175385-anti-phospholipase-a2-receptor-antibody-negative-membranous-nephropathy-in-pregnancy [Last accessed May, 2024].
11. Rovin BH, Adler SG, Barratt J, Bridoux F, Burdge KA, Chan TM, et al. KDIGO 2021 Clinical practice guideline for the management of glomerular diseases. Kidney Int. 2021;100(4):S1-S276.
12. Fu J, Tomlinson G, Feig DS. Increased risk of major congenital malformations in early pregnancy use of angiotensin-converting-enzyme inhibitors and angiotensin-receptor-blockers: a meta-analysis. Diabetes Metab Res Rev. 2021;37(8):e3453.
13. Fakhouri F, Schwotzer N, Cabiddu G, Barratt J, Legardeur H, Garovic V, et al. Glomerular diseases in pregnancy: pragmatic recommendations for clinical management. Kidney Int. 2023;103(2):264–81.
14. Sammaritano LR, Bermas BL, Chakravarty EE, Chambers C, Clowse MEB, Lockshin MD, et al. 2020 American College of Rheumatology Guideline for the Management of Reproductive Health in Rheumatic and Musculoskeletal Diseases. Arthritis Rheumatol. 2020;72(4):529-56.
15. Magee LA, Von Dadelszen P, Rey E, Ross S, Asztalos E, Murphy KE, et al. Less-tight versus tight control of hypertension in pregnancy. N Engl J Med. 2015;372(5):407-17.
16. Tita AT, Szychowski JM, Boggess K, Dugoff L, Sibai B, Lawrence K, et al. Treatment for mild chronic hypertension during pregnancy. N Engl J Med. 2022;386(19):1781-92.
17. Wiles K, Chappell L, Clark K, Elman L, Hall M, Lightstone L, et al. Clinical practice guideline on pregnancy and renal disease. BMC Nephrol. 2019;20(1):401.
18. Holden F, Bramham K, Clark K. Rituximab for the maintenance of minimal change nephropathy - A report of two pregnancies. Obstet Med. 2020;13(3):145-7.
19. Harris C, Marin J, Beaulieu MC. Rituximab induction therapy for de novo ANCA associated vasculitis in pregnancy: a case report. BMC Nephrol. 2018;19(1):152.
20. Bramham K, Chusney G, Lee J, Lightstone L, Nelson-Piercy C. Breastfeeding and Tacrolimus: Serial Monitoring in Breast-Fed and Bottle-Fed Infants. Clin J Am Soc Nephrol. 2013;8(4):563-7.
21. Siligato R, Gembillo G, Cernaro V, Torre F, Salvo A, Granese R, et al. Maternal and fetal outcomes of pregnancy in nephrotic syndrome due to primary glomerulonephritis. Front Med. 2020;7:563094.
22. Marinaki S, Tsiakas S, Skalioti C, Kapsia E, Lionaki S, Vallianou K, et al. Pregnancy in women with preexisting glomerular diseases: a single-center experience. Front Med. 2022;9:801144.
23. Reynolds ML, Oliverio AL, Zee J, Hendren EM, O'Shaughnessy MM, Ayoub I, et al. Pregnancy history and kidney disease progression among women enrolled in cure glomerulonephropathy. Kidney Int Rep. 2023;8(4):805-17.

CHAPTER 11

Lupus Nephritis in Pregnancy

Smita Subhash Divyaveer, Vaishnavi Venkatasubramanian, Vaibhav Tiwari, Manish Rathi

HIGHLIGHTS

- Systemic lupus erythematosus (SLE) during pregnancy can cause obstetric complications such as hypertension, preeclampsia, and thromboembolic events, as well as fetal complications such as preterm delivery, miscarriages, intrauterine growth retardation, and congenital heart block.
- Pregnancy can exacerbate lupus nephritis (LN), leading to progressive kidney disease.
- Patients with active LN should wait at least 6 months after achieving inactive disease before attempting pregnancy.
- Teratogenic medications like mycophenolic acid should be discontinued, with a "wash-out" period of at least 3 months, and replaced with nonteratogenic alternatives such as calcineurin inhibitors or azathioprine.
- Hydroxychloroquine (HCQ) is generally safe to use throughout pregnancy.
- Indicators of LN include hypocomplementemia, elevated dsDNA titers, active urine sediment, and extrarenal lupus symptoms.
- A clinical presentation of hypertension and heavy proteinuria without hematuria is more indicative of preeclampsia, which is typically diagnosed clinically; however, a kidney biopsy should be considered when lupus nephritis or other primary glomerular diseases are suspected.

INTRODUCTION

Systemic lupus erythematosus (SLE) is a multisystem autoimmune disease predominantly affecting women of childbearing age group. When kidneys are involved in SLE, it is called lupus nephritis (LN). It is the most common secondary glomerulonephritis. Clinical spectrum of LN can range from asymptomatic abnormalities to severe organ-threatening manifestations. Just as the severity of the disease can be variable so also the histological activity and/or chronicity may vary. LN can affect the reproductive health of young women in every phase, i.e., prior to conception, after conception, and after parturition in myriad ways. Some of the therapies of LN can adversely affect fertility. Whether disease can affect fertility directly is not yet conclusively proved. When patients of LN conceive, there is a risk of LN flare in pregnancy. Besides, LN may occur for the first time during pregnancy; in either scenario, it has huge impact on maternal as well as fetal outcome. LN can flare in postpartum period as well or the effects of an LN flare may continue in postpartum period. Hence, successful maternal and fetal outcome in patients with LN requires understanding and addressing the nuances of LN in and around pregnancy and it is very pertinent to the practice of obstetrics, nephrology, and rheumatology. In this topic, we shall discuss the effect of LN on prepregnancy, pregnancy, and postpartum period and the management at each stage.

EPIDEMIOLOGY

The reported incidence and prevalence of SLE are quite variable ranging from 1.0 to 23.2 per 100,000 person years and 8 to 241 per 100,000 persons, respectively.[1,2] LN disproportionately affects the nonwhite population of different ethnicity and people from lower socioeconomic condition; therefore, lot of variability is seen in reports from different countries (Hoover et al., 2016). Renal involvement in SLE, i.e., LN also has a very variable incidence[3] ranging from 14 to 75% across different countries. Possible reasons for such variability are genetic predisposition, environmental and geographic factors, socioeconomic factors, and biopsy practices. SLE occurs more often in females with a male-to-female ratio of 1:8 to 1:15 in adults implying a role of hormonal or hormone receptor predilection for the disease.[4,5] However, proportion of SLE patients who develop LN is reported to be more in men in some studies.[6,7] Overall, up to 60% of patients with SLE develop LN at some point of time in their disease course[8] and 5–20% of the patients with SLE progress to end-stage renal disease (ESRD) within 10 years of diagnosis.[1] The prevalence of LN is higher in Asians and Africans than Caucasians.[9] The likelihood of successful pregnancies in patients who have had biopsy-proven LN has improved over last few decades but the estimates form different studies are variable ranging from a dismal less than 50% to 90% according to some reports.[10]

Is fertility affected by lupus nephritis?

Whether SLE per se affects fertility is not conclusively known.[11] There is data to suggest that disease activity of SLE can cause inflammation in ovaries and disturbance of the hypothalamic pituitary ovarian axis.[12] There is some data to suggest that SLE itself may affect ovarian reserve. Many observational studies have reported low anti-Müllerian hormone and some have reported low antral follicle count.[13] Almost half the women with SLE have menstrual irregularities which worsen with presence of disease activity.[14] Factors that can cause infertility or subfertility in SLE patients other than the disease activity itself include presence of renal dysfunction, co-occurrence of antiphospholipid antibody syndrome (APS), advanced maternal age,[15] and psychosocial factors or medication[16] that is needed to treat LN. Patients are advised to delay or avoid conception if they have active LN or when they are on medication such as cyclophosphamide or mycophenolate mofetil. Cyclophosphamide can affect fertility by its effect on oocytes and granulosa cells, particularly if the cumulative doses are high.[17] It has been reported that patients above 24 years of age have higher risk of toxicity than younger ones. Storage of sperms, cryopreservation of oocytes, and gonadotropin-releasing hormone therapy may be considered, although it remains largely experimental and not widely available.[18]

Can lupus nephritis affect outcomes of pregnancy?

Expected outcomes depend on baseline renal function status, histologic class of LN, overall SLE disease activity, occurrence of lupus flare, and comorbidities.

Complications may be maternal, fetal, or both. Maternal complications include flare of SLE and LN, hypertension, preeclampsia, eclampsia, and thromboembolic events. Fetal concerns include miscarriage, premature birth, intrauterine fetal growth retardation, and congenital heart block.[19]

This brings us to the most important section, i.e., prepregnancy planning in patients with LN.

PREPREGNANCY PLANNING IN KNOWN CASE OF LUPUS NEPHRITIS

Prepregnancy Evaluation

A thorough preconception evaluation is crucial for women with LN, aiming to assess the potential maternal and fetal risks of pregnancy, instigate measures to stabilize disease activity, and modify treatments to those least harmful to the fetus.

Typically, women of reproductive age with LN fall into three categories:

1. Women with inactive or quiescent disease
2. Women with active disease
3. Women with LN that has caused severe organ dysfunction and/or damage

Most guidelines recommend disease quiescence for at least 6 months before conception.[20] Waiting time of 6 months reduces the risk of a flare and gives adequate time for stopping teratogenic medication and switching to nonteratogenic pregnancy compatible medication. It also gives time for observation to ensure that disease remains quiescent after change of medication. Disease quiescence can be quantified or measured by the scoring systems that record clinical organ involvement and serological activity. The scoring systems such as SLE Disease Activity Index (SLEDAI) and British Isles Lupus Assessment Group (BILAG) for noting the disease activity are comprehensive and include all organs systems, although there are minor differences among the various scoring systems.[21] The score should be stable to ensure disease quiescence.

Renal remission is generally defined as stabilization or normalization of serum creatinine and reduction in proteinuria to <300–500 mg/day.[22] Longer duration of remission and complete remission (as compared to partial remission) is associated with lesser risk of relapse during pregnancy.[23] Only remission of LN alone is not sufficient; patient must be in complete remission with no manifestation of active SLE.

Active disease at conception is a strong predictor of negative maternal and obstetric outcomes. In those with renal insufficiency, the evaluation should include the potential for a temporary or permanent decline in renal function. Presence of severe renal dysfunction is a contraindication to pregnancy as it is associated with very high risk of maternal and fetal complications.[24] Women with significant organ damage, such as recent events affecting the heart, lungs, kidneys, or having had a stroke, should be advised of the high risks associated with pregnancy and may be advised to consider alternatives like adoption or surrogacy.

The preconception assessment for women with SLE should encompass a review of disease activity, major organ involvement through clinical, laboratory, and histological assessments, and the potential for hypercoagulability or other medical conditions that could affect pregnancy. In patients who have a history of LN, presence of partial remission, i.e., ongoing proteinuria and increased creatinine is associated with adverse pregnancy outcomes as well as a full blown flare of LN. Presence of APLA, hypertension, history of thrombosis, and discontinuation of hydroxychloroquine prior to pregnancy can be associated with flares during pregnancy or adverse pregnancy outcomes. A history of poor obstetric outcomes, such as small for gestational age infants, preeclampsia, stillbirth,

BOX 1: Prepregnancy evaluation in patients with lupus nephritis.

Review prior history	• Severity of LN • LN histology • *Attainment of remission:* Renal function, proteinuria • Hypertension • Prior adverse pregnancy outcomes • Any other extrarenal end organ damage
Clinical and laboratory evaluation	• RFT, urine examination, quantification of proteinuria • CBC, LFT, thyroid function test • Extrarenal SLE features
Disease activity markers	• Complement levels • dsDNA titers
Other risk factors for adverse pregnancy outcomes	• ANA immunoblot especially anti-Ro and anti-La • APLA profile • Coagulation profile • Severe cardiovascular or pulmonary disease: ECG, 2D echocardiography, pulmonary function tests
Review of medications	• Stop teratogenics like RAASi, mycophenolate, and statins • Continue or add HCQs (unless contraindicated) • Folate supplementation • Vitamin D supplementation, if deficient

(ANA: antinuclear antibody; APLA: antiphospholipid antibodies; CBC: complete blood count; HCQ: hydroxychloroquine; LFT: liver function test; LN: lupus nephritis; RFT: renal function test; SLE: systemic lupus erythematosus)

miscarriage, and premature birth, should be meticulously reviewed as these can indicate factors associated with adverse pregnancy outcomes. Prior to pregnancy, antibodies to Ro/La and antiphospholipid (APLA) should be evaluated.

It is, therefore, imperative that planning for pregnancy is done prior to conception. The list of the parameters to be assessed prior to pregnancy is summarized in **Box 1**. Another vital part of planning is counseling regarding follow-up and monitoring during pregnancy as well as maternal and fetal outcomes in individual cases based on these parameters so that patients can make well-informed decision.

Flare of SLE in Pregnancy

Most of the flares of SLE disease activity in pregnancy are renal or hematological, if they occur. True incidence of LN in pregnancy is difficult to estimate but data from observational studies indicates that pregnancy is associated with increased renal involvement. It is widely acknowledged that pregnancy, as well as the postpartum period, is linked to an elevated incidence of SLE flares, though statistics on this vary significantly, with reported rates between range from 25 to 60%.[25,26] Renal flares are more likely to occur if LN is not in complete remission but can occur even in quiescent disease.[10,27] Postpartum, renal disease activity is more prevalent, whereas flares related to nonrenal disease are more likely to occur in the second and third trimesters.

The cause of flares in pregnancy is multifactorial. Clinically, the predominance of LN flares in females, exacerbation by pregnancy or shortly thereafter, association with hormonal treatments and studies in animal models, suggests a huge role of hormonal involvement in the disease mechanism. Pregnancy has significant synergistic effects on the immunologic status. Inflammatory effects of autoantibodies, T cells, cytokines, and chemokines are amplified. The containment of inflammation is suboptimal as indicated by diminished Treg cell response in tissue samples obtained from first trimester spontaneous miscarriages. Hormones such as estrogen and prolactin are likely major influencers in amplification of inflammatory response. There is upsurge of estrogen in final trimester which is believed to enhance immunological response. Some of these factors also may cause flares in postpartum period.

MANAGEMENT OF PREGNANCY IN PATIENTS WITH LUPUS NEPHRITIS

Figure 1 shows the pre-pregnancy, during and after pregnancy considerations in patients with LN.

- The impact of pregnancy on the disease course, both during pregnancy and on long-term kidney function
- How LN affects pregnancy outcomes

The management should be multidisciplinary, as described earlier, aiming to address both of the above issues.

Patients who have had renal involvement should be under close follow-up because of the risk of flares and preeclampsia. As mentioned earlier, pregnancy should be planned when the disease has been quiescent for at least 6 months. Monitoring must be aimed at looking for evidence of new/worsening disease activity, new-onset hypertension, any sign or symptom of preeclampsia, disease activity in other organ systems and fetal well-being. **Table 1** shows the details of clinical and laboratory parameters to be monitored during pregnancy.

FREQUENCY OF VISITS DURING PREGNANCY

Vigilant monitoring of disease activity is essential throughout pregnancy. Routine blood tests for full blood count, kidney function, and electrolytes should be conducted every 4–6 weeks. In planned pregnancies with quiescent disease and stable renal function, blood pressure and urine routine and microscopy once a month and proteinuria quantification, serum creatinine, complement levels C3/C4, and anti-dsDNA every 3 months have been recommended by American College of Rheumatology guidelines. If the LN is active, monthly or more monitoring may be required.[28] Depending on proteinuria levels, urinalysis and urine protein quantification should be checked every 2–4 weeks.

Teratogenic medications must be stopped, transitioning to safer treatments such as calcineurin inhibitors (CNIs) or azathioprine (see section prepregnancy evaluation above). A "washout" period of at least 3 months is recommended during this transition, where disease activity is monitored, and patients are counseled on contraception. Pregnancy can be considered after this washout period if the disease remains inactive.

If antihypertensive treatment is necessary during pregnancy, medications safe for pregnancy like labetalol, nifedipine, or methyldopa should be used. Renin–angiotensin–aldosterone system (RAAS) blockade should be avoided in pregnancy. Alternative antihypertensives should be used instead.[29] The continuation of RAAS blockade agents should be carefully weighed against the risks and benefits, considering kidney function, blood pressure, and proteinuria levels prior to conception. If blood pressure and proteinuria are not well-controlled, RAAS blockade therapy may be

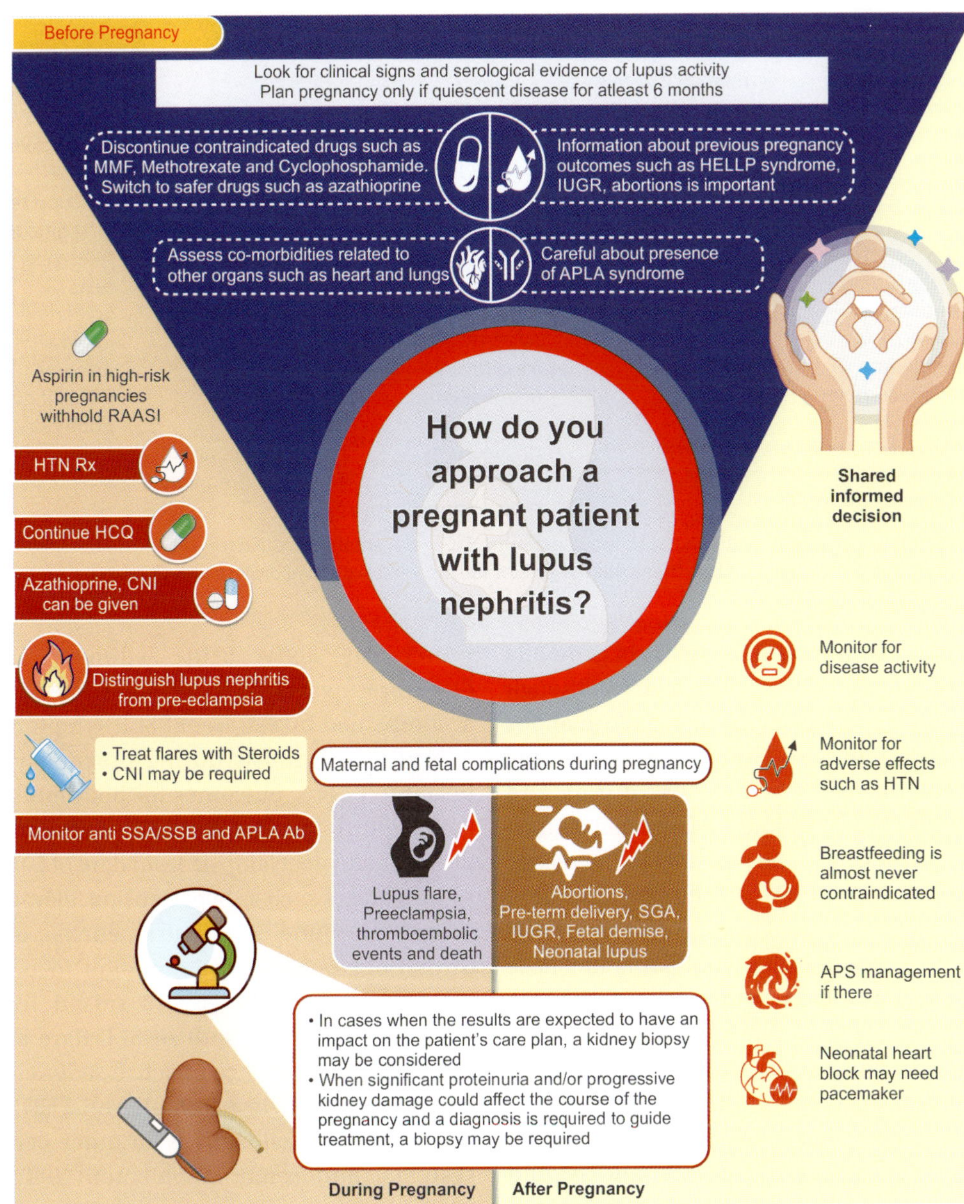

Fig. 1: Approach to pregnancy in a patient with lupus nephritis. (APLA: antiphospholipid antibodies; APS: Antiphospholipid syndrome; CNI: calcineurin inhibition; HCQ: hydroxychloroquine; HELLP: hemolysis, elevated liver enzymes and low platelet; HTN: hypertension; IUGR: intrauterin growth restriction; MMF: mycophenolate mofetil; RAASI: renin-angiotensin-aldosterone system inhibitors; SGA: small for gestational age)

Courtesy: Dr Priti Meena

maintained initially and only ceased upon confirmation of pregnancy to avoid the risk of prolonged cessation while awaiting conception. It is crucial to educate patients about early pregnancy confirmation and immediate cessation of these drugs.

TABLE 1: Monitoring and surveillance during pregnancy in patients with lupus nephritis.

Evidence of new-onset/worsening of LN	*Evidence of new/ worsening SLE disease activity*	*Sign or symptom of preeclampsia*	*Monitoring fetal well-being*	*Routine monitoring as per protocol*
• New-onset or worsening hypertension • New-onset or worsening proteinuria • Rise in serum creatinine • Falling complement levels • Rising dsDNA titers • Occurrence of nephrotic syndrome	• Disease activity scores such as SLEDAI can be used • APLA testing (if not done prior)	• Uric acid levels • Newer biomarkers like sFLT-1/PIGF ratio • New-onset or worsening hypertension • New-onset or worsening proteinuria • Any features of severe preeclampsia	• Obstetric ultrasound for: – Placental blood flow – Intrauterine fetal growth restriction – Anomaly scan • Fetal heart rate monitoring • Daily fetal movement count in advanced pregnancy	• Thyroid function test • Oral glucose tolerance tests • Screening for viral diseases, VDRL (if not done prior)

(APLA: antiphospholipid antibodies; LN: lupus nephritis; PIGF: placental growth factor; sFLT-1: soluble fms-like tyrosine kinase receptor-1; SLE: systemic lupus erythematosus; VDRL: venereal disease research laboratory)

Hydroxychloroquine (HCQ) is generally considered safe during pregnancy, although a slight increase in congenital malformations has been reported. The substantial benefits of HCQ in reducing flare risk during and post-pregnancy should be balanced against this risk. Owing to the potential for increased flare risk upon HCQ discontinuation or dose reduction, continued usage is recommended unless contraindicated.[30] Initiating low-dose aspirin and calcium supplements before the 16th week of gestation is advised to prevent preeclampsia. A multidisciplinary team should oversee regular antepartum maternal and fetal monitoring. Besides routine ultrasound checks in the first and second trimesters, additional fetal surveillance in the third trimester is suggested for patients with stable LN, ideally on a monthly basis from 28 to 34 weeks and then weekly until delivery.

DIAGNOSING LN DURING PREGNANCY

The emergence or exacerbation of LN during pregnancy manifests as increased proteinuria, active urine sediment, and deteriorating renal function, sometimes accompanied by extrarenal SLE symptoms. A new LN diagnosis during pregnancy is linked to poorer outcomes for both mother and child. It can be clinically difficult to differentiate preeclampsia from flare of LN as some features such as hypertension, elevated serum creatinine, proteinuria, edema, and thrombocytopenia[31] are common to both conditions. Hemolysis and raised liver enzymes can occur both in SLE flare and preeclampsia. Presence of active sediments, low complement levels, high anti-DsDNA levels, SLE disease activity in other organ systems, and renal involvement before 20 weeks of gestation are more indicative of LN flare than preeclampsia. Biomarker may be helpful in differentiating the two conditions such as uric acid levels and soluble fms-like tyrosine kinase receptor-1 (sFLT-1)/placental growth factor (PlGF) ratio. Increase in these two parameters occurs in preeclampsia, with the latter can be detectable weeks before the onset of proteinuria

TABLE 2: Comparison of features of lupus nephritis in pregnancy versus preeclampsia.

	Lupus nephritis	***Preeclampsia***
Onset	Anytime in pregnancy or postpartum	After 20 weeks gestation. Less common postpartum
Hypertension	May be present	Always present
Proteinuria	Present, can be nephrotic range	Present, often subnephrotic
Renal function	Reduced in proliferative LN or AKI in nephrotic presentation	Normal or reduced in severe preeclampsia
Urine microscopy	Active sediments are present in proliferative LN	Absent
Serum albumin	Can be normal, slightly low or very low (nephrotic presentation)	May be normal or slightly low
Dyslipidemia	May be present (nephrotic presentation)	Normal
Complement levels	Low or normal	Normal
Anti-DsDNA titers	Often raised	Normal
Other organ involvement	Extrarenal features of SLE may be present	Severe preeclampsia: Liver, central nervous system, HELLP
Uric acid	Normal or low	Raised
sFLT-1/PlGF ratio	Normal	Raised
Resolution after delivery	No, unless treated	Usually resolves after delivery
Recurrence in future pregnancy	Depends on remission, disease activity	Increased risk

(AKI: acute kidney injury; HELLP: hemolysis, elevated liver enzymes, and low platelets; LN: lupus nephritis; PlGF: placental growth factor; sFLT-1: soluble fms-like tyrosine kinase receptor-1; SLE: systemic lupus erythematosus)

or hypertension in preeclampsia.[32] A meta-analysis highlighted the consistent association between low urinary calcium and preeclampsia (<195 mg/day). **Table 2** below summarizes the differences in the two conditions. These disease entities are distinct, necessitating accurate diagnosis for appropriate management—delivery in the case of preeclampsia and immunosuppression for LN flare. It is important to note that there can be superimposed preeclampsia or a cooccurrence of both the conditions and many features of active LN are actually risk factors for preeclampsia.[33] In such circumstances, management of both the entities needs to be done.

Kidney biopsy in pregnant patients should be reserved for situations where the results will significantly influence treatment direction and management.[34] The procedure is generally considered up to the 25th week of gestation to minimize bleeding risks. A comprehensive review suggests that while kidney biopsy during pregnancy carries a small risk of bleeding, it is a relatively safe procedure.[35]

Immediate treatment of LN flares during pregnancy should not be delayed. Management decisions should consider the severity of organ impairment, the duration of pregnancy at the time of the flare, and the risk-benefit ratio of continuing the pregnancy. Treatment options should be personalized, respecting the patient's preferences and values. In cases of severe LN flare early in pregnancy, therapeutic abortion might be considered. The primary aim is to control disease activity swiftly with immunosuppressants while avoiding teratogenic effects, thus improving the chances of a favorable pregnancy outcome. For late-stage pregnancy flares, especially in women with fertility challenges, treating the flare itself might be prioritized. Initial treatment would include intravenous corticosteroids, followed by reduced-dose oral prednisolone, azathioprine, and CNIs, aiming to manage LN sufficiently to prolong pregnancy until fetal maturity is adequate for delivery. Postpartum monitoring is critical due to the heightened risk of disease flares and thromboembolic events within 6 months after delivery. Medications deemed safe during pregnancy are also generally safe for breastfeeding, although evidence for cyclosporine and tacrolimus is limited. Enalapril may be safely used during breastfeeding as it does not significantly pass into breast milk.

For women requiring renal replacement therapy before or during pregnancy, increased hemodialysis frequency to five to seven times weekly is recommended, aiming for over 20 hours to improve clearance and minimize volume shifts. A target predialysis urea level of <20 mmol/L is typically recommended.[36,37]

Given the prothrombotic nature of pregnancy, the risk is exacerbated in women with SLE and antiphospholipid syndrome. The additional complication of proteinuria in LN further increases procoagulant changes. Thromboprophylaxis is advised for pregnant women with significant proteinuria or low serum albumin, with the prescription tailored to the degree of renal impairment. Both low-molecular-weight heparin and unfractionated heparin are considered safe during pregnancy.

DRUGS AND PREGNANCY

Continuing maintenance steroids at the lowest effective dose during pregnancy is standard, as they pose minimal risk to the mother or fetus. Prednisolone is preferred as the placenta metabolizes it, with only about 10% reaching the fetus at maternal doses below 20 mg. Cyclosporine and tacrolimus are not teratogenic, but there is an increased risk of gestational diabetes and hypertension in tacrolimus users, thus glucose tolerance testing is advised at 28 weeks or earlier if risk factors are present. Patients who are on CNIs may require higher doses in pregnancy to maintain their target through CNI concentrations. Limited data exist on the use of biologic medications such as rituximab or belimumab during pregnancy. Since significant IgG transfer across the placenta does not occur until after 15 weeks of gestation, these drugs may be continued through conception.

CONCLUSION

In conclusion, a planned pregnancy taking into account the risk factors and active monitoring during pregnancy and postpartum period can minimize adverse pregnancy outcomes. In those who do have flare during pregnancy, aggressive management while avoid teratogenic drugs is possible to optimize the outcomes.

REFERENCES

1. Anders HJ, Saxena R, Zhao MH, Parodis I, Salmon JE, Mohan C. Lupus nephritis. Nat Rev Dis Primers. 2020;6(1):7.
2. Rees F, Doherty M, Grainge MJ, Lanyon P, Zhang W. The worldwide incidence and

prevalence of systemic lupus erythematosus: a systematic review of epidemiological studies. Rheumatology. 2017;56(11):1945-61.
3. Bastian HM, Roseman JM, McGwin G, Alarcón GS, Friedman AW, Fessler BJ, et al.; LUMINA Study Group. LUpus in MInority populations: NAture vs nurture: Systemic lupus erythematosus in three ethnic groups. XII. Risk factors for lupus nephritis after diagnosis. Lupus. 2002;11(3):152-60.
4. Thomas R, Jawad AS. Systemic lupus erythematosus: rarer in men than women but more severe. Trends Urol Men's Health. 2022;13(5):11-4.
5. Rider V, Abdou NI, Kimler BF, Lu N, Brown S, Fridley BL. Gender bias in human systemic lupus erythematosus: a problem of steroid receptor action?. Front Immunol. 2018; 9:611.
6. Hsu CY, Chiu WC, Yang TS, Chen CJ, Chen YC, Lai HM, et al. Age-and gender-related long-term renal outcome in patients with lupus nephritis. Lupus. 2011;20(11):1135-41.
7. Schwartzman-Morris J, Putterman C. Gender differences in the pathogenesis and outcome of lupus and of lupus nephritis. Clin Dev Immunol. 2012;2012:604892.
8. Maroz N, Segal MS. Lupus nephritis and end-stage kidney disease. Am J Med Sci. 2013;346(4):319-23.
9. Yap DY, Chan TM. Lupus nephritis in Asia: clinical features and management. Kidney Dis. 2015;1(2):100-9.
10. Imbasciati E, Tincani A, Gregorini G, Doria A, Moroni G, Cabiddu G, et al. Pregnancy in women with pre-existing lupus nephritis: predictors of fetal and maternal outcome. Nephrol Dial Transplant. 2009;24(2): 519-25.
11. Stamm B, Barbhaiya M, Siegel C, Lieber S, Lockshin M, Sammaritano L. Infertility in systemic lupus erythematosus: what rheumatologists need to know in a new age of assisted reproductive technology. Lupus Sci Med. 2022;9(1):e000840.
12. Oktem O, Yagmur H, Bengisu H, Urman B. Reproductive aspects of systemic lupus erythematosus. J Reprod Immunol. 2016;117: 57-65.
13. Angley M, Spencer JB, Lim SS, Howards PP. Anti-Müllerian hormone in African-American women with systemic lupus erythematosus. Lupus Sci Med. 2020;7(1):e000439.
14. Dao KH, Bermas BL. Systemic lupus erythematosus management in pregnancy. Int J Womens Health. 2022;14:199-211.
15. Bermas BL, Sammaritano LR. Fertility and pregnancy in systemic lupus erythematosus. Systemic Lupus Erythematosus. Philadelphia: Elsevier; 2021. pp. 497-505.
16. Giambalvo S, Garaffoni C, Silvagni E, Furini F, Rizzo R, Govoni M, et al. Factors associated with fertility abnormalities in women with systemic lupus erythematosus: a systematic review and meta-analysis. Autoimmun Rev. 2022;21(4):103038.
17. Slater CA, Liang MH, McCune JW, Christman GM, Laufer MR. Preserving ovarian function in patients receiving cyclophosphamide. Lupus. 1999;8(1):3-10.
18. Dooley MA, Nair R. Therapy Insight: preserving fertility in cyclophosphamide-treated patients with rheumatic disease. Nat Clin Pract Rheumatol. 2008;4(5):250-7.
19. Wu J, Ma J, Zhang WH, Di W. Management and outcomes of pregnancy with or without lupus nephritis: a systematic review and meta-analysis. Ther Clin Risk Manag. 2018;14:885-901.
20. Parikh SV, Almaani S, Brodsky S, Rovin BH. Update on lupus nephritis: core curriculum 2020. Am J Kidney Dis. 2020;76(2):265-81.
21. Ceccarelli F, Perricone C, Massaro L, Cipriano E, Alessandri C, Spinelli FR, et al. Assessment of disease activity in Systemic Lupus Erythematosus: Lights and shadows. Autoimmun Rev. 2015;14(7):601-8.
22. Wilhelmus S, Bajema IM, Bertsias GK, Boumpas DT, Gordon C, Lightstone L, et al. Lupus nephritis management guidelines compared. Nephrol Dial Transplant. 2016; 31(6):904-13.
23. Buyon JP, Kim MY, Guerra MM, Lu S, Reeves E, Petri M, et al. Kidney outcomes and risk factors for nephritis (flare/de novo) in a multiethnic cohort of pregnant patients with lupus. Clin J Am Soc Nephrol. 2017;12(6): 940.

24. Piccoli GB, Fassio F, Attini R, Parisi S, Biolcati M, Ferraresi M, et al. Pregnancy in CKD: whom should we follow and why?. Nephrol Dial Transplant. 2012;27(suppl_3):iii111-8.
25. Lateef A, Petri M. Managing lupus patients during pregnancy. Best Pract Res Clin Rheumatol. 2013;27(3):435-47.
26. Smyth A, Oliveira GH, Lahr BD, Bailey KR, Norby SM, Garovic VD. A systematic review and meta-analysis of pregnancy outcomes in patients with systemic lupus erythematosus and lupus nephritis. Clin J Am Soc Nephrol. 2010;5(11):2060.
27. Gladman DD, Tandon A, Ibañez D, Urowitz MB. The effect of lupus nephritis on pregnancy outcome and fetal and maternal complications. J Rheumatol. 2010;37(4): 754-8.
28. Hahn BH, Mcmahon MA, Wilkinson A, Wallace WD, Daikh DI, Fitzgerald JD, et al. American College of Rheumatology guidelines for screening, treatment, and management of lupus nephritis. Arthritis Care Res. 2012;64(6):797-808.
29. Buawangpong N, Teekachunhatean S, Koonrungsesomboon N. Adverse pregnancy outcomes associated with first-trimester exposure to angiotensin-converting enzyme inhibitors or angiotensin II receptor blockers: A systematic review and meta-analysis. Pharmacol Res Perspect. 2020;8(5):e00644.
30. Stanhope TJ, White WM, Moder KG, Smyth A, Garovic VD. Obstetric nephrology: lupus and lupus nephritis in pregnancy. Clin J Am Soc Nephrol. 2012;7(12):2089-99.
31. De Jesus GR, De Jesús NR, Levy RA, Klumb EM. The use of angiogenic and antiangiogenic factors in the differential diagnosis of pre-eclampsia, antiphospholipid syndrome nephropathy and lupus nephritis. Lupus. 2014;23(12):1299-301.
32. MacDonald TM, Walker SP, Hannan NJ, Tong S, Tu'uhevaha J. Clinical tools and biomarkers to predict preeclampsia. EBioMedicine. 2022;75:103780.
33. Mecacci F, Simeone S, Cirami CL, Cozzolino M, Serena C, Rambaldi MP, et al. Preeclampsia in pregnancies complicated by systemic lupus erythematosus (SLE) nephritis: prophylactic treatment with multidisciplinary approach are important keys to prevent adverse obstetric outcomes. J Matern Fetal Neonatal Med. 2019;32(8):1292-8.
34. Chen TK, Gelber AC, Witter FR, Petri M, Fine DM. Renal biopsy in the management of lupus nephritis during pregnancy. Lupus. 2015;24(2):147-54.
35. Moroni G, Calatroni M, Donato B, Ponticelli C. Kidney Biopsy in Pregnant Women with Glomerular Diseases: Focus on Lupus Nephritis. J Clin Med. 2023;12(5):1834.
36. Asamiya Y, Otsubo S, Matsuda Y, Kimata N, Kikuchi KA, Miwa N, et al. The importance of low blood urea nitrogen levels in pregnant patients undergoing hemodialysis to optimize birth weight and gestational age. Kidney Int. 2009;75(11):1217-22.
37. Oliverio AL, Hladunewich MA. End-stage kidney disease and dialysis in pregnancy. Adv Chronic Kidney Dis. 2020;27(6):477-85.

CHAPTER

12 Kidney Biopsy in Pregnancy

Sabina Yusuf, Suceena Alexander

HIGHLIGHTS

- Initial reports of renal biopsy in pregnancy described a high complication rate but subsequent reports indicate low complication rates varying from 2 to 4% in some studies similar to nonpregnant subjects.
- Consequences to the mother and fetus of post biopsy hemorrhage, if it was to occur, could be serious.
- Risks of renal biopsy are partly counterbalanced by a high probability of therapeutic interventions as seen in various studies.
- While considering a patient for biopsy, the risks must be carefully balanced with the benefits of identifying the pathological diagnosis.
- A biopsy can be safely performed in patients with adequate BP control and normal coagulation parameters in the first and early second trimesters. After 30 weeks of gestation, the risks of biopsy often outweigh the benefits of establishing a diagnosis and are typically not advisable.

INTRODUCTION

Since its introduction in the 1950s, closed renal biopsy has revolutionized our understanding of pathology in kidney diseases and has become an indispensable tool for management of patients. It provides specific diagnostic and prognostic information and facilitates informed management decisions. An early prospective study on the impact of renal biopsy in clinical management showed that the pathological diagnosis provided by renal biopsy resulted in altered patient management in 50–80% of cases.[1] Nevertheless, the use of renal biopsy during pregnancy continues to be a subject of debate and generates concern for nephrologists. This chapter intends to examine the advantages and disadvantages of kidney biopsy during pregnancy, employing a literature review to provide guidance to physicians on the most effective utilization of this crucial diagnostic procedure.

RISKS OF RENAL BIOPSY IN PREGNANCY

Possible factors that may contribute to complications during biopsy procedures in pregnant women include a physiologically increased blood flow to the kidneys and the presence of an enlarged gravid uterus, which can make it challenging to perform the biopsy in the typical prone position. Additionally, using alternative positions such as lying on the side or sitting can further complicate the procedure.[2,3]

Expectant mothers undergoing kidney biopsy may face an increased likelihood of experiencing maternal or fetal complications due to the procedure. Additionally, there is an added concern regarding potential harm to the developing fetus. In the event of substantial bleeding resulting from the biopsy, there is a risk of compromising blood supply to the placenta and safeguarding the fetus from radiation exposure during angiography may prove challenging.

A BRIEF REVIEW OF THE LITERATURE

In 1944, Nils Alwall of Lund, Sweden, pioneered the clinical application of renal needle biopsy for diagnosing patients. Alwall initially achieved success in obtaining renal tissue through an aspiration technique in his first 13 patients. However, when one of the patients succumbed to complications, he discontinued the method and refrained from publishing his findings until 1952. Subsequent to Alwall's efforts, Paul Iversen and Claus Brun from Copenhagen published their initial series of renal biopsies in 1951, and Robert Kark from Chicago also contributed to advancing the technique.[4,5] 4 years later, Dieckmann reported for the first time the use of percutaneous renal biopsy in pregnant patients. Dieckmann, Potter, and McCartney[6] published, in 1957, the first important analysis of this technique in patients with toxemia of pregnancy. The diagnostic criteria for renal biopsies during pregnancy mirrored those for the nonpregnant population. However, the main objective was to distinguish between different causes of hypertension in the latter stages of pregnancy. During this period, there was a belief that identifying the distinct pathological lesions associated with preeclampsia would warrant the termination of pregnancy. Simultaneously, the observation of other lesions might prompt specific therapeutic interventions, potentially enabling the continuation of pregnancy to a stage where fetal survival could be enhanced. While multiple papers were published on the complications of renal biopsy in pregnancy, one of the most widely referenced papers is by Schewitz et al.[7] who described the bleeding complications to be significantly high, gross hematuria in 16.7%, perirenal hematoma in 4.4%, and maternal fatality in one patient. Further subsequent evaluation of this review and other shreds of evidence highlighting the complications of biopsy in pregnancy recognized several concerns about interpreting the results of these studies which included biopsies done in the upright position, via transperitoneal route or while patients were still hypertensive and prior bleeding tendencies related to preeclampsia. Indeed, it was realized that complications may be considerably less proven in further studies. **Table 1** lists the major studies done on this subject over the years.

In a retrospective study by Chen et al., conducted between 1990 and 1999, renal biopsies performed on pregnant patients were examined. All participants underwent renal biopsy before reaching 30 weeks of gestation, with indications including renal dysfunction of unknown origin or symptomatic nephrotic syndrome. Except for one patient who encountered gross hematuria, there were no significant complications noted.[8] Another study by Kuller et al. reviewed the clinical progress of 18 patients who underwent renal biopsy during pregnancy.[9] Seven renal hematomas were identified post biopsy, leading to two patients requiring blood transfusions. Despite four intrauterine fetal deaths in the series, it was presumed that none resulted from the biopsy procedure. The authors concluded that renal biopsy during pregnancy should be regarded

TABLE 1: Studies analyzing the safety and effectiveness of renal biopsy in pregnancy.

Authors	***Period***	***Biopsies***	***Complications***	***Effect on management***
Packham et al.[21]	1965–1985	111 biopsies antepartum	Complication rate 4.5% (1 perirenal hematoma, 1 macroscopic hematuria, 3 loin pain, and 3 insufficient tissue)	Definitive histological diagnosis in majority
Kuller et al.[9]	1989–2000	18 biopsies, 15 antepartum, 3 postpartum	7 hematomas, 2 requiring transfusion, 4 IUDs (none related to biopsy)	10 received a histological diagnosis that allowed pregnancy to be prolonged
Chen et al.[8]	1990–1999	15 biopsies antepartum before 30 weeks excluding patients with toxemia	• No major complications • Microscopic hematuria in all • Gross hematuria in 1	• Histopathological diagnosis in 100% • 11/15 received steroid therapy after biopsy
Day et al.[12]	1983–2004	20 biopsies antepartum (median gestational age 20 weeks), 75 biopsies postpartum	No major complications 1/20 hematuria	• 9/20 immediate change in therapy after biopsy • Glomerular disease diagnosed in 65% postpartum
Chen et al.[16]	2001–2012	11 pregnant women with SLE (median gestational age 16 weeks)	No complications	10/11 change in management after biopsy
Castro et al.[11]	2016	19 biopsies, 8 antepartum (mean gestational age 21 weeks), 4 postpartum	• No major complications • 2/8 minor complication (hematoma in 1, hematuria in 1)	Change in management in 6/8 (75%) after biopsy

(IUD: intrauterine device; SLE: systemic lupus erythematosus) as a potentially morbid procedure and recommended consideration only when it presents an opportunity for diagnosis beyond severe preeclampsia in patients distant from term.

In one of the largest systematic reviews of studies on renal biopsies during pregnancy, major complications were documented in 2% of cases.[10] These complications encompassed significant bleeding leading to large perirenal hematomas necessitating blood transfusion, as well as incidents of placental abruption, preterm delivery, and fetal death. Apart from microhematuria, an additional 5% of cases had minor complications, such as smaller hematomas not requiring transfusion and macrohematuria lasting several hours accompanied by intense loin pain. Adverse events related to biopsies were categorized based on the pregnancy stage at which they occurred: "early" pregnancy (0–21 weeks), the "gray phase" (23–28 weeks), and "late" pregnancy (28 weeks to term). The "gray phase," specifically the period between 23 and 26 weeks of gestation, was notable for recording all severe biopsy-related complications.

IMPACT ON MANAGEMENT OF KIDNEY DISEASE IN PREGNANCY

While considering the risks of renal biopsy in pregnancy, it will be worthwhile to review the benefits of this controversial procedure. There are only few papers examining the influence on the therapy of kidney disease made by performing a renal biopsy in pregnancy. In the review by Piccoli et al.[10] therapy was initiated or modified as a result of biopsy findings in 66% cases. Iris De Castro et al.[11] conducted a retrospective study to investigate the outcome of nephrotic syndrome in pregnancy and identified that renal biopsy changed the management in 6 out of the 8 individuals who underwent biopsy in pregnancy. Day et al.[12] published the presentation and outcomes of 20 pregnant women who developed renal disease and underwent a renal biopsy within 20 weeks of pregnancy. Among these, 19 patients were diagnosed with glomerular disease, and in 9 cases, there was an immediate alteration in therapy, primarily involving the initiation or escalation of immunosuppressive medication, based on the insights derived from renal histology. In a series by Chen et al.,[8] focusing on pregnant women with undetermined renal disease, a conclusive diagnosis was achieved in 100% of cases after biopsy, underscoring the high diagnostic value of renal biopsy performed during pregnancy.

Hence, when contemplating renal biopsy in a pregnant patient, it is crucial to address two key questions: (1) Is it safe to perform renal biopsy, taking into account the individual patient's clinical status, gestational age, and the likelihood of harm from the procedure relative to the benefits of obtaining a definitive diagnosis? (2) Will the information gleaned from renal biopsy influence the management of the mother or the course of the pregnancy?

WHEN TO CONSIDER RENAL BIOPSY IN PREGNANCY

In light of the above knowledge, renal biopsy may be considered in selected women before 28 weeks of gestation (preferably before 23 weeks). This should be done if the urine is sterile, the kidneys are of normal size, blood pressure is well controlled, and there is no evidence of coagulopathy or thrombocytopenia before the biopsy. The primary manifestations should be such that the information obtained from the renal biopsy is expected to result in a prompt therapeutic action that will allow the pregnancy to advance with fetal viability.

During the initial 3 months of pregnancy, a renal biopsy may be suggested if there is evidence of active sediments in the urine, nephrotic syndrome, unexplained kidney dysfunction, or renal dysfunction in the setting of a systemic disease or positive autoimmune serology. An early diagnosis will provide guidance for therapy and enable the assessment of the potential risks and advantages associated with continuing the pregnancy. During the second trimester, it is advisable to first eliminate the possibility of preeclampsia and a physiological proteinuria. A renal biopsy is usually suggested for individuals who have unexplained nephrotic range proteinuria, a progressive decline in glomerular filtration rate (GFR) that remains unexplained, kidney dysfunction in the presence of an active systemic disease, or instances in which pursuing a treatment without a clear diagnosis is not suitable or the patient fails to respond to empirical treatment. If these criteria are not met, renal biopsy may be done after pregnancy if indications remain. Beyond 28 weeks, the increased risks of kidney biopsy are likely to outweigh the benefits of continuing the pregnancy before proceeding to a low-risk renal biopsy in the postpartum period.

Renal biopsy should be avoided in the presence of untreated urinary tract infection (UTI) or asymptomatic bacteriuria, uncontrolled blood pressure, or uncorrected coagulopathy. In circumstances where a biopsy is not expected to alter the course of treatment or if the patient has shown improvement with initial medication, it may be suitable to delay the kidney biopsy until after pregnancy, provided that the indications for the biopsy persist.

A WORD ON LUPUS NEPHRITIS

During pregnancy, nephrologists frequently encounter two challenging questions in managing patients with systemic lupus erythematosus (SLE): (1) Does the presence of increasing proteinuria and hypertension indicate a lupus flare? (2) Does the presence of increasing proteinuria and hypertension suggest preeclampsia? This distinction is crucial because lupus nephritis typically requires immunosuppression, while severe and superimposed preeclampsia often necessitates delivery, even if it is far from the term. In the early stages of pregnancy, these symptoms typically indicate a lupus flare; however, beyond 24–26 weeks, distinguishing between flare and preeclampsia becomes diagnostically and therapeutically challenging.

While falling complement levels and rising dsDNA levels may point toward a lupus flare, they may not always provide a definitive diagnosis. Renal biopsy should be considered in the management of SLE during pregnancy if laboratory evaluations are inconclusive, if proteinuria is significant and associated with a rise in creatinine suggesting a possible class change, and if it is likely to lead to a modification in immunosuppressive treatment.[13] In the first and second trimesters of pregnancy in SLE patients, renal biopsy can facilitate the initiation of disease-specific treatment, allowing for targeted therapy rather than empirical treatment. Postpartum, immunosuppressive agents contraindicated during pregnancy can be introduced. Empirical treatment may be considered in specific clinical circumstances, such as patients presenting with active urine sediment, proteinuria, and serological abnormalities, either with a confirmed diagnosis of lupus nephritis based on a previous kidney biopsy or for those who decline the procedure.[14]

Use of anticoagulation in the presence of heavy proteinuria or APLA-positive cases with risk of venous thromboembolism remain controversial areas for empirical treatment and would benefit a personalized approach.

Currently, there is a limited amount of data available about the use of renal biopsy in pregnant women with SLE. In an initial investigation on the assessment of lupus nephritis during pregnancy, renal biopsies were conducted on three women with SLE while they were pregnant.[15] Additionally, the fourth biopsy was done in the postpartum period. The findings from these biopsies were deemed highly valuable in providing guidance to these patients and suggesting appropriate treatment approaches. In another study, Chen et al. found proliferative lupus nephritis in 91% of 11 pregnant women with SLE who underwent a renal biopsy to assess a suspected flare of lupus nephritis. Specifically, they observed five cases with ISN/RPS Class III and five cases with ISN/RPS Class IV. Except for one person, everyone had a management modification based on insights obtained from a kidney biopsy. There were no observable complications resulting from the biopsy for either the mother or the fetus. These case series highlight the importance of renal biopsy in helping guide the management of lupus nephritis in pregnancy.

EVADING THE RISK

Conducting a renal biopsy in individuals with urinary abnormalities or changes in renal function before contemplating pregnancy can be advantageous for diagnosing and determining the appropriate treatment strategy. Selecting an optimal timing for conception during a period of stable remission in the underlying condition can reduce the likelihood of pregnancy-related complications and obviate the need for a biopsy during gestation.

Ongoing research in the use of biomarkers for diagnosing and monitoring various glomerular diseases holds significant promise. This potential benefit is particularly noteworthy in a patient population facing the complexity of clinical diagnoses and the limitations of kidney biopsy under certain circumstances. Whenever possible, integrating biomarkers into diagnostic assessments may bring clarity to complex diagnostic scenarios arising in the context of kidney disease during pregnancy.[17-19] Actively exploring novel biomarkers with high diagnostic accuracy in the pregnant chronic kidney disease population should be a focal point of research and has the potential to alter the indications for renal biopsy in pregnancy in the future.

POSTPARTUM RENAL BIOPSY

In instances where concerns about bleeding complications or contraindications deter women from undergoing a kidney biopsy during pregnancy, and if persistent symptoms persist postpartum, a kidney biopsy should be considered. It is advisable to wait approximately 4–6 weeks for the complete resolution of clinical and histological features of preeclampsia before evaluating the necessity of a kidney biopsy for diagnosing primary glomerular disease.[20] However, the most appropriate timing should be determined by the clinical condition; if there is suspicion of rapidly progressive glomerular disease, an urgent biopsy should be pursued.

The decision to perform a renal biopsy during pregnancy necessitates careful consideration of the risks and benefits for both the mother and the fetus. While severe bleeding complications are rare, their potential impact on the mother and fetus can be severe. Nonetheless, in cases where a precise diagnosis is crucial and less invasive diagnostic tests have proven inconclusive, a renal biopsy proves highly beneficial for promptly obtaining a diagnosis and determining the appropriate course of action.

The summary of the chapter is provided in **Figure 1**.

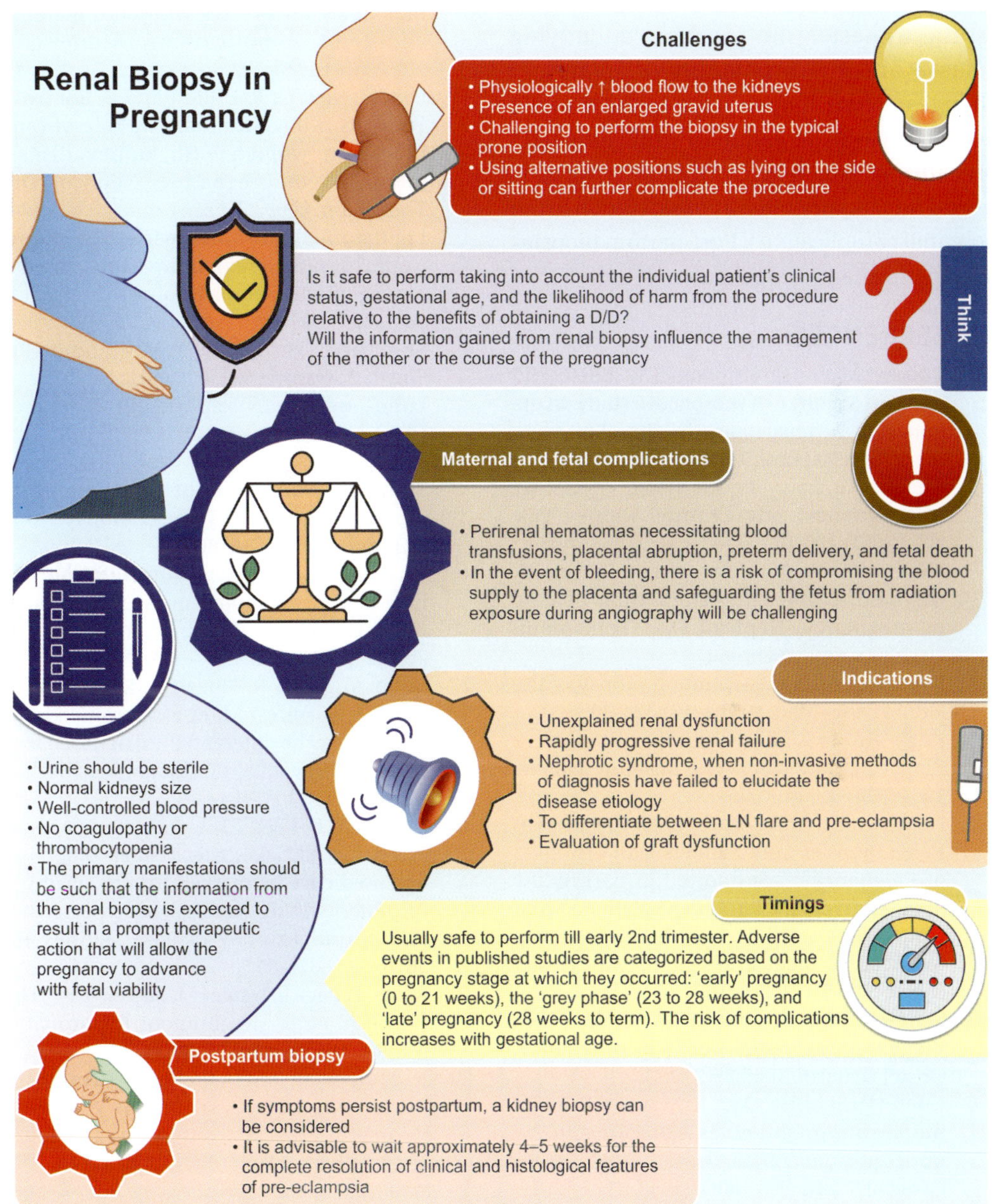

Fig. 1: Pictogram of renal biopsy in pregnancy. (D/D: differential diagnoses; LN: lupus nephritis)
Courtesy: Priti Meena

CONCLUSION

In conclusion, kidney biopsy to be performed before conception if pregnancy is planned in kidney disease patients. If kidney diseases are discovered or aggravate during pregnancy, the risks and benefits to be considered based on the trimester, the probable underlying disease and the probability of treatment changes. Renal biopsies are relatively safe before 23 weeks of gestation when adequate precautions are taken. Anytime after this period, will require careful consideration to the potential complications. Post-partum biopsies to be performed 4-6 weeks after delivery.

REFERENCES

1. Turner MW, Hutchinson TA, Barré PE, Prichard S, Jothy S. A prospective study on the impact of the renal biopsy in clinical management. Clin Nephrol. 1986;26(5):217-21.
2. Cheung KL, Lafayette RA. Renal Physiology of Pregnancy. Adv Chronic Kidney Dis. 2013;20(3):209-14.
3. Hladunewich MA, Bramham K, Jim B, Maynard S. Managing glomerular disease in pregnancy. Nephrol Dial Transplant. 2017;32(suppl_1):i48-i56.
4. Iversen P, Brun C. Aspiration biopsy of the kidney. Am J Med. 1951;11(3):324-30.
5. Kark Robert M, Muehrcke Robert C. Biopsy of kidney in prone position. Lancet. 1954;263(6821):1047-9.
6. Dieckmann WMJ, Potter EL, McCartney CP. Renal Biopsies from Patients with "Toxemia of Pregnancy"**. Supported in part by the 50th Anniversary Fund for Eclampsia and United States Public Health Service grant No. 3166 for medical research. Am J Obstet Gynecol. 1957;73(1):1-16.
7. Schewitz LJ, Friedman IA, Pollak VE. Bleeding after renal biopsy in pregnancy. Obstet Gynecol. 1965;26(3):295.
8. Chen HH, Lin HC, Yeh JC, Chen CP. Renal biopsy in pregnancies complicated by undetermined renal disease. Acta Obstet Gynecol Scand. 2001;80(10):888-93.
9. Kuller JA, D'Andrea NM, McMahon MJ. Renal biopsy and pregnancy. Am J Obstet Gynecol. 2001;184(6):1093-6.
10. Piccoli GB, Daidola G, Attini R, Parisi S, Fassio F, Naretto C, et al. Kidney biopsy in pregnancy: evidence for counselling? A systematic narrative review. BJOG Int J Obstet Gynaecol. 2013;120(4):412-27.
11. De Castro I, Easterling TR, Bansal N, Jefferson JA. Nephrotic syndrome in pregnancy poses risks with both maternal and fetal complications. Kidney Int. 2017;91(6):1464-72.
12. Day C, Hewins P, Hildebrand S, Sheikh L, Taylor G, Kilby M, et al. The role of renal biopsy in women with kidney disease identified in pregnancy. Nephrol Dial Transplant. 2008;23(1):201-6.
13. Lightstone L, Hladunewich MA. Lupus Nephritis and Pregnancy: Concerns and Management. Semin Nephrol. 2017;37(4):347-53.
14. Stanhope TJ, White WM, Moder KG, Smyth A, Garovic VD. Obstetric Nephrology: Lupus and Lupus Nephritis in Pregnancy. Clin J Am Soc Nephrol. 2012;7(12):2089.
15. Krane NK, Thakur V, Wood H, Meleg-Smith S. Evaluation of lupus nephritis during pregnancy by renal biopsy. Am J Nephrol. 1995;15(3):186-91.
16. Chen TK, Gelber AC, Witter FR, Petri M, Fine DM. Renal biopsy in the management of lupus nephritis during pregnancy. Lupus. 2015;24(2):147-54.
17. Rolfo A, Attini R, Nuzzo AM, Piazzese A, Parisi S, Ferraresi M, et al. Chronic kidney disease may be differentially diagnosed from preeclampsia by serum biomarkers. Kidney Int. 2013;83(1):177-81.
18. Bramham K, Seed PT, Lightstone L, Nelson-Piercy C, Gill C, Webster P, et al. Diagnostic and predictive biomarkers for pre-eclampsia in patients with established hypertension and chronic kidney disease. Kidney Int. 2016;89(4):874-85.
19. Ronco P, Beck L, Debiec H, Fervenza FC, Hou FF, Jha V, et al. Membranous nephropathy. Nat Rev Dis Primers. 2021;7(1):69.
20. Hladunewich MA, Myers BD, Derby GC, Blouch KL, Druzin ML, Deen WM, et al. Course of preeclamptic glomerular injury after delivery. Am J Physiol Renal Physiol. 2008;294(3):F614-620.
21. Packham D, Fairley KF. Renal biopsy: indications and complications in pregnancy. BJOG Int J Obstet Gynaecol. 1987;94(10):935-9.

CHAPTER

13

Diabetic Kidney Disease in Pregnancy

Sreejith Parameswaran, Jayasurya R

HIGHLIGHTS

- All women with diabetic nephropathy should be offered prepregnancy counseling to:
  - Inform them of potential adverse outcomes
  - Enable optimization of glycemic and hypertension control
  - Improve pregnancy outcomes
- Metformin and sulfonylureas are mostly considered safe during pregnancy, but oral hypoglycemic agents are less effective than insulin for achieving adequate glycemic control.
- Diabetic nephropathy is linked to higher rates of preeclampsia and other maternal complication.
- Women with diabetic nephropathy have high rates of neonatal complications, including perinatal mortality.
- Women with diabetic nephropathy may be more susceptible to pregnancy-related acceleration of the disease.

INTRODUCTION

The worldwide prevalence of diabetes mellitus (DM) has steadily increased over the past three decades, and India is a significant contributor to this burden. Chronic kidney disease (CKD) prevalence worldwide has increased by about 30% in 30 years. Diabetic nephropathy (DN) is the most common cause, accounting for 31% of CKD in India. With the age of onset of diabetes being lower in India compared to elsewhere, with at least 50% of people with diabetes developing it below 40 years of age, the number of women of reproductive age with DM is also increasing. The incidence of gestational diabetes is also increasing. Diabetes, with or without diabetic kidney disease (DKD), is associated with multiple adverse maternal and fetal outcomes. Those with overt DKD have the worst outcomes with high risks of preterm delivery, small for gestational age infants, and preeclampsia. Also, pregnancy in women with overt DN can lead to worsening of kidney function.[1-3]

In this chapter, we discuss the effects of diabetes and DKD on pregnancy and the effects of pregnancy on the progression of DKD.

Physiologic Changes in Kidney During Pregnancy

In the first 20 weeks of pregnancy, the glomerular filtration rate (GFR) increases by approximately 50%, there is an increase in renal plasma flow of up to 80%. GFR, renal plasma flow, and renal volume decrease toward nonpregnant levels by the third trimester of pregnancy. Hemodynamic changes in normal pregnancy include increased blood volume, decreased vascular resistance, and increased cardiac output. There is a decrease in blood pressure (BP), reaching nadir by 20 weeks of gestation. In normal pregnancy, proteinuria can occur mainly after 20 weeks of gestation and up to 300 mg/day of protein excretion is considered normal.[4,5]

EFFECTS OF DIABETES AND KIDNEY DISEASE ON PREGNANCY

Effects of Diabetes without Overt Nephropathy on Pregnancy: Maternal and Fetal Impacts

Women with diabetes who are normoalbuminuric have a considerable increase (threefold to fourfold) in albuminuria after 20 weeks of gestation compared to women without diabetes. Usually, proteinuria reverses in these women after pregnancy. In women with moderately increased albuminuria (microalbuminuria), the increase in protein excretion is even more exaggerated. 20–30% of these women may develop nephrotic range proteinuria.

The most common maternal complications in type 1 DM and type 2 DM are preeclampsia, preterm delivery, and the need for cesarean section. The most common causes of obstetric interventions and preterm delivery are macrosomia, fetal distress, and preeclampsia. Fetal survival rates in pregnancies of women with diabetes and DKD have improved to >95%. Babies born to diabetic mothers have a higher prevalence of congenital malformations, fetal macrosomia (birthweight >4,000 g), being large for gestational age (>90th percentile of birth weight), stillbirth, and infant death. Major congenital malformations are two to three times more common in babies born of diabetic mothers compared to nondiabetic mothers. Cardiovascular anomalies, urogenital malformations, and neural tube defects are described. Higher incidence of birth injuries, including Erb's palsy and shoulder dystocia, is reported. The increased risk of stillbirth can be up to four times higher compared to nondiabetic pregnancies.[6]

Effects of Diabetic Nephropathy with Preserved Renal Function on Pregnancy

In women with overt DN, the physiologic increase in GFR often fails to occur. In women with DN with creatinine clearance above 70 mL/min, deterioration of kidney function is uncommon during pregnancy.[1] Proteinuria increases during the third trimester of pregnancy. The average increase in proteinuria can be as high as 3 grams between the first and third trimesters. Nephrotic range proteinuria can occur in >50% of cases. In the majority, proteinuria reverses to prepregnancy levels after delivery. Worsening of hypertension is another common complication in women with overt DN. Incidence of hypertension ranged between 11% in the first trimester and 83% at the time of delivery.[1,2]

Effects of Diabetic Nephropathy with Decreased Renal Function on Pregnancy

Worsening of proteinuria and development of nephrotic syndrome can occur similarly to those with preserved renal function and will usually reverse postpartum. However, pregnancy can worsen renal function in this group.

In a study by Purdy et al., 27% of 11 women had transient worsening of renal function, 27% had a stable renal function, and 45% had a permanent decline in renal function.

In a study of 49 nondiabetic women with CKD, prepregnancy GFR <40 mL/min and prepregnancy proteinuria >1 g/day were associated with more significant decline in GFR after delivery, shorter time to end-stage renal disease (ESRD), and low infant birth weight.[1,2]

EFFECTS OF PREGNANCY ON DIABETIC KIDNEY DISEASE

Pregnancy is expected to affect the progression of kidney disease because of the possible effects of hyperfiltration, hypertension, and preeclampsia. In patients with gestational diabetes, there is an increased prevalence of moderately increased albuminuria (microalbuminuria). Also, an increased risk of type-2 diabetes and hypertension is seen in women with a history of gestational DM. A systematic review of multiple small studies showed that despite a temporary decline in kidney function during pregnancy, the rate of progression of kidney disease is unaffected by gestation. DCCT (Diabetes Control and Complications Trial) study compared women with type 1 diabetes who became pregnant with those who never had a pregnancy and did not find an increased incidence of microalbuminuria or overt nephropathy. Multiple other small studies showed similar results.[2] But in the subgroup with GFR <40 mL/min/1.73 m^2 and proteinuria >1 g/day, an increased risk of disease progression during pregnancy is shown. One case-control study showed a high incidence of DN in women with a history of type-1 DM prepregnancy who developed preeclampsia on long-term follow-up.[1,2]

TREATMENT OF DIABETES IN PRESENCE OF DKD IN PREGNANCY

More significant blood glucose fluctuations, including lower fasting and higher postprandial levels, are seen during pregnancy. Rigid glycemic control is needed to reduce maternal and fetal complications. In type-1 diabetes, insulin requirement increases toward term; peak increases being at 9 and 37 weeks.[2] Insulin is the mainstay of treatment in both type-1 and type-2 DM, though oral hypoglycemics like metformin may be continued in women with pregestational type-2 DM and reasonable glycemic control. Both long- and short-acting insulin analogs are recommended to ensure optimum glycemic control. Self-monitoring of fasting and postprandial blood glucose levels is recommended. The recommended target range is fasting blood glucose 70–95 mg/dL and 1-hour postprandial glucose 110–140 mg/dL or 2-hour postprandial glucose 100–120 mg/dL, according to the American Diabetes Association (ADA) and the American College of Obstetricians and Gynecologists (ACOG). These targets should be relaxed if hypoglycemic events occur. HbA1C level is slightly lower in pregnancy due to increased red blood cell turnover. Ideally, the HbA1C target is <6%, but the target may be relaxed to <7% if needed to avoid hypoglycemia.[3,6-8]

PREECLAMPSIA IN DIABETES

Women with diabetes and DKD have a higher risk for the development of preeclampsia. Preeclampsia is a condition that involves the activation of the endothelium, thrombotic mechanisms, and the involvement of multiple organs, including the liver, brain, placenta, and kidney. Preeclampsia can be diagnosed without proteinuria in the presence of other clinical features of severity. The incidence of preeclampsia is 2–5% in unaffected women and 7–10% in gestational diabetes, which increases to 15–20% in diabetic women, with risk increasing with worsening nephropathy. In women with DN, the level of prepregnancy microalbuminuria is a strong predictor of preeclampsia. Preeclampsia is shown to be associated independently with HbA1C levels in pregnancy. Diagnosis of preeclampsia is often difficult in women with DKD because of the presence of hypertension and preexisting proteinuria. The development of preeclampsia often exacerbates preexisting proteinuria, and this should be considered when there is a sudden increase in proteinuria level. In women with proteinuric CKD, superimposed preeclampsia is diagnosed when there is new-onset hypertension (systolic BP >140 mm Hg and/or diastolic BP >90 mm Hg) or maternal organ dysfunction after 20 weeks of gestation. Angiogenic markers (placental growth factor ± soluble fms-like tyrosine kinase 1/sFlt-1) can be used as adjuncts in diagnosing superimposed preeclampsia. Low-dose aspirin (75–150 mg/day) is found to reduce the risk for severe, early onset preeclampsia, especially when started early, before 16 weeks of gestation. It is recommended to start aspirin therapy between 12 and 28 weeks of gestation. In women with DKD and low calcium intake, calcium supplementation is advised with at least 1 g/day of elemental calcium.[1,6,7]

MANAGEMENT OF HYPERTENSION DURING PREGNANCY

Hypertension in diabetic pregnant women increases risks for adverse maternal and fetal outcomes. Hence, optimum BP control is advised. ACOG recommends initiation or titration of antihypertensive therapy in BP >140/90 mm Hg in chronic hypertension. As recommended by ADA, target BP levels are 120–130/80–85 mm Hg. Angiotensin-converting enzyme (ACE) inhibitors and angiotensin receptor blockers (ARBs) are contraindicated in pregnancy because of their association with congenital malformations when given in the first trimester. Also, atenolol, mineralocorticoid receptor antagonists, and nitroprusside should be avoided during pregnancy. Antihypertensives which are safe in pregnancy include methyldopa, nifedipine, hydralazine, diltiazem, clonidine, and prazosin. First-line options are labetalol, nifedipine, and methyldopa. Diuretics should be used only in the presence of significant volume overload.[6,8]

PREGNANCY AFTER KIDNEY TRANSPLANT IN DIABETIC KIDNEY DISEASE

In patients with advanced CKD, it is beneficial to delay pregnancy until after kidney transplantation. In the general cohort, no increased 20-year mortality or 20-year decrease in graft function is demonstrated with pregnancy after kidney transplantation. Graft survival is likely to be the same in subgroups with diabetes, but cardiovascular and overall mortality are greater. Serum creatinine levels of >1.4 mg/dL and an increase in serum creatinine during pregnancy and preeclampsia are associated with a higher risk for postpartum graft dysfunction. Higher rates of preterm delivery, preeclampsia, and low birth weight are seen in pregnancy after renal transplantation. Age >35 years is associated with negative pregnancy outcome.[1] In the literature on pregnancy after a combined kidney-pancreas transplant, the outcome was slightly worse compared to pregnancy after kidney transplant alone, about infections during pregnancy and graft loss to be reframed. However, glycemic control is optimum after a pancreas transplant. The optimum time for pregnancy is 1 year after the kidney transplant, with stable dosage of immunosuppressives. Special attention is needed in the adjustment of immunosuppressive drug dosage to account for changes in clearance during pregnancy, management of nausea and vomiting, which may prevent absorption of drugs, management of infections, treatment of rejection, and control of hypertension.[1,2,7]

RENAL REPLACEMENT THERAPY IN PREGNANCY

Hemodialysis is the preferred mode of renal replacement therapy (RRT) in pregnancy. Hemodialysis should be started when maternal urea concentration is >17–20 mmol/L to reduce the risk of preterm delivery. Fluid balance, biochemical parameters, BP, and uremic symptoms should also be considered when initiating RRT. Improved pregnancy outcomes are noted with intensified dialysis regimes of >20 hours/week.[2,7]

FOLLOW-UP OF DIABETIC KIDNEY DISEASE PATIENTS AFTER PREGNANCY

Diligent care of women with DKD should continue in the postpartum period. Glycemic and BP control will need optimizing. ACE inhibitors can be restarted postpartum if necessary but are preferably done a few weeks after delivery. Drugs like labetalol, methyldopa, and nifedipine can be continued as required. Insulin resistance decreases after delivery. So, insulin requirement substantially decreases after delivery, and monitoring for hypoglycemia is needed. Statins should be withheld during lactation.[6]

PREPREGNANCY COUNSELING

Prepregnancy counseling is necessary for all women with type-1 and type-2 diabetes with or without DN who plan for pregnancy. Appropriate reproductive counseling helps to reduce the risks for congenital malformations, preterm delivery, perinatal complications, perinatal mortality, and small for gestational age birth weight. It is recommended to start reproductive counseling from the adolescent age for all with type-1 or type-2 diabetes. They should be informed about the association of poor glycemic control with poor maternal and fetal outcomes. Achieving glycemic control as close to normal, without hypoglycemia, is advised to reduce maternal and fetal complications risks, ideally with an HbA1C level of <6.5%. Optimization of nutrition and screening for diabetes complications is needed before conception. Women with impaired renal function should be informed about the risks of the progression of renal disease. Patients should be counseled regarding the risk for the development and progression of retinopathy. The dilated eye examination should be conducted before pregnancy or in the first trimester, followed up every trimester, up to 1-year postpartum. Review of the medication list and stopping potentially harmful drugs, including ACE inhibitors, ARBs, and statins, in the prepregnancy period is important.[3,6]

Figure 1 Summarizes the key points on how to manage diabetic kidney disease during pregnancy.

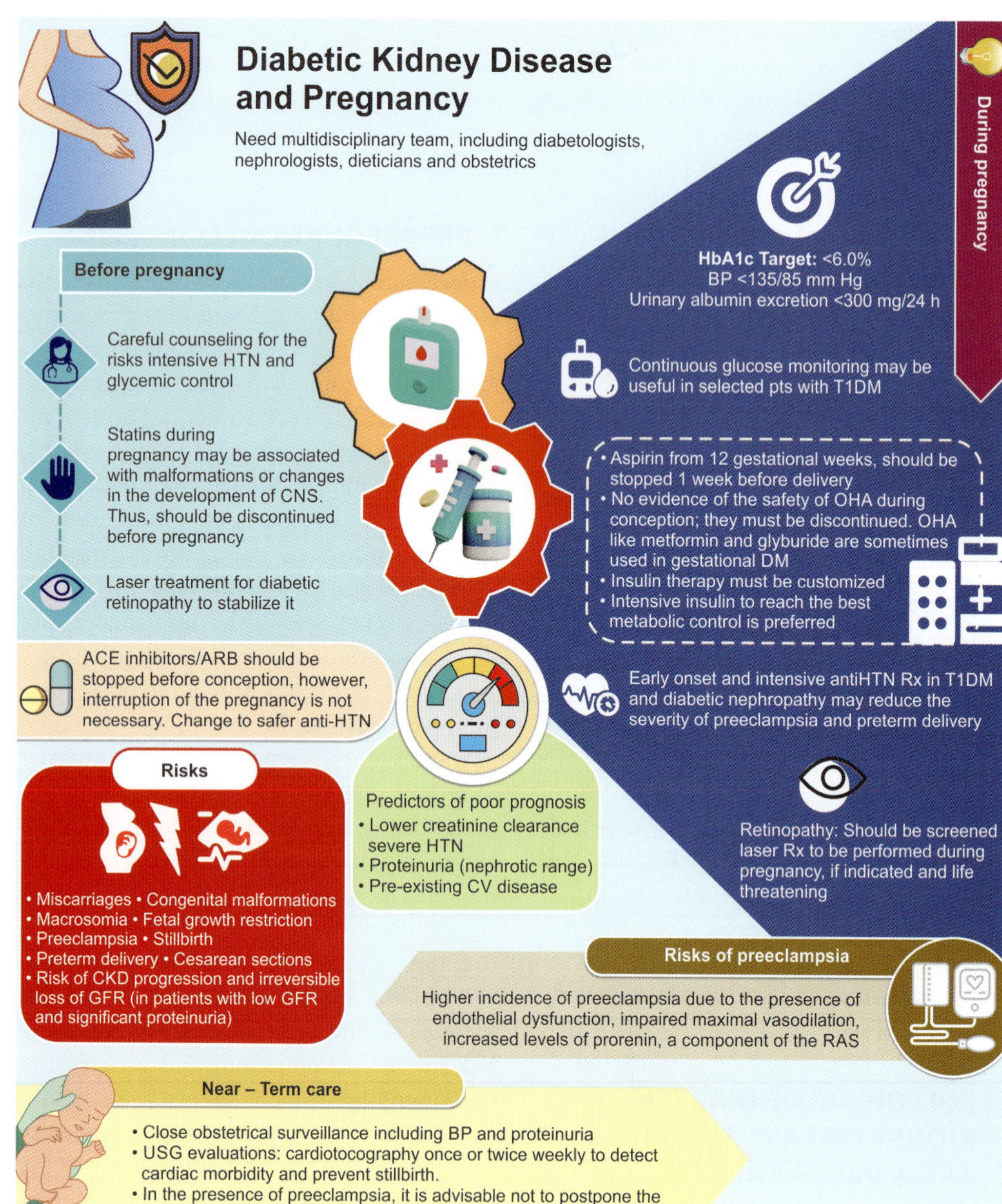

Fig. 1: Summarizes the key points on how to manage diabetic kidney disease during pregnancy. (CNS: central nervous system; CV: cardiovascular; HTN: hypertension; OHA: oral hypoglycemic drugs; RAS: renin angiotensinogen system; Rx: treatment; T1DM: type 1 diabetes)

Courtesy: Dr Priti Meena

CONCLUSION

Diabetes with or without DKD during pregnancy is associated with adverse maternal and fetal outcomes. Understanding possible complications and optimizing management, starting from the preconception period with adequate preparation of the individual for pregnancy and extending to the postpartum period, is essential for optimum outcomes.

REFERENCES

1. Powe CE, Thadhani R. Diabetes and the kidney in pregnancy. Semin Nephrol. 2011;31(1):59-69.
2. Bramham K, Rajasingham D. Pregnancy in diabetes and kidney disease. J Ren Care. 2012;38 (Suppl 1):78-89.
3. American Diabetes Association. 14. Management of Diabetes in Pregnancy: Standards of Medical Care in Diabetes—2021. Diabetes Care. 2021;44(Suppl 1): S200-10.
4. Gonzalez Suarez ML, Kattah A, Grande JP, Garovic V. Renal Disorders in Pregnancy: Core Curriculum 2019. Am J Kidney Dis. 2019;73(1):119-30.
5. Cheung KL, Lafayette RA. Renal physiology of pregnancy. Adv Chronic Kidney Dis. 2013;20(3):209-14.
6. Seshan SV, Reddi AS. Albuminuria and Proteinuria. In: Lerma EV, Batuman V (Eds).; Diabetes and Kidney Disease. Cham, Switzerland: Springer; 2022. pp. 243-62.
7. Wiles K, Chappell L, Clark K, Elman L, Hall M, Lightstone L, et al. Clinical practice guideline on pregnancy and renal disease. BMC Nephrol. 2019;20:401.
8. ElSayed NA, Aleppo G, Aroda VR, Bannuru RR, Brown FM, Bruemmer D, et al., on behalf of the American Diabetes Association. 15. Management of Diabetes in Pregnancy: Standards of Care in Diabetes— 2023. Diabetes Care. 2023;46(Suppl 1):S254-66.

CHAPTER 14

Contraception in Kidney Disease

Urmila Anandh, Anand Chellappan

HIGHLIGHTS

- Pregnancy in a patient with kidney disease is associated with adverse maternal and fetal prognosis.
- Pregnancy and contraception counseling should begin early to allow for optimization of the patient and prevent unintended pregnancies.
- The choice of contraception depends on individual patient preferences and the underlying comorbidities.
- Progestin-containing contraceptives appear to be safe and effective in patients with chronic kidney disease.
- Follow-up of patients initiated on contraception is vital.

INTRODUCTION

The State of World Population Report 2022 estimates that nearly 121 million unintended pregnancies occur every year of which more than 60% end in abortion, representing a global failure to uphold a basic human right.[1] In light of an increasing global prevalence of chronic kidney disease (CKD), it is not uncommon for every nephrologist, physician, or gynecologist to face the scenario of pregnancy in a patient with kidney disease. Pregnancy in a patient with kidney disease holds the potential for unfavorable medical ramifications including adverse maternal and fetal outcomes. The choice of motherhood is an inherent aspect of a woman's autonomy. However, prioritizing the right to motherhood over one's health and well-being warrants reconsideration and proper guidance. If such pregnancies occur without prior optimization, it could result in disastrous complications for the mother and the child. Hence, it requires adequate preparedness on the part of the medical community, meticulous management, and vigilant preventive efforts. A detailed understanding of the utility and application of contraceptive measures is therefore essential.

SEXUAL FUNCTION IN KIDNEY DISEASE

Chronic kidney disease is associated with decreased fertility in both males and females. Overall, it has been estimated that the pregnancy rate in patients on dialysis is 1% of that of the general population and that in kidney-transplanted women it is around 10%.[2] An impaired hypothalamic–pituitary–gonadal axis is believed to play a key role among others. The prevalence of infertility among patients with end-stage kidney disease

(ESKD) is around 92%. The loss of fertility is presumed to be progressive across the stages of CKD. In CKD, there is a loss of pulsatile release of gonadotropin hormone-releasing hormone (GnRH) from the hypothalamus, resulting in impaired luteinizing hormone (LH) and follicle stimulating hormone (FSH) cyclicity. This leads to lower estrogen levels which in turn results in the inhibition of the LH surge culminating in anovulation. Elevated prolactin levels also inhibit ovulation. It is believed to result from decreased renal clearance and decreased sensitivity to dopaminergic inhibition of prolactin secretion. Menstrual irregularities are common in women with CKD. These include amenorrhea, polymenorrhagia, and oligomenorrhea. CKD often results in functional menopause which may be reversed by kidney transplantation or increasing the frequency of hemodialysis. CKD patients have a lower level of the anti-Müllerian hormone, a marker of ovarian reserve. They have markedly high rates of sexual dysfunction resulting from a loss of libido, failure of vaginal lubrication, orgasmic impairment, and or vaginismus.

WHY IS CONTRACEPTION REQUIRED IN PATIENTS WITH KIDNEY DISEASE?

Providing counseling and prescribing appropriate contraception options to patients with kidney disease become imperative for the following reasons:

- Patients with kidney disease are often on medications that have teratogenic potential. Prenatal exposure to renin-angiotensin system inhibitors [angiotensin-converting enzyme (ACE) inhibitors (ACEi) and angiotensin receptor blockers (ARB)] could result in renal dysfunction, oligohydramnios, death, arterial hypotension, intrauterine growth retardation, respiratory distress syndrome, pulmonary hypoplasia, hypocalvaria, limb defects, persistent patent ductus arteriosus, or cerebral complications in the baby. The fetopathy caused by exposure to ACEi or ARBs could have long-term complications as well. Immunosuppressive agents are often used for the management of autoimmune disorders, glomerular disease, and postrenal transplant. Mycophenolate mofetil (MMF) could result in pregnancy loss and congenital malformations, including limb and organ abnormalities, cleft lip, and palate. Cyclophosphamide use during pregnancy is associated with pregnancy loss and congenital malformations. Rituximab is associated with neonatal B-cell depletion. Valganciclovir used for cytomegalovirus (CMV) prophylaxis in kidney transplant recipients is fetotoxic. Switching to an alternative medication and adequate optimization is often recommended before planning pregnancy in such patients. Effective contraceptive measures help in preventing unintended pregnancies and aid in the optimization of such patients who wish to conceive.
- Pregnancy in a patient with kidney disease is associated with adverse maternal and fetal outcomes (preeclampsia, fetal growth restriction, preterm delivery, fetal demise). The severity of renal disease, hypertension, and proteinuria are major determinants of the outcome. Pregnancy also portends a risk of flare of the underlying kidney disease like lupus nephritis. More than 40% of patients with moderate-to-severe kidney disease experience an irreversible decline in glomerular filtration rate (GFR) and around

10% experience an accelerated decline in renal function during pregnancy.[3]

- Although fertility rates are reduced in patients with CKD, pregnancy is possible in all stages including while on maintenance dialysis. There is also data to suggest that intensive hemodialysis including nocturnal hemodialysis could result in restoration of normal menstrual cycles and improved conception rates in dialysis patients. The infertility rates among CKD patients are difficult to ascertain due to poor CKD screening in the general population. Successful kidney transplantation restores fertility within few months. Hence, although it is acknowledged that patients with kidney disease may have low fertility rates, it should not dissuade the treating nephrologists/gynecologists from counseling regarding and advocating appropriate contraceptive measures.

WHEN AND HOW TO INITIATE DISCUSSION REGARDING CONTRACEPTION?

Discussion regarding pregnancy and conception could be initiated in the following situations:

- In general, pregnancy and contraception counseling should begin in the early stages of kidney disease. Patients with normotension and preserved or mildly deranged kidney function do well with >95% live births, of which 75% are of appropriate size for the gestational age. The prognosis is worse for patients with moderate (serum creatinine ≥1.4–2.8 mg/dL) to severe (serum creatinine ≥2.8 mg/dL) renal dysfunction. Proteinuria >1 g/day portends a poor prognosis. CKD affects 3–6% of women of childbearing age in high-income countries, and the prevalence is estimated to be 50% higher in low- and middle-income countries.[4] Regrettably, women are often hesitant to discuss pregnancy due to fears of judgment and concerns over prioritizing pregnancy over their health. It hence appears prudent to initiate the conversation at the earliest opportunity.
- Women on dialysis should be counseled regarding the high risk associated with pregnancy and should be advised to delay conception if transplantation is an option.
- Women with glomerular diseases not in remission should be counseled regarding the possibilities of worsening proteinuria and progression of the disease during pregnancy. Patients with lupus nephritis should be counseled to postpone pregnancy until the disease is quiescent for at least 6 months and the patient is switched to nonteratogenic medications.
- Kidney transplant recipients, patients with glomerular disease, and those on immunosuppression and teratogenic medications should be advised contraception until safe nonteratogenic medications are instituted. Patients with a kidney transplant are generally advised not to conceive for 1–2 years until the graft function is stable without any ongoing rejection or infection episodes.
- Contraception could be offered immediately after delivery or termination of pregnancy in a patient with kidney disease considering the high risk of subsequent pregnancies.

According to the United States Renal Data System (USRDS) data, pre-ESKD nephrology care is lacking. Around 30% of patients received no pre-ESKD nephrology care. Discussion regarding contraception is often inadequate since this is generally not a high priority for the treating nephrologist during a typical outpatient visit. In a national survey undertaken by Sachdeva et al., it was found that only 46% of the nephrologists or their staff counseled female dialysis patients regarding contraception.[5] In a cross-border survey of adult nephrologists by the women's health working group of Cure Glomerulonephropathy (CureGN), it was found that more than 65% of the respondents lacked confidence in managing women's health issues, including menstrual disorders, preconception counseling, pregnancy management, and menopause.[6] Only around 37.1% of respondents from the United States and 27.1% of respondents from Canada felt confident or very confident in counseling regarding contraception. The respondents felt that interdisciplinary guidelines established by obstetrics and nephrology, continuing education seminars or case-based discussions, and access to nephrologists with special interest or training in women's health would help improve their ability to counsel and manage women with CKD. Hence, there is a large unmet need to address this knowledge and practice gap concerning women's health.

ASSESSING ELIGIBILITY FOR CONTRACEPTION

At this point, there is a paucity of data to guide contraceptive methods in patients with kidney disease and should be based on the individual preference and the underlying comorbidities. The World Health Organization (WHO) has provided a Medical Eligibility Criterion (MEC) for contraception based on two complementary considerations: First, the effect the contraceptive method has on the disease, and second, the effect of the disease on the efficacy of the contraceptive method used. The safety of a particular contraceptive is classified into one of the four categories as mentioned in **Box 1**. The categorization would differ based on the contraceptive method and the underlying comorbidities. It is based on evidence from studies on a wide range of diseases including diabetes, systematic lupus erythematosus (SLE), and kidney transplantation. However, CKD is not one of them. This is also available as a digital tool/app which could be accessed by the patients from their mobile devices **(Fig. 1)**.

BOX 1: Medical eligibility criteria (MEC) for contraceptive use.

MEC categories for contraceptive eligibility

1. A condition for which there is no restriction for the use of the contraceptive method
2. A condition where the advantages of using the method generally outweigh the theoretical or proven risks
3. A condition where the theoretical or proven risks usually outweigh the advantages of using the method
4. A condition that represents an unacceptable health risk if the contraceptive method is used

Source: WHO 2015.

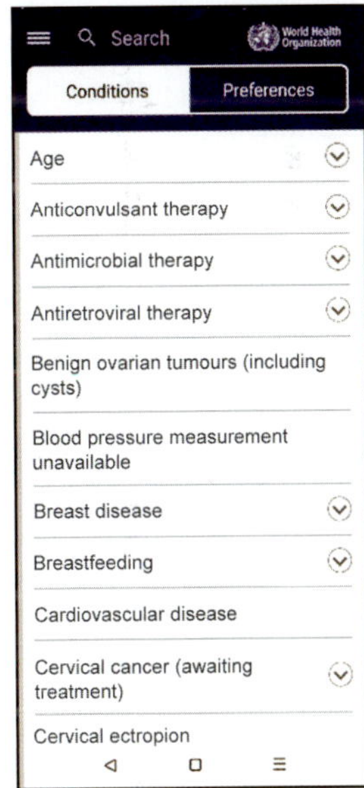

Fig. 1: WHO app to evaluate medical eligibility criteria for contraceptive use.

Guideline Recommendations

UK renal association clinical practice guideline on pregnancy and renal disease (2019)[12]

- We recommend advice on safe and effective contraception is offered to all women of reproductive age with CKD (1D)
- We recommend safe and effective contraception is offered to women of reproductive age who are taking teratogenic medication, have active glomerulonephritis, are within one year of renal transplantation or acute graft rejection, and for any woman who does not wish to conceive (1D)

CONTRACEPTIVE METHODS[7-9]

The contraceptive methods can be broadly classified into temporary and permanent methods as shown in **Box 2**.

BOX 2: Contraceptive methods.

Temporary

- *Barrier methods*:
  - Condoms—male and female
  - Diaphragm
  - Cervical caps
  - Vaginal sponges
- *Hormonal methods*:
  - Estrogen-containing hormonal contraception
    - Combined oral contraceptives
    - Combined transdermal patch
    - Combined vaginal ring
    - Combined injectable contraceptives
  - Progestin-containing hormonal contraception
    - Progestin-only contraceptives
    - Progestin-only subdermal implants
    - Injectable progestin-only contraceptive
- *Intrauterine devices (IUDs):*
  - Non-medicated IUDs
  - Medicated IUDs
- *Emergency contraception:*
  - Emergency contraceptive pill
  - Copper IUD

Permanent

- Vasectomy
- Tubectomy

Hormonal Methods

Hormonal methods are described in **Table 1**.

Combined Injectable Contraceptives

Combined injectable contraceptives are newly developed contraceptives that contain either 25 mg of depot medroxyprogesterone acetate and 5 mg of estradiol cypionate or 50 mg of norethisterone enanthate and 5 mg of estradiol valerate. They provide the ease of less frequent administration and are subject to fewer individual variations.

Guideline Recommendations

UK renal association clinical practice guideline on pregnancy and renal disease (2019)

- We recommend that the progesterone only-pill, a progesterone subdermal implant, and the progesterone intrauterine system are safe and effective for women with CKD (1C)

Combined Vaginal Ring

Content: Ethinyl estradiol (2.7 mg) and progestin (Etonogestrel 11.7 mg).

Mechanism of action: Inhibit the release of GnRH blocking ovulation, alter the endometrium, cause thickening of cervical mucus.

Advantages: Highly effective with a failure rate of 7% with typical use and 0.3% with perfect use.

Disadvantages: Vaginal irritation and discharge, Thrombotic and cardiovascular risk, worsens albuminuria, progestin-containing contraceptives increase the concentration of calcineurin inhibitors while CNIs reduce the efficacy of Progestin containing contraceptives.

Absolute contraindications: SLE with antiphospholipid antibodies, cardiovascular

TABLE 1: Various methods of contraception commonly used.

Method	Mechanism of action	Advantages	Disadvantages	Contraindications
Hormonal methods				
Combined oral contraceptive				
Content: Ethinyl estradiol (10–35 µg/day) and progestin (any of levonorgestrel, desogestrel, gestodene or norgestimate, norelgestromine, etonogestrel, drospirenone, or dienogest)	Inhibit the release of GnRH blocking ovulation, alter the endometrium, cause thickening of cervical mucus	Highly effective with a failure rate of 7% with typical use and 0.3% with perfect use	Thrombotic and cardiovascular risk, worsens albuminuria, must be taken correctly every day at the same time, progestin-containing contraceptives increase the concentration of CNIs while CNIs reduce the efficacy of progestin-containing contraceptives	• *Absolute contraindications:* SLE with antiphospholipid antibodies, cardiovascular disease, venous thromboembolism, breast cancer, smokers >35 years of age, impaired liver function. • *Relative contraindications:* SLE, diabetes mellitus, hypertension, hyperlipidemia, proteinuric glomerular disease
Estrogen-containing hormonal contraception				
Content: Ethinyl estradiol (6 mg) and progestin (norelgestromine 600 µg)	Inhibit the release of GnRH blocking ovulation, alter the endometrium, cause thickening of cervical mucus	Highly effective with a failure rate of 7% with typical use and 0.3% with perfect use	Thrombotic and cardiovascular risk, worsens albuminuria, avoids first-pass metabolism resulting in higher circulating levels and higher adverse effects, progestin-containing contraceptives increase the concentration of CNIs while CNIs reduce the efficacy of progestin-containing contraceptives	• *Absolute contraindications:* SLE with antiphospholipid antibodies, cardiovascular disease, venous thromboembolism, breast cancer, smokers >35 years of age, impaired liver function. • *Relative contraindications:* SLE, diabetes mellitus, hypertension, hyperlipidemia, proteinuric glomerular disease
Progestin-only OCP				
Content: Ethinyl estradiol (2.7 mg) and progestin (etonogestrel 11.7 mg)	Inhibits the release of GnRH blocking ovulation, reduce the endometrial thickness, modify the composition of cervical mucus, affects tubal motility	• Does not affect coagulation and blood pressure, unlike combined oral contraceptives. • The failure rate of 9–13% with typical use and 0.3% with perfect use (less effective than combined oral contraceptives)	Weight gain, spotting, and irregular menses, interaction with CNIs (progestin-containing contraceptives increase the concentration of CNIs while CNIs reduce the efficacy of progestin-containing contraceptives)	• *Absolute contraindications:* None • *Relative contraindications:* SLE (±Antiphospholipid antibody syndrome), diabetes mellitus, hypertension

Contd...

Contd...

Method	**Mechanism of action**	**Advantages**	**Disadvantages**	**Contraindications**
Progestin-only subdermal implants				
Content: Etonogestrel or levonorgestrel	Inhibit the release of GnRH blocking ovulation, reduce the endometrial thickness, modify the composition of cervical mucus, affects tubal motility	Failure rate of 0.1%, long-acting (3 years) and reversible	Weight gain, spotting, and irregular menses, interaction with CNIs (progestin-containing contraceptives increase the concentration of CNIs while CNIs reduce the efficacy of progestin-containing contraceptives), reduction in bone mineral density	• *Absolute contraindications:* Thromboembolic disease • *Relative contraindications:* SLE (± Antiphospholipid antibody syndrome), diabetes mellitus, hypertension, cardiovascular disease, hypercholesterolemia, immunocompromised states
Injectable progestin-only contraceptive				
Content: Depot-medroxy-progesterone acetate (DMPA150 mg) or norethisterone enanthate (NET-EN, 200 mg)	Inhibits the release of GnRH blocking ovulation, reduce the endometrial thickness, modify the composition of cervical mucus, affects tubal motility	The failure rate of 4–6% with typical use and 0.2% with perfect use, long-acting (2–3 months) and reversible	Weight gain, reduction in bone mineral density	• *Absolute contraindications:* Breast cancer, coagulation disorders • *Relative contraindications:* SLE (±Antiphospholipid antibody syndrome), diabetes mellitus, hypertension, cardiovascular disease, osteoporosis, history of fractures
Nonmedicated copper-containing IUDs				
Content: T-shaped flexible devices containing copper	Copper ions are toxic to the sperm and induce local modifications in the endometrium and the cervical mucus preventing fertilization	Very low failure rate 0.1–0.6%, useful as an emergency contraceptive if inserted within 120 hours of unprotected sexual intercourse, long-acting (5–10 years), no drug interactions, safer in patients with thromboembolic risk, hypertension, and weight gain	Higher risk of pelvic infections in the initial 20 days after placement, increased chances of extrauterine pregnancy, expulsion of the IUD, uterine perforation (rare)	• *Absolute contraindications:* None *Relative contraindications:* Immunocompromised states including complicated kidney transplant recipients (risk outweighs benefit), peritoneal dialysis patients

Contd...

Contd…

Method	Mechanism of action	Advantages	Disadvantages	Contraindications
Medicated IUDs				
Content: T-shaped flexible devices containing levonorgestrel	Thickens cervical mucus, prevents movement of sperms, and impairs ovulation	Very low failure rate 0.1–0.6%, high compliance, long-acting (3–5 years)	Higher risk of pelvic infections in the initial 20 days after placement, increased chances of extrauterine pregnancy, expulsion of the IUD, uterine perforation (rare)	• *Absolute contraindications:* None • *Relative contraindications:* SLE (±Antiphospholipid antibody syndrome), hypertension, immunocompromised states including complicated kidney transplant recipients (risk outweighs benefit), peritoneal dialysis patients, uterine malformations
Barrier methods				
Types: Male and female condoms, diaphragms, cervical caps, sponges	Prevent direct contact between spermatozoa and the ovum	No adverse effects, condom is the only contraceptive method that protects against sexually transmitted disease	High failure rate which is dependent on the correct positioning of the device (Male condom: 2–15%; female condom: 5–21%; diaphragm: 6–16%; cervical cap: 6–16%; sponges: 9–16%), diaphragms and cervical caps can increase the risk of urinary tract infections (especially with spermicide use)	–

(CNIs: calcineurin inhibitors; GnRH: gonadotropin hormone-releasing hormone; IUDs: intrauterine devices; OCP: oral contraceptive pills; SLE: systemic lupus erythematosus) disease, venous thromboembolism, breast cancer, smokers > 35 years of age, impaired liver function.

Relative contraindications: SLE, diabetes mellitus, hypertension, hyperlipidaemia, proteinuric glomerular disease.

Emergency Contraception

Emergency contraception include high-dose progestin and copper intrauterine devices (IUDs)

High-dose Progestin
Types: Levonorgestrel (1.5 mg) or ulipristal acetate (selective progesterone receptor modulator, dose 30 mg).

Mechanism of action: Thickening the cervical mucus and interfering with ovulation: Before the peak of LH they inhibit follicular maturation and prevent ovulation; ulipristal acetate inhibits ovulation even after the onset of the LH peak, delaying ovulation for at least 5 days.

The efficacy of progestin ranges between 54 and 99% within the first 72 hours of sexual intercourse. The adverse effects are similar to progestin-containing oral contraceptives. However, vomiting is more frequent. It is safe for kidney disease but not recommended in patients with severe liver disease.

Permanent Contraception

Permanent contraception or sterilization includes vasectomy in males and salpingectomy or tubal ligation in females. These are irreversible methods of contraception. Tubal ligation may be performed immediately after delivery or after an interval period. The failure rate of tubal ligation is around 0.5%, while that of vasectomy is 0.01% at 5 years. For the initial 3 months after vasectomy, the patient should be advised to use an alternative contraceptive method. The risks associated with this procedure are those associated with any abdominal surgery including infections and bleeding.

Termination

Termination of pregnancy or abortion is not a method of contraception since conception has already occurred. Abortion can be considered if the pregnancy is unintended and implies a risk to the maternal health and may be performed up to the legally permitted gestational age. Abortion could be done by surgical or medical methods. Surgical methods include curettage or dilatation and evacuation. Medical methods include intravaginal mifepristone in the first trimester or intravaginal misoprostol with or without mifepristone in the second trimester. There is limited evidence on the use of these methods in patients with kidney disorders.

MONITORING A PATIENT ON CONTRACEPTION

Patients initiated on any method of contraception should be followed up periodically to ensure compliance with the prescribed method and to check for adverse effects. Estrogen/progestin-containing contraceptive pills have been shown to cause a mild increase in blood pressure by activating the renin-angiotensin system.[10] They are also known to cause albuminuria by a mechanism that is not clearly understood. Hence, blood pressure and proteinuria assessment during follow-up is essential, especially in these patients.

CONTRACEPTION DURING THE POSTPARTUM PERIOD AND LACTATION

Progestin-containing contraceptive methods or copper IUDs are the preferred contraceptive methods in the postpartum period

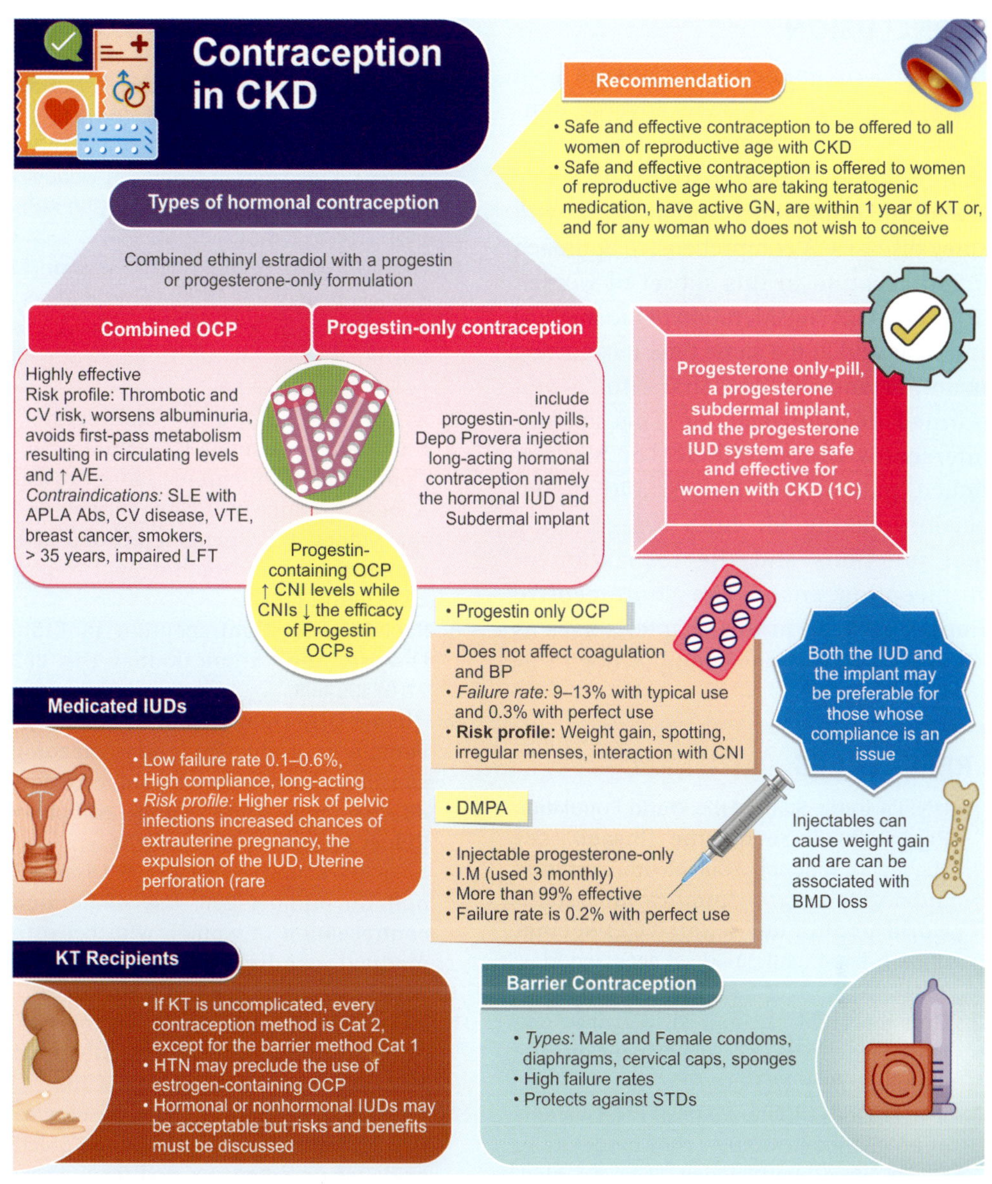

Fig. 2: Contraception in CKD. (A/E: adverse effects; APLA: antiphospholipid antibodies; BMD: bone mineral density; BP: blood pressure; CNI: calcineurin inhibitors; CV: cardiovascular; DMPA: depot medroxyprogesterone acetate; GN: glomerulonephritis; IUD: intrauterine device; KT: kindney transplantation; OCP: oral contraceptive pills; STDs: sexually transmitted diseases; VTE: venous thromboembolism)

Courtesy: Dr Priti Meena

including lactation.[11] Long-acting methods are preferable over short-acting methods. Given the increased risk of thromboembolism, estrogen-containing contraceptives should be avoided in the immediate postpartum period and should be preferably delayed for at least 6 weeks in high-risk patients. **Figure 2** summarizes contraception in CKD.

CONCLUSION

Unplanned pregnancies in patients with kidney disorders can have adverse consequences for the mother and the fetus. Tailored family planning strategies are of paramount importance for patients with kidney diseases. A comprehensive approach to contraception in this subset of women involves careful consideration of the medical conditions and at the same time recognizing the importance of personal choice and informed decision-making. This chapter underscores the confluence of medical science, patient preferences, and shared decision-making for both safeguarding renal functions and the realization of contraception goals. The contraceptive compass outlined in this chapter serves as a valuable guide to navigating through this complex process.[12]

REFERENCES

1. UNFPA India. State of the World Population Report 2022: Seeing the Unseen. Key Highlights. [online]. Available from: https://india.unfpa.org/en/publications/state-world-population-report-2022-seeing-unseen-key-highlights [Last accessed May, 2024].
2. Dumanski SM, Ahmed SB. Fertility and reproductive care in chronic kidney disease. J Nephrol. 2019;32(1):39-50.
3. Avid D, Ones CJ, Ohn J, Ayslett PH. Outcome of pregnancy in women with moderate or severe renal insufficiency. N Engl J Med. 1996;335(4):226-32.
4. Maule SP, Ashworth DC, Blakey H, Osafo C, Moturi M, Chappell LC, et al. CKD and Pregnancy Outcomes in Africa: A Narrative Review. Kidney Int Rep. 2020;5(8):1342-9.
5. Sachdeva M, Barta V, Thakkar J, Sakhiya V, Miller I. Pregnancy outcomes in women on hemodialysis: a national survey. Clin Kidney J. 2017;10(2):276-81.
6. Hendren EM, Reynolds ML, Mariani LH, Zee J, O'shaughnessy MM, Oliverio AL, et al. Confidence in women's health: A cross border survey of adult nephrologists. J Clin Med. 2019;8:176.
7. Attini R, Cabiddu G, Montersino B, Gammaro L, Gernone G, Moroni G, et al. Contraception in chronic kidney disease: a best practice position statement by the Kidney and Pregnancy Group of the Italian Society of Nephrology. J Nephrol. 2020;33(6):1343-59.
8. Sachdeva M. Contraception in Kidney Disease. Adv Chronic Kidney Dis. 2020; 27(6):499-505.
9. Chang DH, Dumanski SM, Ahmed SB. Female reproductive and gynecologic considerations in chronic kidney disease: adolescence and young adulthood. Kidney Int Rep. 2022;7(2):152-64.
10. Allen RH, Kaunitz A, Bartz D. ACOG practice bulletin number 206: Use of hormonal contraception in women with coexisting medical conditions. Obstet Gynecol. 2019;133(2):E128-50.
11. Woodhams EJ, Gilliam M. In the clinic. Contraception. Ann Intern Med. 2012; 157(7):ITC4-1-ITC4-15; quiz ITC4-16.
12. Wiles K, Chappell L, Clark K, Elman L, Hall M, Lightstone L, et al. Clinical practice guideline on pregnancy and renal disease. BMC Nephrol. 2019; 20(1):1-43.

CHAPTER

15 Pregnancy in Chronic Kidney Disease

Sabarinath S, Renu Singh, Narayan Prasad

HIGHLIGHTS

- Diagnosing pregnancy in chronic kidney disease (CKD) is challenging as measuring urinary beta-human chorionic gonadotropin (β-hCG) in advanced CKD can be unreliable and may yield false negatives. Confirmatory pregnancy diagnosis requires serial monitoring of β-hCG in conjunction with ultrasound.
- Women with any form of underlying CKD have:
  - A 10-fold increased risk of preeclampsia
  - A five-fold increased risk of preterm delivery and small-for-gestational-age infants
  - An almost three-fold increased risk of cesarean delivery
- Failure to see a physiologic increase in glomerular filtration rate (GFR) and/or a fall in serum creatinine during pregnancy may suggest underlying CKD or acute kidney injury (AKI).
- The greatest risk for estimated GFR (eGFR) decline after delivery is observed in patients with eGFR <40 mL/min/1.73 m^2 and 24-hour urine protein >1 g/day.
- Superimposed preeclampsia is difficult to diagnose in patients with preexisting hypertension, elevated serum creatinine, and/or proteinuria; it requires monitoring features of maternal organ dysfunction due to preeclampsia.
- The target blood pressure (BP) during pregnancy for women with CKD is 135/85 mm Hg or less. Persistent hypertension and inadequate BP control are associated with poorer outcomes.

INTRODUCTION

Globally, chronic kidney disease (CKD) is estimated to affect 6% of women of reproductive age and 3% of pregnancies. Women with CKD are at high risk for adverse outcomes in pregnancy.[1] A meta-analysis revealed that women with any form of underlying CKD had an approximately 10-fold increased risk of preeclampsia, a 5-fold increased risk for preterm delivery and small-for gestational-age infants, and an almost 3-fold increased risk for cesarean delivery.[2] Also, there is a risk of progression in underlying CKD if there is uncontrolled hypertension, especially in advanced renal failure. This chapter overviews multiple aspects and the impact of pregnancy on CKD outcomes as well as pregnancy outcomes in CKD **(Fig. 1)**.

DEFINING CHRONIC KIDNEY DISEASE IN PREGNANCY

The kidney undergoes several physiological and anatomical changes during pregnancy. The glomerular filtration rate (GFR) increases by 50% due to renal vasodilatation and increased renal plasma flow. Owing to this hyperfiltration and associated increase in

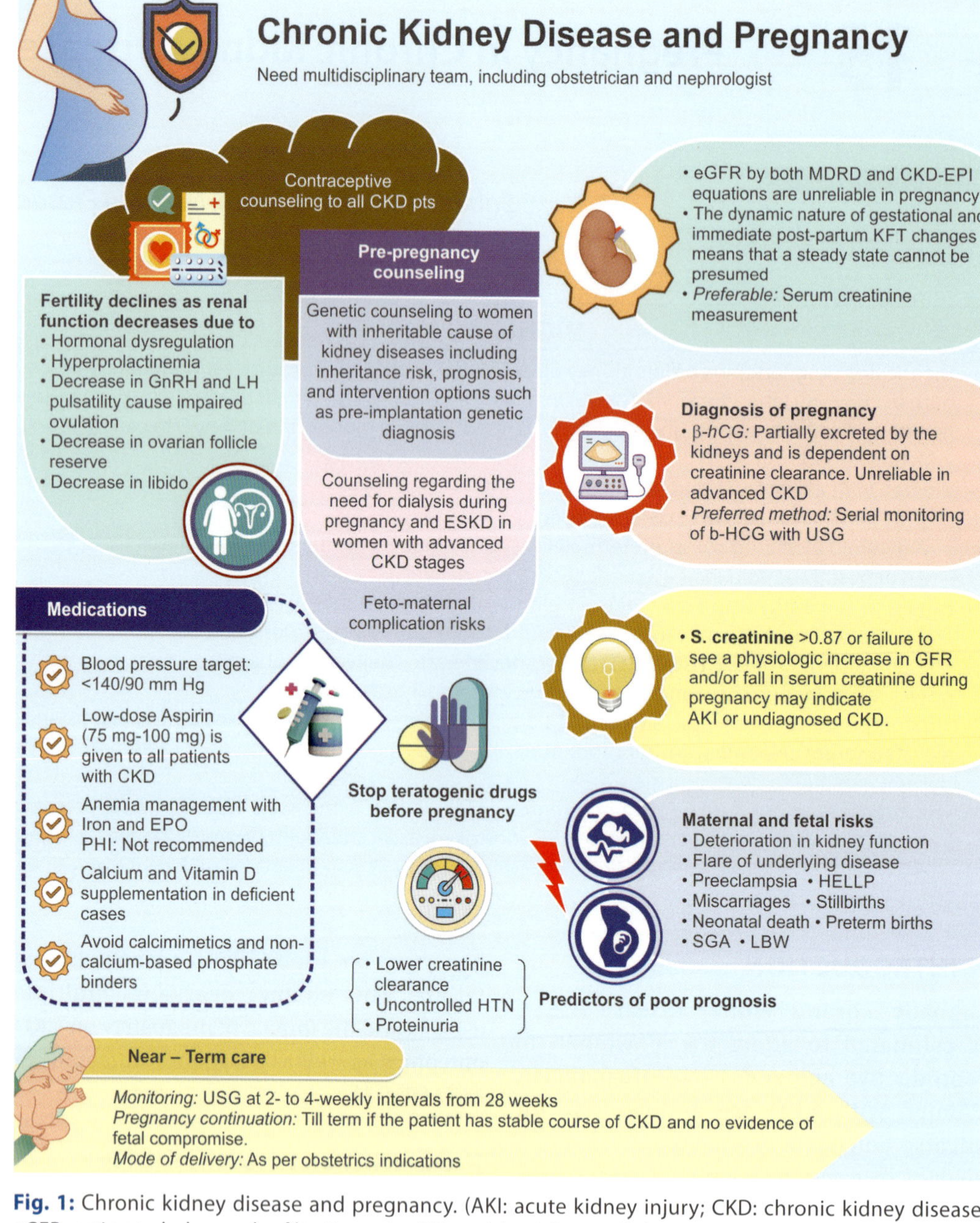

Fig. 1: Chronic kidney disease and pregnancy. (AKI: acute kidney injury; CKD: chronic kidney disease; eGFR: estimated glomerular filtration rate; EPI: epidemiology collaboration; EPO: erythropoietin; ESKD: end-stage kidney disease; GnRH: gonadotropin hormone-releasing hormone; HELLP: hemolysis, elevated liver enzymes, low platelet count; HTN: hypertension; LBW: low birthweight; LH: luteinizing hormone; MDRD: modified diet in renal disease; PHI: prolyl hydroxylase inhibitor; SGA: small-for-gestational age; USG: ultrasound; β-hCG: beta-human chorionic gonadotropin)

Courtesy: Dr Priti Meena.

glomerular basement membrane permeability, up to 300 mg proteinuria in 24 hours is considered physiologic.[3] Also, systemic vascular resistance decreases in healthy pregnancy, lowering the mean arterial pressure to a nadir at 24 weeks of gestation and returning to the baseline near term.[4] Defining CKD in pregnancy is challenging, especially when prepregnancy kidney function is unknown. In a meta-analysis, Wiles and Bramham showed that the upper-normal creatinine levels might be 0.86 mg/dL in the first trimester, 0.81 mg/dL in the second trimester, and 0.87 mg/dL in the third trimester.[5] A serum creatinine >0.87 may indicate AKI or undiagnosed CKD. In addition, a failure to see a physiologic increase in GFR and/or fall in serum creatinine during pregnancy may indicate underlying CKD or AKI. Estimated glomerular filtration rate (eGFR) derived by both modified diet in renal disease (MDRD) and Chronic Kidney Disease Epidemiology Collaboration (CKD-EPI) equations are unreliable in pregnancy as they underestimate GFR up to 20%.[6] Also, the dynamic nature of gestational and immediate postpartum changes in renal function means that a steady state cannot be presumed, prohibiting the use of eGFR. Hence, it is preferable to monitor serum creatinine in pregnancy.

MATERNAL AND FETAL OUTCOMES IN CHRONIC KIDNEY DISEASE

Previously, CKD was considered a contraindication to pregnancy, but with evolving shreds of evidence, many pregnant patients with CKD have successful maternal and fetal outcomes.

Unlike the general population, pregnancy in CKD is considered high risk, as the diseased kidneys may be unable to adapt to physiological changes, leading to perinatal complications.

In cases of mild renal function impairment, pregnancy is generally successful without altering the course of maternal renal disease, provided BP is normal and there is no proteinuria. However, in women with moderate or severe renal function impairment, there is a significant risk to fetal outcomes and long-term maternal renal function.

Pregnancy is rare when serum creatinine exceeds 3 mg/dL, as these women may have amenorrhea or anovulatory cycles. If pregnancy occurs, about a third may progress to end-stage renal disease (ESRD) within 1 year postpartum. Additionally, women with a GFR below 60 mL/min are at a higher risk of developing preeclampsia, and nephrotic proteinuria is common. It could be associated with increased maternal mortality and a higher incidence of cesarean deliveries.

A meta-analysis found no significant difference in kidney outcomes between pregnant women with stage 1–3 CKD and those without CKD-complicated pregnancy.[2] More recent studies reported an increase in live birth rates, even in those with advanced CKD.

The following three parameters are more important in predicting outcomes rather than specific kidney disease etiology:

1. Proteinuria before conception
2. Presence of hypertension
3. eGFR/serum creatinine before conception

The greatest risk for eGFR decline after delivery was noted in patients with eGFR <40 mL/min/1.73 m^2 and 24-hour urine protein >1 g/day.[7] CKD etiology has less influence on outcomes than CKD stage, proteinuria, hypertension, and preeclampsia. An exception is systemic lupus erythematosus

TABLE 1: Maternal and fetal outcomes according to the severity of kidney function.

	Maternal kidney outcomes	*Fetal outcomes*
CKD stages 1–2	Progression to ESRD is 10%, the greatest risk if eGFR is <40 mL/min/min^2 and proteinuria is >1 g/day	• Live birth—most pregnancies • Preterm delivery—50%
CKD stage 3	Progression to ESRD in 30%, up to 50% in those with uncontrolled hypertension	• Live birth—most pregnancies • Preterm delivery—60%
CKD stages 4 and 5	Progression to ESRD is highly likely during or soon after pregnancy	• Live birth—most pregnancies • Preterm delivery—90%

(CKD: chronic kidney disease; ESRD: end-stage renal disease)

(SLE) nephritis, in which outcomes are poorer than for women with comparable renal impairment from other causes, particularly if associated with antiphospholipid antibodies. The maternal kidney outcomes and the fetal outcomes according to the stage of CKD are given in **Table 1**.

PREPREGNANCY CARE

Contraception

Contraceptive counseling should be given to all patients with CKD (including those on dialysis) who are not planning for pregnancy, who are taking teratogenic medications, who have active glomerulonephritis, and who are within 1 year of renal transplantation or acute graft rejection. Estrogen-containing contraceptive preparations are not advisable because of thrombotic episodes, risk of hypertension, and cervical cancer.[8] Progesterone-only contraception (progesterone-only pill, progesterone subdermal implant, and progesterone intrauterine system) is safe for women with CKD. Although there is no robust data to support this, women on immunosuppressive therapy have been advised against intrauterine devices due to fear of pelvic inflammatory disease and failure rates (due to inhibition of uterine inflammation, which is believed to contribute to the underlying contraceptive mechanism).

Fertility Assessment

Fertility is affected by CKD and declines as renal function decreases. Hormonal dysregulation with hyperprolactinemia and decrease in gonadotropin-releasing hormone and luteinizing hormone (LH) pulsatility in CKD lead to impaired ovulation. Also, the decrease in ovarian follicle reserve due to the above hormonal imbalance and the decrease in libido in advanced CKD stages contribute to infertility.[9] A woman who has had previous exposure to cyclophosphamide should have an early investigation for fertility. There is no strong evidence that hormonal manipulation has additional adverse outcomes unless they develop ovarian hyperstimulation syndrome, which may further compromise kidney function. In assisted conception, the single-embryo transfer technique is recommended to reduce complications associated with multifetal pregnancies in women with CKD.

Preconception Counseling

The preconception counseling should be offered by a multidisciplinary team including an obstetrician and a nephrologist. They should be advised regarding the increased risk of antenatal complications, including preeclampsia, preterm delivery,

TABLE 2: Maternal and fetal risk during pregnancy in CKD patients.

Maternal risk	*Fetal risk*
Worsening of hypertension with risk of stroke	Fetal growth restriction due to placental insufficiency
Worsening of proteinuria with risks of thrombosis	Preterm delivery
Accelerated decline in GFR	Inheritance of a kidney disorder
Superimposed preeclampsia	Teratogenicity of some drugs prescribed for kidney disease

(CKD: chronic kidney disease; GFR: glomerular filtration rate)

and fetal growth restriction compared to women without CKD, although a successful pregnancy is feasible for most women.[2]

The counseling should include the following points:

- Women with CKD who were taking renin-angiotensin inhibitors should be stopped before planning pregnancy.
- Women with CKD stages 4–5 should be counseled regarding the need for dialysis during pregnancy and even developing ESRD.
- Those with suspected renal disease are offered genetic counseling, including inheritance risk, prognosis and options, including preimplantation genetic diagnosis.

The maternal and fetal risks should be clearly emphasized **(Table 2)**.

DIAGNOSING PREGNANCY

Diagnosing pregnancy in women with CKD can be challenging, particularly in advanced CKD, as they have abnormal menstrual cycles and anovulatory cycles. Beta-human chorionic gonadotropin (β-hCG) is partially excreted by the kidneys and is dependent on creatinine clearance. Hence, measuring urinary β-hCG in advanced CKD is unreliable and might be falsely negative. Serial monitoring of β-hCG in conjunction with ultrasound is confirmatory for pregnancy diagnosis.[10,11]

PREGNANCY CARE

General Considerations

All women are offered screening for the most common fetal aneuploidies in pregnancy. Screening options include first- and/or second-trimester maternal serum measurements (β-hCG, pregnancy-associated plasma protein-A, etc.) in combination with ultrasound fetal nuchal translucency scan. Pregnancy-associated plasma protein-A measurement is unreliable in advanced CKD or ESRD and falsely elevated in women receiving heparin.

The following parameters have to be carefully evaluated in pregnant CKD patients apart from routine antenatal care.

Proteinuria

Proteinuria is exacerbated in pregnancy due to glomerular hyperfiltration and increased plasma blood flow and also due to stopping renin-angiotensin system blockade. Measuring the spot urine protein-creatinine ratio is useful. Isolated non-nephrotic proteinuria may develop de novo during pregnancy. The following are the differential diagnoses:

- Superimposed preeclampsia (after 20 weeks of gestation)
- Gestational proteinuria (non-nephrotic proteinuria, no pregnancy complications, which usually resolve after delivery)

- Rarely, patients may develop primary glomerular disease before or during pregnancy and may remain postpartum.

It is important to note that serum albumin falls below 3 g/dL even in healthy pregnancy as a result of volume expansion. Also, a rise in serum cholesterol and pedal edema is expected in healthy pregnancies. In patients with nephrotic range proteinuria and serum albumin value <2.5 g/dL, and those with high-risk conditions (e.g., membranous nephropathy), anticoagulation is recommended to prevent the risk of venous thromboembolic disease.[12] The anticoagulant choices include low-molecular-weight heparin dosed appropriately for GFR and unfractionated heparin for women on dialysis. Diltiazem may have a small benefit in reducing proteinuria but no strong evidence among pregnant patients.

Hypertension

Hypertension in pregnancy is defined as BP of 140/90 mm Hg or greater. Pregnant CKD patients do not exhibit the first-trimester fall in BP, and in many women, BP increases as the pregnancy progresses. The target BP during pregnancy for women with CKD is 135/85 mm Hg or less. The persistence of hypertension and inadequate control have been associated with poorer outcomes. The first-line medications used to control hypertension in pregnancy are methyldopa, labetalol, and nifedipine. Angiotensin-converting enzyme (ACE) inhibitors and angiotensin receptor blockers (ARBs) are contraindicated due to fetotoxicity like intrauterine growth restriction, renal dysplasia, oligohydramnios, and fetal death. Women with renal or cardiac indications can continue ACE inhibitors till the time of conception, provided they are counseled to undertake regular pregnancy testing and stop at a positive pregnancy test.[13] Due to the paucity of evidence supporting ARBs' safety, these agents are usually discontinued in advance of pregnancy. Aldosterone antagonists should be avoided in pregnancy, and atenolol is associated with fetal growth restriction. Diuretics are avoided during pregnancy because any reduction in maternal plasma volume may have adverse effects on uteroplacental or kidney perfusion. Diuretics are used for the treatment of pulmonary edema where substantial peripheral edema leads to skin breakdown. The drugs and dosages used in pregnant hypertensive CKD patients are given in **Table 3**.

Diagnosing Preeclampsia in CKD Patients

All women with any degree of CKD are considered at high risk for preeclampsia. Roughly one in four women with chronic

TABLE 3: Antihypertensives for pregnant CKD patients.

Drug	***Dose***	***Maximum dose per day***
Methyldopa	250 mg PO BD up to maximum of 1,000 mg PO every 8 hours	3,000 mg
Labetalol	100 mg PO BD up to 800 mg PO every 8 hours	2,400 mg
Nifedipine	*Short-acting*: 10 mg PO every 8 hours *Extended release*: 30–90 mg PO QD	120 mg
Hydralazine	10–50 mg PO every 6 hours	200 mg

(CKD: chronic kidney disease)

BOX 1: Criteria for diagnosing preeclampsia in a CKD patient.

- A diagnosis of superimposed preeclampsia is considered
- In a woman with nonproteinuric CKD, if she develops new hypertension (systolic BP >140 mm Hg and/or diastolic BP >90 mm Hg) and proteinuria (uPCR >30 mg/mmol or uACR >8 mg/mmol) or maternal organ dysfunction after 20 weeks' gestation
- In a woman with proteinuric CKD if she develops new hypertension (systolic BP >140 mm Hg and/or diastolic BP >90 mm Hg) or maternal organ dysfunction after 20 weeks' gestation
- In a woman with chronic hypertension and proteinuria, if she develops maternal organ dysfunction after 20 weeks' gestation

(CKD: chronic kidney disease; uACR: urine albumin–creatinine ratio; uPCR: urine protein–creatinine ratio)

hypertension will develop superimposed preeclampsia **(Box 1)**.

Superimposed preeclampsia is challenging to diagnose in a patient with preexisting hypertension, elevated serum creatinine, and/or proteinuria. In such cases, the following features of maternal organ dysfunction due to preeclampsia can provide clues to diagnosis:

- New proteinuria [urine protein–creatinine ratio (uPCR) >30 mg/mmol or albumin-creatinine ratio (ACR) >8 mg/mmol]
- AKI (serum creatinine ≥90 µmol/L in a woman with previously normal creatinine concentrations)
- Liver involvement (alanine aminotransferase or aspartate aminotransferase >40 IU/L) with or without right upper quadrant or epigastric pain
- Neurological complications (eclampsia, altered mental status, blindness, stroke, clonus, severe headache, persistent visual scotomata)
- Hematological complications (platelet count <150,000/µL, disseminated intravascular coagulation, hemolysis)
- Uteroplacental dysfunction (fetal growth restriction, abnormal umbilical artery, Doppler waveform analysis, stillbirth)

Novel biomarkers like soluble FMS-like tyrosine kinase (sFlt), placental growth factor (PlGF), and serum placental protein may help in differentiating and predicting preeclampsia in women with CKD. A recent meta-analysis has shown sFlt:PlGF ratio as a predictive and diagnostic marker of preeclampsia in both low- and high-risk patients. This could detect preeclampsia with a sensitivity of 80% and specificity of 92%.[14]

Medications in Pregnancy

Low-dose aspirin (75–100 mg) is given to all patients with CKD. Limited studies suggest that low-dose aspirin is of benefit in reducing the risk of superimposed preeclampsia and perinatal death in patients with an underlying kidney disease.[15] Mycophenolate mofetil is stopped before pregnancy, as use in pregnancy is associated with an increased risk of spontaneous miscarriage and fetal abnormality. A 3-month interval is advised before conception to allow conversion to a pregnancy-safe alternative and ensure stable disease/kidney function. Teratogenic medications like methotrexate and cyclophosphamide are not taken in pregnancy because of their teratogenic effect. Sirolimus and everolimus are avoided in pregnancy due to insufficient safety data. The use of immunosuppressive agents like azathioprine, ciclosporin, tacrolimus, and hydroxychloroquine is safe in pregnancy.

Anemia Management

The most common cause of anemia in pregnancy is iron deficiency, which is estimated to affect >40% of pregnancies. Oral iron is cheap and accessible, although the intravenous route may offer better bioavailability and tolerability in pregnancy, in women with CKD.[16] Erythropoietin concentrations increase approximately two-fold during pregnancy. As women with CKD may have insufficient capacity for a gestational increase in erythropoietin, supplementation with synthetic erythropoietin may be required, even in the context of mild or moderate renal impairment. For women who require erythropoietin before pregnancy, an increased dose requirement should be anticipated during pregnancy. Being a large molecule, it does not cross the placenta.[16] Hypoxia-inducible factor (HIF) activators, that is, prolyl hydroxylase inhibitors (PHI), are the new group of drugs for renal anemia. Being a small molecule, these drugs can be transferred to the fetus via the placenta. HIF has multiple direct and indirect effects on developmental and physiological processes. Hence, this group of drugs is not recommended for use in pregnancy due to lack of clinical safety and efficacy data.[17]

CKD–Mineral and Bone Disorder Management

Calcium and vitamin D supplementation can be given to those who are vitamin D deficient. It is better to avoid calcimimetics and non-calcium-based phosphate binders during pregnancy, given insufficient data.

Renal Biopsy

It is not indicated to perform a kidney biopsy unless a histological diagnosis will change management in pregnancy. Complications are more common in the late second and third trimesters of pregnancy compared with those in general nephrology practice. A systematic review reported bleeding complications in 7% of biopsies performed in pregnancy compared with 1% performed postpartum.[18] The indications to perform kidney biopsy in a pregnant patient are as follows:

- New-onset nephrotic syndrome
- Unexplained kidney injury with abnormal urinary sediments (in the first and early second trimesters when the risks are lower)
- When a histologic diagnosis changes management in the pregnancy
- Suspected acute rejection in a renal transplant recipient

Fetal Monitoring

Early pregnancy ultrasound between 11 and 14 weeks is advised to estimate accurately the expected date of delivery (dating scan). A morphology scan is performed at 18–20 weeks of gestation to screen for fetal anomalies and check placental function and position (anomaly screening). Ultrasound scans should be offered at 2- to 4-weekly intervals from 28 weeks of gestation in women with CKD to assess fetal growth and amniotic fluid volume, with Doppler studies of umbilical artery blood flow. Absent end-diastolic flow on umbilical artery velocimetry is an indication for the need for delivery.

TIMING OF DELIVERY

The pregnancies should be continued till term if the patient has a stable course of CKD and no evidence of fetal compromise. Also, the mode of delivery (vaginal or cesarean) should be determined by the obstetric issue rather than the CKD. The indications for delivery are as follows:

- Inability to control BP
- Worsening renal function
- Eclampsia
- Worsening thrombocytopenia, worsening transaminitis

- Failure of fetal growth
- Absent or reversed end-diastolic flow on cardiotocography

A global clinical assessment rather than a specific parameter should be considered while assessing the delivery timing.

SPECIAL CONSIDERATIONS

IgA nephropathy: Though the outcome of pregnancy in IgA nephropathy patients was generally positive and comparable to other causes of CKD, a Swedish cohort study described an increased risk of preterm birth [adjusted odds ratio (OR), 2.69], preeclampsia (adjusted OR, 4.29), and small for gestational age (adjusted OR, 1.84), but no reduction in live birth rates.[19] Patients with CKD stage 1 or 2 do not experience accelerated kidney function decline, but proteinuria may increase in the third trimester.

Diabetic kidney diseases (DKDs)*:* Women with DKD likely have worse pregnancy outcomes than women with other causes of CKD and comparable kidney function. (e.g., preeclampsia 42%, preterm before 34 weeks 21%, neonatal care admission 49%).[20] The outcome of DKD during pregnancy depends on the usual factors of severity of kidney impairment and hypertension

Lupus nephritis: Higher levels of pro-inflammatory cytokines and fewer T regulatory cells in SLE may result in implantation defects and recurrent fetal loss. Hence, pre-pregnancy counselling is important before planning a pregnancy in a lupus patient. Active lupus nephritis at conception (or during pregnancy) is associated with worse fetal and maternal outcomes. Pregnancy can be allowed if the disease is under complete remission for 6 months. Lupus nephritis flares are described in 30% of women during pregnancy and in 15% of women immediately postpartum. Anti-Ro positivity has a 2% risk of the fetus developing congenital heart block. Hydroxychloroquine reduces risk by 50%.

Reflux nephropathy: Of those patients with reflux nephropathy, 20% will develop symptomatic urinary tract infection (UTI) during pregnancy, with a 6% incidence of pyelonephritis. Regular urine culture should be performed throughout pregnancy, and treatment should be given for confirmation. Vesicoureteric reflux may be a familial disorder, estimated to affect 20% of infants with a positive parental family history, compared with a 1–2% frequency in the general population.[21]

Pregnancy in ESRD Patients

The incidence of pregnancy in ESRD women is as low as 2.2%, as LH surge is suppressed because of increased prolactin levels. However, the intensification of hemodialysis has increased the conception rate to 16% and the live birth rate from 23% to 87%.[22]. Significant elevations of β-hCG with a doubling of values every 48–72 hours are indicative of true pregnancy in hemodialysis (HD) patients, which should be confirmed with a sonology scan. A Canadian cohort study showed improvement in birth weight and length of gestation in patients who received prolonged HD (40 h/wk) when compared with those who received 17 h/wk. Intensive HD improves urea clearance, lowers peripheral vascular resistance, and ameliorates fluctuation in volume status. Daily dialysis offers the advantage of decreased risk of hypotension owing to decreased fluid removal per session, allows high protein intake to meet calorie needs, and increases solute clearance, thereby decreasing

BOX 2: Managing hemodialysis (HD) in a pregnant patient.

The highlights of HD management in a pregnant patient are listed below.

- Dialysis prescription should be individualized (5–7 times/week of 8–10 h/session).
- Use of a biocompatible nonreusable dialyzer.
- Unfractionated heparin can be used as it cannot cross the placenta.
- Graded increase in dialysis dose based on biochemical parameters and residual renal function.
- Maternal serum urea target <48 mg/dL correlates with delivery after 32 weeks of gestation and birth weight greater than 1.5 kg.
- Weekly hours of HD: Based on midweek predialysis serum urea, BP control, weight gain in a week, polyhydramnios and uremic symptoms. The dialysis duration for a patient with 1 L urine output can be managed with 20 h/week, and anuric patients need 36 h/week.
- *UF removal:*
  - Physiological weight gain in the first trimester: 1–1.5 kg; then 300–500 mg/week thereafter.
  - This should be factored in dry weight assessment and fluid removal.
  - Residual renal function should be taken into account.
  - With daily HD, fluid gain should be minimal.
- Target BP goal <140/90 mm Hg; after HD, avoid intradialytic hypotension (not below 120/70 mm Hg).
- *HCO_3*: 25 mM is preferred to avoid superimposed metabolic alkalosis along with underlying respiratory alkalosis of pregnancy.
- Intensive dialysis may lead to hypophosphatemia; addition of phosphorus to dialyze may be necessary.
- Persistent elevation of BP despite optimal fluid removal—suspect preeclampsia.
- In patients who are newly starting on HD after 20 weeks, it should be a "gentle HD start" and not an intensive HD start, with intensification of HD as per maternal and fetal well-being, residual renal function and serum biochemistry over the course of pregnancy.

Nutritional support:

- Erythropoiesis stimulating agent dose is typically doubled in pregnancy.
- Intravenous iron to supplement the extra 700–1,000 mg of elemental iron.
- Protein intake of 1.8 g/kg per day and folate dose of 5 mg/day.
- Calcium supplementation: Oral 2 g/day with a standard 2.5 mEq/L dialysate.

placental urea, thus reducing fetal osmotic diuresis and resulting in complications such as polyhydramnios.[23] The important aspects to be noted while dialyzing a pregnant patient are listed in **Box 2**.

The indications to initiate HD include:

- Urea >17 mmol/L
- Serum creatinine of 3.5–5.0 mg/dL
- GFR <20 mL/min

In addition, uncontrolled BP, volume overload, and uremic symptoms are other indications. HD should be initiated when there is a disturbance in the fetal growth profile or polyhydramnios.[24]

INDIAN STUDIES

A retrospective analysis conducted in India, involving 51 pregnancies, revealed a significant increase in the risk of prematurity when the diastolic BP was ≥90 mm Hg at conception (OR 8.3, confidence interval 1.6–41.5). Notably, all pregnancies with a diastolic BP exceeding 100 mm Hg resulted in preterm delivery.[25] Hypertension worsened in 35.5% of women during pregnancy, leading to preterm termination in 13 cases due to uncontrolled BP. Additionally, 32.5% experienced a deterioration in serum creatinine, with the percentage increase inversely correlated with the baseline creatinine clearance. Another study covering 14 years and examining the outcomes of 30 pregnancies found comparable results across various types of glomerulonephritis.[26] Disease progression during pregnancy occurred in six patients, while 90% of women developed hypertension, with 40% experiencing mild hypertension and 43.3% requiring drug therapy for severe hypertension. Obstetrical complications included a high incidence of preterm delivery (85%) and cesarean section (30%). The overall fetal survival rate was 77%. A study conducted at Sanjay Gandhi Postgraduate Institute of Medical Sciences (SGPGI) involving 51 pregnancies in women with CKD showed a faster average decline in GFR 6 weeks postdelivery in patients with GFR <60 mL/min/1.73 m^2, particularly in stage 3 (n = 13, 20.2 mL/min) and stage 4 (n = 6, –15.8 mL/min), compared to –15.1 mL/min in patients with GFR ≥60 mL/min/ 1.73 m^2. In stage 4 CKD, 50% of patients required dialysis, while none in earlier stages did. Preeclampsia occurred in 17.6%, with a higher incidence (36.84%) in patients with GFR <60 mL/min. Among the 51 pregnancies, 15 ended in stillbirth and 36 resulted in live births, with 21.56% being delivered preterm, and 13.72% weighing <2,500 g.[27] **Figure 1** summarizes the key points of the Chapter.

CONCLUSION

To conclude, managing a pregnancy in a CKD patient needs a multidisciplinary approach and a meticulous follow-up with an obstetrician and nephrologist to have a better maternal and fetal outcome.

REFERENCES

1. Webster P, Lightstone L, McKay DB, Josephson MA. Pregnancy in chronic kidney disease and kidney transplantation. Kidney Int. 2017;91(5):1047-56.
2. Zhang JJ, Ma XX, Hao L, Liu LJ, Lv JC, Zhang H. A systematic review and meta-analysis of outcomes of pregnancy in CKD and CKD outcomes in pregnancy. Clin J Am Soc Nephrol. 2015;10(11): 1964-78.
3. Higby K, Suiter CR, Phelps JY, Siler-Khodr T, Langer O. Normal values of urinary albumin and total protein excretion during pregnancy. Am J Obstet Gynecol. 1994; 171(4):984-9.
4. Chapman AB, Abraham WT, Zamudio S, Coffin C, Merouani A, Young G, et al. Temporal relationships between hormonal and hemodynamic changes in early human pregnancy. Kidney Int. 1998;54(6):2056-63.
5. Wiles K, Bramham K. Serum Creatinine in Pregnancy: A Systematic Review. Kidney Int Rep. 2018;4:408-19.
6. Ahmed SB, Bentley-Lewis R, Hollenberg NK, Graves SW, Seely EW. A comparison of prediction equations for estimating glomerular filtration rate in pregnancy. Hypertens Pregnancy. 2009;28:243-55.
7. Imbasciati E, Gregorini G. Pregnancy in CKD stages 3 to 5: Fetal and maternal outcomes. Am J Kidney Dis. 2007;49:753-62.
8. Brynhildsen J. Combined hormonal contraceptives: prescribing patterns, compliance, and benefits versus risks. Ther Adv Drug Saf. 2014;5:201-13.
9. Wiles K, Anckaert E, Holden F, Grace J, Nelson-Piercy C, Lightstone L, et al. Anti-Müllerian hormone concentrations in women with chronic kidney disease. Clin Kidney J. 2019;14(2):537-42.
10. Doubilet PM, Benson CB, Bourne T, Blaivas M, Society of Radiologists in Ultrasound Multispecialty Panel on Early First Trimester Diagnosis of Miscarriage and Exclusion of a Viable Intrauterine Pregnancy, Barnhart KT, Benacerraf BR, et al. Diagnostic criteria for nonviable pregnancy early in the first trimester. N Engl J Med. 2013;369(15):1443-51.
11. Spencer K, Enofe O, Cowans NJ, Stamatopoulou A. Is maternal renal disease

a cause of elevated free beta-hCG in first trimester aneuploidy screening? Prenat Diagn. 2009;29(11):1045-9.
12. Hui D, Hladunewich MA. Chronic kidney disease and pregnancy. Obstet Gynecol. 2019;133(6):1182-94.
13. Bateman BT, Patorno E, Desai RJ, Seely EW, Mogun H, Dejene SZ, et al. Angiotensin-converting enzyme inhibitors and the risk of congenital malformations. Obstet Gynecol. 2017;129:174-84.
14. Agrawal S, Cerdeira AS, Redman CW, Vatish M. Meta-Analysis and systematic review to assess the role of soluble FMS-Like tyrosine kinase-1 and placenta growth factor ratio in prediction of preeclampsia. Hypertension. 2018;71(2):306-16.
15. Rolnik DL, Wright D, Poon LC, O'Gorman N, Syngelaki A, de Paco Matallana C, et al. Aspirin versus Placebo in Pregnancies at High Risk for Preterm Pre-eclampsia. N Engl J Med. 2017;377:613-22.
16. Albaramki J, Hodson EM, Craig JC, Webster AC. Parenteral versus oral iron therapy for adults and children with chronic kidney disease. Cochrane Database Syst Rev. 2012;1:CD007857.
17. Maxwell PH, Eckardt K-U. HIF prolyl hydroxylase inhibitors for the treatment of renal anaemia and beyond. Nat Rev Nephrol. 2016;12:157-68.
18. Piccoli GB, Daidola G, Attini R, Parisi S, Fassio F, Naretto C, et al. Kidney biopsy in pregnancy: evidence for counselling? A systematic narrative review. BJOG. 2013;120:412-27.
19. Jarrick S, Lundberg S, Stephansson O, Symreng A, Bottai M, Höijer J, et al. Pregnancy outcomes in women with immunoglobulin A nephropathy: a nation-wide populationbased cohort study. J Nephrol. 2021;34(5):1591-8.
20. Klemetti MM, Laivuori H, Tikkanen M, Nuutila M, Hiilesmaa V, Teramo K. Obstetric and perinatal outcome in type 1 diabetes patients with diabetic nephropathy during 1988-2011. Diabetologia. 2015;58:678-86.
21. Scott JE, Swallow V, Coulthard MG, Lambert HJ, Lee RE. Screening of newborn babies for familial ureteric reflux. Lancet. 1997;350:396-400.
22. Hladunewich MA, Hou S, Odutayo A, Cornelis T, Pierratos A, Goldstein M, et al. Intensive hemodialysis associates with improved pregnancy outcomes: a Canadian and United States cohort comparison. J Am Soc Nephrol. 2014;25(5):1103-9.
23. Piccoli GB, Minelli F, Versino E, Cabiddu G, Attini R, Vigotti FN, et al. Pregnancy in dialysis patients in the new millennium: a systematic review and meta-regression analysis correlating dialysis schedules and pregnancy outcomes. Nephrol Dial Transplant. 2016;31(11):1915-34.
24. Sato JL, De Oliveira L, Kirsztajn GM, Sass N. Chronic kidney disease in pregnancy requiring first-time dialysis. Int J Gynaecol Obstet. 2010;111(1):45-8.
25. Misra R, Bhowmik D, Mittal S, Kriplani A, Kumar S, Bhatla N, et al. Pregnancy with chronic kidney disease: outcome in Indian women. J Womens Health (Larchmt). 2003;12(10):1019-25.
26. Chopra S, Suri V, Aggarwal N, Rohilla M, Keepanasseril A, Kohli HS. Pregnancy in chronic renal insufficiency: single centre experience from North India. Arch Gynecol Obstet. 2009;279(5):691-5.
27. Singh R, Prasad N, Banka A, Gupta A, Bhadauria D, Sharma RK, et al. Pregnancy in patients with chronic kidney disease: Maternal and fetal outcomes. Indian J Nephrol. 2015;25(4):194-9.

CHAPTER 16

Dialysis in Pregnancy

Kiran Munir, Mala Sachdeva

HIGHLIGHTS

- Patients on dialysis are much less likely to become pregnant and more likely to have complicated pregnancies compared to those with normal kidney function.
- Hypertensive disorders, including uncontrolled hypertension, preeclampsia, and HELLP (hemolysis, elevated liver enzymes, low platelet) syndrome, are encountered in pregnant patients receiving dialysis.
- Major fetal issues for pregnant females on dialysis can include high rates of neonatal death/stillbirth, preterm birth, and low birth weight.
- Patients are seen frequently and we suggest at least monthly during the early first trimester, every two weeks in the second trimester, and weekly in the third trimester.
- Hemodialysis, peritoneal dialysis, or home hemodialysis are all options for women trying to conceive and all pregnant patients on dialysis.
- More frequent and/or longer dialysis sessions can:
  - Decrease the risk of polyhydramnios
  - Help control hypertension
  - Increase birth weight and gestational age
  - Improve maternal nutrition
  - Increase the chances of live birth
- For patients without residual kidney function, at least 36 hours of dialysis per week is suggested, however may not be feasible.
- Some experts recommend targeting a lower blood urea nitrogen level.

INTRODUCTION

Caring for women of childbearing age on dialysis is becoming more common. This can be attributed to improved dialysis techniques, more intense prescriptions, improved anemia management, better blood pressure and volume control, or even advances in fertility treatments. Nephrologists should remember to ask these women about their future pregnancy plans. Ideally, contraception should be discussed with them to prevent unplanned pregnancies. If possible, pregnancy should be delayed until after kidney transplantation. Still, there are a number of women who conceive while they are on dialysis and some women with advanced chronic kidney disease who conceive and progress to requiring dialysis during pregnancy. In this chapter, we discuss the history of pregnancy and dialysis, followed by a discussion of how best to dialyze a pregnant woman.

HISTORY OF PREGNANCY AND DIALYSIS

In 1965, the first United States case report was published where a 33-year-old, 32-week pregnant patient was dialyzed four times within 3 weeks and then delivered.[1] In 1968, the second United States case report was published where a pregnant woman was dialyzed 5 days per week for 8 hours a day from the 30th to 37th week of pregnancy and then delivered.[2] Both deliveries resulted in viable infants. The first international case report was published in Italy in 1971, where a pregnant woman was dialyzed two times a week for a total of 24 hours per week.[3] After this, numerous case series and surveys were published worldwide. The first case series reporting sixteen successful pregnancies in women on hemodialysis was published by the European Dialysis and Transplant Association in 1980.[4] In the late 1990s and 2000s, Saudi Arabia, the United States, Belgium, Brazil, Australia and New Zealand, and Canada all reported their experiences with dialyzing pregnant women. Successful and unsuccessful pregnancies were discussed.[5-11] More recently, in a review in 2016, compared to 2000–2008, from 2000–2014 there was an increase in a number of pregnancies in dialysis patients, reaching >600 reported pregnancies.[12] A 2019 study also showed that the pregnancy rate in the United States has been increasing, reaching 40.9 per thousand person-years in women aged 20–24.[13]

INITIAL STEPS

Upon finding out that a dialysis patient is pregnant, the patient should be referred to a high-risk maternal-fetal medicine obstetrician to receive intense counseling on the risks and benefits of the pregnancy, their risk of poorer maternal and fetal outcomes, and the options to terminate or continue the pregnancy. For the mother, pregnancy can result in poorer outcomes which could include increased risk of miscarriage, placental abruption, premature rupture of membranes, preeclampsia/eclampsia, uncontrolled hypertension, anemia, infections, premature delivery, cesarian sections, or even maternal death. For the fetus, the poor outcomes include intra-uterine growth restriction, respiratory abnormalities, lower birth weight infants, small for gestational age, premature delivery, increased neonatal intensive care unit stays, or even neonatal death.[14,15]

After counseling, should a patient decide to proceed with the pregnancy, a number of changes should be made to their medications and the dialysis prescription.

INITIAL MEDICATION ADJUSTMENTS

A thorough review of medications should be performed. Teratogenic medications should be discontinued. These include discontinuation of angiotensin-converting enzyme (ACE) inhibitors and angiotensin receptor blockers (ARBs), renin blockers, mineralocorticoid receptor antagonists, mycophenolate mofetil, or any other fetotoxic medications. Labetalol, nifedipine, hydralazine, and methyldopa can be anti-hypertensive substitutes if needed.

INDICATIONS AND TIMING FOR INITIATION OF DIALYSIS IN A PREGNANT WOMAN

The reasons to start dialysis in a pregnant patient are similar to a nonpregnant female dependent on when the nephrologist, obstetrician, and patient agree that the benefits of dialysis will outweigh the burden and risks. Acidemia, bone mineral disease, anemia, residual kidney function, along with volume management, hypertension, and uremic symptoms such as severe anorexia constitute the plethora of laboratories and clinical symptoms which are closely monitored as the patient progresses to advanced CKD. Management of these components is key in delaying the need for dialysis and dialysis should be initiated when medical management is no longer effective.

Initiation of dialysis, however, may sometimes be earlier in pregnant women if acidosis cannot be controlled medically or if blood urea nitrogen (BUN) level continues to increase. BUN levels >50 mg/dL have been associated with poorer fetal outcomes. Retrospective studies have recommended to target lower BUN levels.[16] One study showed a correlation of lower predialysis BUN levels of 48–49 mg/dL or less with increased birth weight and gestational age of delivery.[17] More recently, there was a recommendation that achieving an average midweek BUN <35 mg/dL led to better fetal outcomes.[18] With frequent, longer dialysis in pregnant women, it has been noted that their pre-dialysis BUN levels fall below even 30 mg/dL, hence this is an achievable target.

During pregnancy, patients' serum bicarbonate levels decrease to 20–21 mEq/L due to increased minute ventilation. Maintaining serum bicarbonate somewhere between 18 and 20 mEq/L can be a common practice in pregnant woman. Oral bicarbonate therapy is frequently added to maintain this. If serum bicarbonate is unable to be maintained despite maximal oral therapy, initiation of dialysis should be considered as acidemia can adversely affect fetal bone growth, circulation, and may even lead to fetal demise.

MODALITY CHOICES

Dialysis modalities during pregnancy can include in-center intermittent hemodialysis or home therapies such as peritoneal dialysis and home hemodialysis. Generally, if a woman is on hemodialysis, peritoneal dialysis, or home hemodialysis/nocturnal dialysis at the time of conception, that same modality is continued. If dialysis is initiated during pregnancy, many nephrologists prefer hemodialysis due to the ease of placing a tunneled dialysis catheter or vascular access to start dialysis. Patient preference, comorbid conditions, and environmental and social factors should also be considered.

Reports of using peritoneal dialysis (PD) during pregnancy date back to the 1980s.[19-21] There are no comparisons of utilizing chronic ambulatory peritoneal dialysis (CAPD) with automated peritoneal dialysis (APD) during pregnancy. If a female has significant residual urine output, she may be considered for PD. Benefits of PD during pregnancy include a continuous, more hemodynamically stable therapy. This, however, needs to be balanced with the gravid abdomen in late pregnancy, requiring changes in the PD prescription such as longer therapy times, increasing the number of cycles, and decreasing dwell volumes to decrease the sensation of abdominal fullness for the pregnant woman.

A 2019 study reported more pregnancies in patients on hemodialysis than PD.[13] This was consistent with prior studies. A registry of pregnancy in dialysis patients in 1998 similarly showed less conception on PD than on hemodialysis.[8] One hypothesis the authors cited may be that the hypertonic peritoneal dialysate prevents fertilization or even transfer of the ovum to the fallopian tube. Still, no significant difference in outcomes is noted between the two modalities in terms of infant survival, frequency of prematurity, or low birth weight babies for women who conceived on both modalities.

Nocturnal hemodialysis pregnancies have been reported as well. Typically, these women were on 7–8 hours per day treatments for 5–7 nights per week.[22] Outcomes remained good on these therapies.

INTENSITY OF DIALYSIS

Providing intensive hemodialysis is a common approach for the pregnant woman on hemodialysis. The goal of dialysis is to reduce interdialytic weight gains, intradialytic hypotension, uremic toxin build up, and electrolyte derangements during the pregnancy. For many nephrologists, this means having discussions with their patients on increasing the time and frequency of their dialysis sessions. Intensified dialysis prescriptions have been shown to improve blood pressure and volume management, and lead to better fetal outcomes such as increased live birth rates and later gestational age of delivery. For those on hemodialysis, the prescribed time can be >36 hours per week if possible.[11] In a national survey conducted in 2017 on pregnancy outcomes in women on hemodialysis, physicians reported prescribing an average of 4–4.5 hours for 6 days/week for a composite of 23±7 h/week for their pregnant patient on dialysis.[23] An optimal start would be changing from 3 days a week to 6 days a week and from 3 to 3.5 hours a session to 4–5-hour treatments each session if >36 hours is not feasible. Dialysate flow rates and blood flow rates are as standard similar to nonpregnant patients, but one may need to gradually increase the blood flow rates during a typical dialysis session.

TARGET WEIGHT ADJUSTMENT

With more frequent dialysis, caution should be taken to prevent excessive fluid removal which can lead to intradialytic hypotension and thus placental hypoperfusion. Weekly monitoring and adjustment of dry weight should be performed, accounting for mother's weight gain and fetal weight gain. Target weight can increase approximately 0.5 kg per week during the second and third trimesters, necessitating continuous weekly adjustments. When adjusting the dry weight, it is important to also evaluate the patient and make adjustments based on their blood pressure measurement trends obtained pre-, intra-, and postdialysis sessions, interdialytic weight gains, and physical examination dictating the presence or absence of volume overload.

MEDICATION MANAGEMENT DURING THE PREGNANCY

Frequent dialysis may also lead to lower levels of serum potassium and phosphorus levels. Liberalizing potassium and phosphorus in the women's diet and eliminating phosphorus binders is recommended. In fact, addition of potassium or phosphorus supplements is common. If the patient remains hypokalemic, higher dialysate potassium baths can be used.

Pregnancy in females with CKD will need close monitoring of their iron panel and hemoglobin levels to ensure hemoglobin levels remain at target, for optimal delivery of oxygen for fetal growth. Erythropoietin stimulating agents (ESAs) and iron therapy are considered safe for pregnant patients. ESAs can be utilized to maintain hemoglobin levels during pregnancy. If epoetin alpha is used, the use of a single-dose vial rather than a multi-dose vial is preferred due to the multidose vial containing benzyl alcohol which is contraindicated in both pregnant and lactating women due to fetal neurotoxic effects. Intravenous iron is allowed during pregnancy and is preferred over the oral route similarly to the nonpregnant dialysis patient.

Since water-soluble vitamins are lost with dialysis, extra supplementation of folic acid should be given during pregnancy. Dosages of up to 5 mg per day of folic acid can be administered.

The risk of preeclampsia is increased in pregnant dialysis women. Although not studied in the end-stage kidney disease (ESKD) population, aspirin can be started as a preventative measure if there is no usual contraindication.[24]

Heparin can be used with dialysis to decrease the risk of clotting. Contraindications to heparin would be the same as any patient and could include a recent bleeding event or thrombocytopenia. Toward the end of pregnancy, heparin is usually stopped in case emergent surgery is needed. Most of the time, for dialysis patients who get intensified dialysis prescriptions, BUN is usually low, thus eliminating the need for DDAVP at the time of delivery if a cesarian section is done.

DIALYSIS ACCESS

If dialysis is started before arm access is placed, access of choice by many nephrologists would be a graft which we can cannulate within 1 week of placement. This minimizes the presence of hemodialysis catheters and hence reduces the risk of infection.

LABORATORY MONITORING

Continuation of standard monthly blood work during dialysis should be performed as usual, including clearances, complete blood counts, iron studies, calcium, phosphorus, parathyroid levels, and electrolytes. Nutrition should be assessed with serum albumin level. By the 20th week of pregnancy, hemolysis laboratories including haptoglobin and lactate dehydrogenase and hepatic function tests should be added and checked every 2 weeks to allow for any early detection of HELLP (hemolysis, elevated liver enzymes, low platelet count) syndrome. Of note, because creatinine is cleared during dialysis, it cannot be used diagnostically as a criterion for preeclampsia. Likewise, proteinuria or 24-hour urine collections cannot be utilized as many dialysis women are oliguric or anuric.

TIMING AND MODE OF DELIVERY

If the woman has not delivered earlier, in the high-risk ESKD population, obstetricians tend to plan elective delivery around 37 weeks. After this time, the benefits of prolonging pregnancy may outweigh the risks. Induction versus cesarean section is decided by the obstetrician based on the history of prior pregnancies and need at the time of delivery.

In an Indian series of pregnant women with CKD, three out of five patients had viable fetuses, whereas the remaining two patients had fetuses with intrauterine growth retardation and low birth weight.[25]

Figure 1 summarizes the chapter hemodialysis during pregnancy.

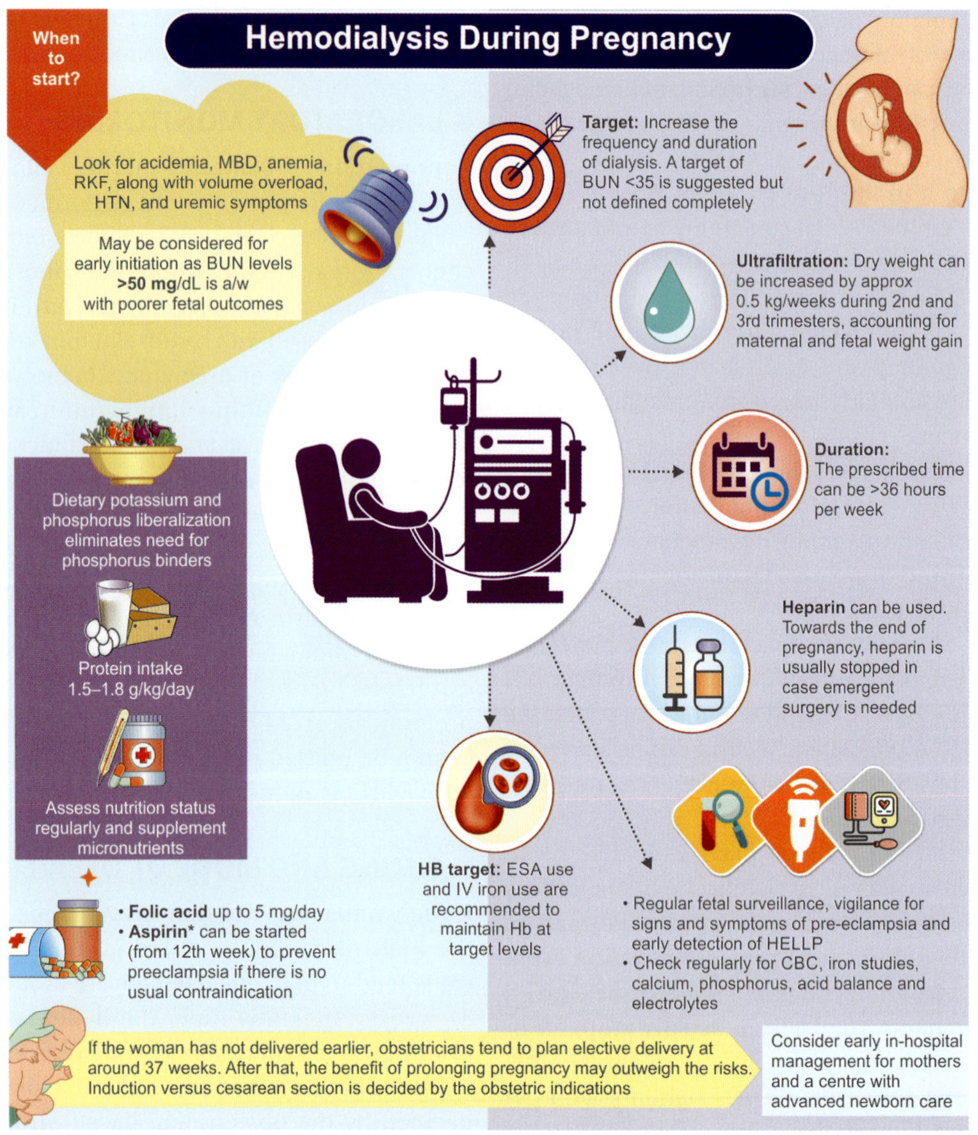

Fig. 1: Hemodialysis during pregnancy. (BUN: blood urea nitrogen; CBC: complete blood count; ESA: erythropoietin stimulating agent; HELLP: hemolysis, elevated liver enzymes, low platelet; RKF: residual kidney function; HTN: hypertension in pregnancy; MBD: metabolic bone disease)

Note: *Not studied in ESKD patients

Courtesy: Dr Priti Meena

CONCLUSION

Encountering a pregnant woman on dialysis is becoming more common. Live birth rates of women on dialysis in the United States seem to be increasing. Maternal and fetal outcomes can be improved with close monitoring, timely initiation of dialysis, and intensive dialysis prescriptions. Preeclampsia remains a major complication of pregnancy and one must monitor for signs and symptoms of preeclampsia or HELLP syndrome which can occur. A good multidisciplinary team approach involving internists, obstetricians, nephrologists, nutritionists, and social work can lead to successful pregnancies.

REFERENCES

1. Herwig KR, Merill JP, Jackson RL, Oken DE. Chronic renal disease and pregnancy. Am J Obstet Gynecol. 1965;92:1117-21.
2. Orme BM, Ueland K, Simpson DP, Scribner BH. The effect of hemodialysis on fetal survival and renal function in pregnancy. Trans Am Soc Artif Intern Organs. 1968;14:402-4.
3. Confortini P, Galanti G, Ancona G, Giongo A, Bruschi E, Lorenzini E. Full term pregnancy and successful delivery in a patient on chronic haemodialysis. Proc Eur Dial Transplant Assoc. 1971;8:74-80.
4. Registration Committee of the European Dialysis and Transplant Association. Successful pregnancies in women treated by dialysis and kidney transplantation. Report from the Registration Committee of the European Dialysis and Transplant Association. Br J Obstet Gynaecol. 1980;87:839-45.
5. Souqiyyeh MZ, Huraib SO, Saleh AGM, Aswad S. Pregnancy in chronic hemodialysis patients in the Kingdom of Saudi Arabia. Am J Kidney Dis. 1992;19:235-8
6. Hou S. Frequency and outcome of pregnancy in women on dialysis. Am J Kidney Dis. 1994;23:60-3.
7. Bagon JA, Vernaeve H, Muylder XD, Lafontaine JJ, Martens J, Van Roost G. Pregnancy and dialysis. Am J Kidney Dis. 1998;31:756-65.
8. Okundaye I, Abrinko P, Hou S. Registry of pregnancy in dialysis patients. Am J Kidney Dis. 1998;31:766-73.
9. Luders C, Castro MCM, Titan SM, De Castro I, Elias RM, Abensur H, et al. Obstetric outcome in pregnant women on long term dialysis: a case series. Am J Kidney Dis. 2010;56:77-85.
10. Shahir AK, Briggs N, Katsoulis J, Levidiotis V. An observational outcome study from 1966–2008, examining pregnancy and neonatal outcomes from dialyzed women using data from ANZDATA Registry. Nephrology. 2013;18:276-84.
11. Hladunewich MA, Hou S, Odutayo A, Cornelis T, Pierratos A, Goldstein M, et al. Intensive hemodialysis associates with improved outcomes: a Canadian and United States cohort comparison. J Am Soc Nephrol. 2014;25:1-7.
12. Piccoli GB, Minelli F, Versino E, Cabiddu G, Attini R, Vigotti FN, et al. Pregnancy in dialysis patients in the new millennium: A systematic review and meta-regression analysis correlating dialysis schedules and pregnancy outcomes. Nephrol Dial Transplant. 2016;31:1915-34.
13. Shah S, Christianson AL, Meganathan K, Leonard AC, Schauer DP, Thakar CV. Racial Differences and Factors Associated with Pregnancy in ESKD Patients on Dialysis in the United States. J Am Soc Nephrol. 2019;30(12):2437-48.
14. Tangren J, Nadel M, Hladunewich MA. Pregnancy and end-stage renal disease. Blood Purif. 2018;45:194-200.
15. Manisco G, Poti M, Maggiulli G, DiTullio M, Losappio V, Vernaglion L. Pregnancy in end-stage renal disease patients on dialysis: how to achieve a successful delivery. Clin Kidney J. 2015;8:293-9.
16. Holley JL, Reddy SS. Pregnancy in dialysis patients: A review of outcomes, complications, and management. Semin Dial. 2003;16: 384-88.
17. Asamiya Y, Otsubo S, Matsuda Y, Kimata N, Kikuchi KAN, Miwa N, et al. The importance of low blood urea nitrogen levels in pregnant patients undergoing hemodialysis to optimize birth weight and gestational age. Kidney Int. 2009;75:1217-22.
18. Luders C, Titan SM, Kahhale S, Francisco RP, Zugaib M. Risk Factors for Adverse Fetal Outcome in Hemodialysis Pregnant Women. Kidney Int Rep. 2018;3(5): 1077-88.

19. Redrow M, Cherem L, Elliott J, Mangalat J, Mishler RE, Bennett WM, et al. Dialysis in the management of pregnant patients with renal insufficiency. Medicine (Baltimore). 1988;67:199-208.
20. Cattran DC, Benzie RJ. Pregnancy in a continuous ambulatory peritoneal dialysis patient. Perit Dial Bull. 1983;3:13-14.
21. Kioko EM, Shaw KM, Clarke AD, Warren DJ. Successful pregnancy in a diabetic patient treated with continuous ambulatory peritoneal dialysis. Diabetes Care. 1983;6: 298-300.
22. Barua M, Hladunewich M, Keunen J, Pierratos A, McFarlane P, Sood M, et al. Successful pregnancies on nocturnal home hemodialysis. Clin J Am Soc Nephrol. 2008;3(2):392-6.
23. Sachdeva M, Barta V, Thakkar J, Sakhiya V, Miller I. Pregnancy outcomes in women on hemodialysis: a national survey. Clin Kidney J. 2017;10(2):276-81.
24. American College of Obstetricians and Gynecologists. ACOG Committee Opinion No. 743: Low-Dose Aspirin Use During Pregnancy. Obstet Gynecol. 2018;132(1):e44-e52.
25. Choudhary S, Mishra VV, Shinde S, Patel H, Aggarwal R, Gandhi K. Chronic Kidney Disease with Pregnancy: Hemodialysis can be considered for Better Maternal and Fetal Outcomes. J South Asian Feder Obst Gynae. 2021;13(1):11-4.

CHAPTER 17

Kidney Transplantation and Pregnancy

Namrata Parikh, Prasoon Verma, Silvi Shah

HIGHLIGHTS

- Chronic kidney disease is associated with disruption of hypothalamic gonadal axis, but kidney transplant restores fertility.
- Pregnancy in a kidney transplant recipient is challenging due to risk of deterioration of kidney function, a higher risk of adverse maternal outcomes of preeclampsia and hypertension, and a higher risk of adverse fetal complications of premature birth, low birth weight, and small for gestational age infants.
- The factors associated with poor pregnancy outcomes include presence of hypertension, serum creatinine greater than 1.4 mg/dL, and proteinuria.
- The recommended maintenance immunosuppression during pregnancy in patients with kidney transplant is calcineurin inhibitors (tacrolimus/cyclosporine), azathioprine, and low dose prednisone.
- Sirolimus and mycophenolate mofetil should be stopped 6 weeks prior to conception.
- Pregnancy in a kidney transplant recipient should be managed in a multidisciplinary team consisting of transplant nephrologist, maternal fetal medicine, and a neonatologist.

INTRODUCTION

One of the consequences of chronic kidney disease (CKD), which is often underrecognized but associated with reduced quality of life, is impaired reproductive function and infertility. Several contributory factors have been identified, but the most important is the disruption of the hypothalamic-pituitary-ovarian axis by the uremic milieu.[1] Other associated factors include functional response, abnormal endometrial morphology, reduced ovarian reserve, and loss of libido. Measures to improve fertility include assisted reproduction technology, intensification of dialysis prescriptions, and kidney transplantation. According to data from the United States Organ Transplant Procurement Network (OPTN), in 2022, 9,953 women underwent kidney transplantation.[2] Of these, approximately 37% were in the childbearing age group of 18–49 years. Hence, it becomes very relevant to discuss the implications of transplantation on pregnancy outcomes and the impact of pregnancy on the allograft function.

TRANSPLANTATION AND FERTILITY

It has been described that the hypothalamic-pituitary axis can resume normal function within 6 months of successful kidney transplantation.[3] Moreover, pregnancy may have undesirable outcomes on allograft function, and traditionally, guidelines have advocated against pregnancy for at least 2 years after transplantation. More recently, it has been suggested that in the absence of recent rejection or infectious complication, pregnancy may be considered at 1 year post-transplantation.[4] While the ideal time for conception remains a matter of debate, the American Society of Transplantation Consensus Conference on Reproductive Issues and Transplantation concluded that preconception counseling should form a part of pretransplant evaluation and that this should be revisited throughout the post-transplant period.[4] Counseling should be offered to both prospective parents and should include information about potential risks to allograft as well as implications on maternal and fetal health.

Of note, the 2016 US Medical Eligibility Criteria for Contraceptive Use suggests that pregnancy within 2 years of solid organ transplantation may be associated with an increased risk for adverse health events. The same criteria have listed most methods of contraception as category 2, meaning "advantages of using the method generally outweigh the theoretical or proven risks" for patients with uncomplicated post-transplant course.[5] Hence, women should make an informed decision about contraception preference for at least the first year after transplantation, and this should ideally be done before transplantation during the evaluation process.

RECOMMENDED CRITERIA FOR PREGNANCY POST-KIDNEY TRANSPLANTATION

The 2005 AST consensus conference summary has provided certain criteria for determining timing for pregnancy post-transplantation **(Box 1)**.

BOX 1: Criteria for pregnancy in kidney transplant recipients to determine the timing of pregnancy.

- No rejection in the past one year
- Adequate and stable graft function (creatinine <1.5 mg/dL) or no or minimal proteinuria (<500 mg/24 hours)
- No acute infections that might impact the fetus
- Maintenance immunosuppression at stable dosing, which is safe during pregnancy
- Blood pressure at goal

Special circumstances that may impact recommendations on the timing of pregnancy include a history of rejection within the 1st year, maternal age, comorbid factors that may impact pregnancy and graft function, and established medical non-compliance. Pregnancies outside the guidelines need to be evaluated on a case-by-case basis. In addition, the Society for Maternal–Fetal Medicine has suggested recommendations for baseline evaluation before pregnancy in solid organ transplant recipients.[6] These include:

- Multidisciplinary consultation with transplant surgery, nephrology, maternal–fetal medicine, and other medical subspecialists as required
- Post-transplant history, including episodes of acute rejection or potentially fetotoxic infections
- Comprehensive medical history, including medical comorbidities and indication for solid organ transplant
- Medication history, including maintenance immunosuppressive regimen
- Assessment of vaccination status
- Complete physical examination including blood pressure assessment
- Baseline laboratory evaluation (including complete metabolic panel, complete blood count, hemoglobin A1c, and urine protein/creatinine ratio)

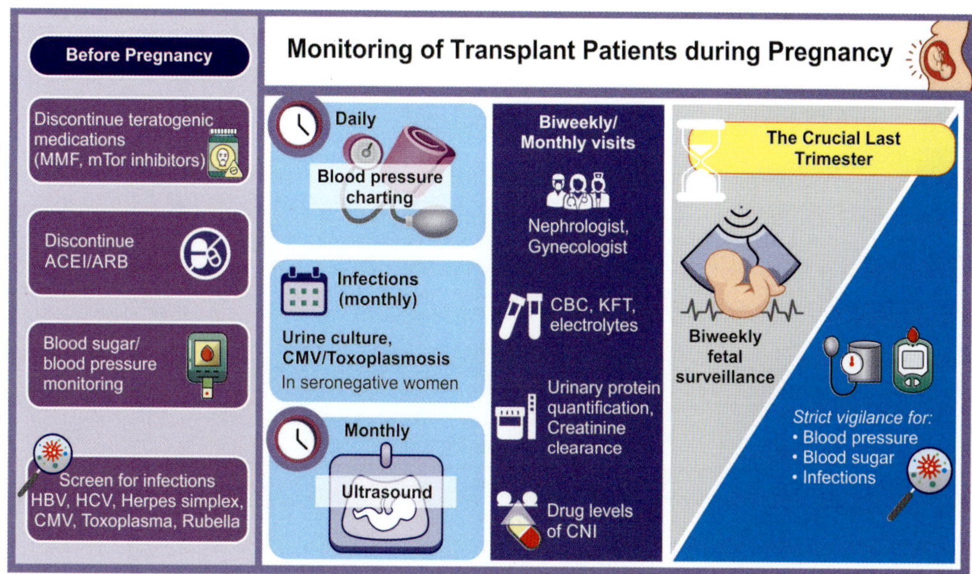

Fig. 1: Monitoring of transplant patients during pregnancy. (ACEI: angiotensin-converting enzyme inhibitors; ARB: angiotensin receptor blocker; CMV: cytomegalovirus; CNI: calcineurin inhibitors; HBV: hepotitus B virus; HCV: hepotitus C virus; MMF: mycophenolate mofetil)

Courtesy: Dr Priti Meena

- Type and screen because of risk for post-transplant red blood cell alloimmunization
- Evaluation of psychosocial status

Figure 1 shows monitoring of transplant patient during pregnancy.

MANAGEMENT OF TRANSPLANT IMMUNOSUPPRESSION

Immunosuppression before, during, and after pregnancy must be carefully planned to mitigate the risk of teratogenicity while at the same time avoiding adverse effects on graft function. **Table 1** lists the safety profile of common immunosuppression medications used in kidney transplant recipients.[7]

Note that most transplantation protocols incorporate mycophenolate mofetil or mycophenolic acid, which is contraindicated in pregnancy and requires switching over to an alternative antimetabolite, such as azathioprine, at least 6 weeks before conception. For mTOR inhibitors such as sirolimus and everolimus, the limited data available is conflicting, and the current recommendation is to stop at least 6–12 weeks before conception.

EFFECT OF PREGNANCY ON ALLOGRAFT FUNCTION

In normal pregnancies, the estimated glomerular filtration rate (eGFR) increases by approximately 50% due to increased cardiac output, hyperfiltration, intrarenal vasodilatation, and reduced systemic vascular resistance.[9] In kidney transplant recipients, the creatinine clearance increases by up to 30% in the first trimester, decreases slightly in the second trimester, and then returns to normal in the third trimester.[10] Failure of the serum creatinine to fall in the first trimester may indicate acute kidney injury (AKI) and may need evaluation of

TABLE 1: Safety profile of immunosuppressive medications during pregnancy and breastfeeding.[8]

Drugs that may be used:		
Drug	***Pregnancy and breastfeeding***	
Prednisone	Safe	
Azathioprine	Safe	
Tacrolimus	Safe	
Cyclosporine	Safe	
Drugs that are contraindicated:		
Drug	***Teratogenic potential***	***Breastfeeding***
Mycophenolate mofetil/ mycophenolic acid	Congenital facial and limb defects, atrial septal defect, tracheoesophageal fistula	Not recommended—known teratogen
Sirolimus	Toxicity in animal studies	Not recommended—lack of safety evidence
Everolimus	Toxicity in animal studies	Not recommended—lack of safety evidence
Belatacept	No data	No data

graft function. A landmark prospective study by Davidson et al. showed that protein excretion increases throughout pregnancy and can even exceed 500 mg/day by the third trimester.[11] However, this should be interpreted cautiously and causes like urinary tract infection and preeclampsia should be ruled out.

ACUTE KIDNEY INJURY IN KIDNEY TRANSPLANT RECIPIENTS

A study of over 5 million hospitalizations resulting in delivery showed that pregnant kidney transplant recipients had 11-fold higher odds of developing AKI during hospitalization compared to pregnant women with no known kidney disease.[12] Conventional definitions of AKI have not been validated in pregnancy. Moreover, as mentioned above, serum creatinine usually falls in the first trimester, making it even more challenging to diagnose AKI in pregnant kidney transplant recipients and may lead to delayed diagnosis. This highlights the importance of a multidisciplinary approach to pregnancy in kidney transplant recipients with regular follow-up.

The causes of AKI in kidney transplant recipients are a combination of causes of AKI in pregnancy and causes of allograft dysfunction. Pregnancy-related complications like preeclampsia, hemolysis, elevated liver enzymes, low platelets (HELLP) syndrome, thrombotic microangiopathy, hemolytic uremic syndrome, etc. are more likely to be the cause of AKI in the second and third trimester of pregnancy. However, several transplant-specific factors may contribute to AKI and are listed in **Table 2**.

PREGNANCY OUTCOMES IN KIDNEY TRANSPLANT RECIPIENTS

Pregnancy has several important implications on the mother's health, allograft

TABLE 2: Causes of AKI in kidney transplant recipients.

Prerenal (Solitary functioning kidney in kidney transplant recipients with impaired autoregulation is more susceptible)	• Volume depletion due to hyperemesis gravidarum • Use of calcineurin inhibitors which cause arteriolar vasoconstriction • Opportunistic infections due to immunocompromised status—sepsis, infectious diarrhea, refluxing transplant ureter causing pyelonephritis, etc.
Renal	*Immunological causes*: • Cellular or antibody medicated rejection • Transplant glomerulopathy • Recurrence of or de novo glomerulonephritis *Medication*: • Calcineurin inhibitors • Antibiotics *Infectious causes*: • Polyomavirus nephropathy • Systemic cytomegalovirus infection • Pyelonephritis • Sepsis *Pregnancy-related complications*: • Preeclampsia • HELLP syndrome • Acute fatty liver of pregnancy • Disseminated intravascular coagulation *Vascular*: • Renal artery/vein thrombosis • Allograft thrombosis • Thrombotic microangiopathy • Progression of underlying kidney disease
Postrenal	• Hydronephrosis due to ureteral obstruction • Neurogenic bladder • Injury to ureters during cesarean section • Abdominal compartment syndrome in the setting of multiple transplants or multifetal gestation • Malignancy like post-transplant lymphoproliferative disease (may also have intrinsic kidney involvement)

(AKI: acute kidney injury; HELLP: hemolysis, elevated liver enzymes, low platelet)
Source: Modified from Yadav et al.[13]

function, and the developing fetus. **Table 3** shows data regarding pregnancy outcomes from the Transplant Pregnancy Registry International (TPRI—a voluntary registry of pregnancy outcomes in solid organ transplant recipients) and two important meta-analyses.

IMPACT ON MATERNAL HEALTH

Hypertension and Preeclampsia

Hypertension is a well-known consequence of CKD and is frequently encountered in the post-transplant population. Studies have estimated that the prevalence of

TABLE 3: Summary of pregnancy outcomes in kidney transplant recipients.

Outcome	*TPRI annual report, 2017*	*Deshpande et al. (meta-analysis)*	*Shah et al. (meta-analysis)*
Hypertension in pregnancy (%)	48.0	54.2	24.2*
Preeclampsia (%)	31.0	27.0	21.5
Acute rejection during pregnancy (%)	1.0	4.2	9.4
Postpartum rejection (%)	1.3	NR	NR
Graft loss within 2 years of pregnancy (%)	5.6	8.1	9.2
Preterm birth (<37 weeks) (%)	51	45.6	43.1
Live births (%)	75.0	73.5	72.9
Miscarriages (%)	18.0	14.0	15.4
Neonatal deaths (%)	1.4	NR	3.8
Stillbirths (%)	2.0	2.5	5.1
Birth defects (%)	4.5	NR	NR

*Only pregnancy-induced hypertension reported
(NR: not reported: TPRI: Transplant Pregnancy Registry International)
Source: Modified from Kumar et al.[14]

hypertension in kidney transplant recipients is around 50–80%.[15] Hence, it follows that hypertensive disorders of pregnancy are more frequently encountered in kidney transplant recipients. While preeclampsia complicates around 4–5% of pregnancies in the general population,[10] this risk is increased up to six-fold in kidney transplant recipients, with the prevalence ranging from 20 to 30% **(Table 3)**. Moreover, diagnosis is often challenging because of the presence of confounding factors. Many of these women have pre-existing proteinuria, which can be made worse by hyperfiltration. Moreover, using calcineurin inhibitors is associated with hyperuricemia, which reduces the reliability of serum uric acid as a marker of preeclampsia. Uterine artery Dopplers may be helpful in early diagnosis. Worsening of hypertension with an increase in serum creatinine and proteinuria may also be seen in acute rejection, which needs to be differentiated from preeclampsia.

A best practice position statement by the Italian Society of Nephrology has stressed strict control of hypertension with an "ideal" target of <130/80 mm Hg. Blood pressure <140/90 mm Hg is acceptable.[16] Hypertension in these patients should be managed with β-blockers, calcium-channel blockers, methyldopa, or hydralazine. Drugs like angiotensin-converting enzyme inhibitors and angiotensin receptor blockers must be avoided owing to teratogenic potential. As in all high-risk pregnancies, aspirin should be offered to all kidney transplant recipients for its protective role against preeclampsia.

EFFECTS ON GRAFT FUNCTION

In the absence of risk factors, pregnancy by itself is not associated with the worsening of graft function in kidney transplant recipients. Evidence suggests that the risk of worsening graft function and graft loss is higher in the presence of:[10]

- Pre-existing hypertension
- Baseline serum creatinine ≥1.4 mg/dL
- An episode of rejection within 1–2 years before pregnancy
- Baseline proteinuria ≥500 mg/24 hours

RISK OF GRAFT REJECTION

Although pregnancy is considered an immunosuppressed state, there is evidence to suggest that there is no change in the maternal immune response on the systemic level and that maternal responses to the allogeneic fetus are only suppressed at the maternal-fetal interface.[4] Moreover, the fetal antigens themselves may trigger the maternal immune system. Hence, reducing the transplant immunosuppression can lead to graft rejection. The incidence of acute rejection in pregnancy is not more than that in the nonpregnant kidney transplant population without risk factors **(Table 3)**. Risk factors include higher baseline serum creatinine, rejection before pregnancy, and reduction in baseline immunosuppression medication dose.[10] Further, it can be quite challenging to distinguish rejection from preeclampsia, as discussed above, and diagnosis may be delayed due to a physiological fall in serum creatinine early in pregnancy. Ultrasound-guided allograft biopsy is considered safe before 25 weeks. High-dose corticosteroids may be used for the treatment of rejection, but there is limited data regarding the use of thymoglobulin, intravenous immunoglobulins, rituximab, and plasmapheresis.

MATERNAL INFECTIONS

There is an increased incidence of maternal infections, particularly urinary tract infections, in pregnant kidney transplant recipients. This is due to a combination of factors, including the use of immunosuppressive medications, anatomy of the transplant ureter, and pregnancy-related dilation of renal collecting ducts and ureters. Hence, regular screening for urinary tract infections should be carried out with dipstick testing and urine cultures. European best practice guidelines for renal transplantation suggest that urine cultures should be performed monthly and that all asymptomatic infections should be treated.[17]

It is also widely recognized that cytomegalovirus (CMV) infection is commonly encountered in kidney transplant recipients. In pregnant women, CMV infection is associated with vertical transmission and may lead to fetal anomalies such as microcephaly, hearing loss, developmental delay, and perinatal morbidity. There is limited data regarding the safety and efficacy of antiviral agents like ganciclovir in pregnancy. Moreover, data is lacking to guide monitoring and timing of pregnancy after CMV infection. Hence, the Society of Maternal-Fetal Medicine has suggested that solid organ transplant recipients should ideally complete any indicated antiviral prophylaxis or treatment before pursuing pregnancy.[6]

IMPACT ON FETAL HEALTH

Preterm Birth, Fetal Growth Restriction, and Low Birth Weight

The incidence of preterm birth in infants born to kidney transplant recipients is high **(Table 3)**, and up to 50% of these women have preterm delivery. This is in significant contrast to the incidence of 5–15% in the general population. Medical conditions causing maternal and fetal complications (most commonly maternal hypertension) are the most frequent causes of preterm deliveries. Pregnancy in kidney transplant recipients is also associated with an increased incidence of intrauterine growth restriction and ranges from 20 to 30%, 2–3 times higher that seen in the general population.[18] A United Kingdom national cohort study that studied 105 pregnancies in 101 kidney transplant recipients reported that there was a 13-fold higher risk of preterm deliveries, 12-fold higher risk of low birth weight babies, and five-fold higher risk of small for gestation babies as compared to the general population.[19] Preterm births and low birth weight are associated with significant morbidity and mortality and have short- and long-term implications. Women contemplating pregnancy after a kidney transplant should be counseled on the higher risk of adverse fetal outcomes.

Stillbirth and Perinatal Mortality

As seen from **Table 3**, the live birth rate in kidney transplant recipients is like that in the general population (70–75%). However, the miscarriage rate ranges from 11 to 26% (compared to 8–9%). Factors associated with increased perinatal mortality include serum creatinine >1.3 mg/dL, proteinuria >500 mg per day, diastolic blood pressure >90 mm Hg, and more than one kidney transplant.[19]

LABOR AND DELIVERY

Delivery by cesarean section is not indicated for these patients in the absence of obstetric indications. The allograft itself is not obstructive to delivery, and spontaneous labor can be allowed up to 38–40 weeks, if there are no obstetrical complications. A registry-based retrospective cohort study including 1,435 kidney transplant recipients suggested that a trial of labor was not associated with adverse pregnancy outcomes and was associated with decreased neonatal morbidity.[20] However, for reasons not fully understood, the likelihood of cesarean section is higher in kidney transplant recipients compared to the general population (up to five-fold higher).[19] One of the most frequently implicated factors is fetal distress. When contemplating delivery by cesarean section, involving the transplant surgical team may be beneficial. Overall, the incidence of injury to the allograft is <1%. Medication used for analgesia and anesthesia should consider the pharmacokinetics of the agent used and potential drug–drug interactions with the immunosuppression.

BREASTFEEDING

As seen in **Table 1**, immunosuppressive drugs such as azathioprine, tacrolimus, cyclosporine, and prednisone are considered safe in breastfeeding women. Infant exposure to these drugs via breast milk is low (tacrolimus: <1% of maternal dose; prednisone: <0.1% of maternal dose; azathioprine: undetectable).[8,10] Data is limited for exposure to mycophenolate, sirolimus, everolimus, and belatacept through breastmilk, and hence, these drugs should be avoided in lactating women.

In an Indian study, 16 kidney transplant patients who had become pregnant were evaluated.[21] Among these patients, eight had abortions, six had full-term deliveries, and two had preterm deliveries. Two individuals experienced the onset of gestational hypertension, which was identified for the first time at 20 weeks of gestation. One patient experienced graft rejection 2 months after undergoing an abortion, while another patient developed cholestasis of pregnancy starting from the 7th month of gestation.

CONCLUSION

Chronic kidney disease leads to infertility, which can be reversed through successful kidney transplantation. Women of childbearing age should receive counseling about contraception and the implications of pregnancy on maternal, fetal, and transplant outcomes. Pregnancy in kidney transplant recipients should be considered high risk and requires multidisciplinary follow-up. Prerequisites include stable allograft function with no recent rejection or infection and modifying immunosuppression to a pregnancy and lactation-safe regimen.

Figure 1 shows important points for monitoring of a kidney transplant patient during pregnancy.

FUNDING

SS is supported by the National Institutes of Health K23 career development award, under Award Number 1K23HL151816-01A1. The content is solely the responsibility of the authors and does not necessarily represent the official views of the National Institutes of Health. The funders of the study had no role in writing the report, and the decision to submit the report for publication.

COMPETING INTERESTS

All the authors have no disclosures and competing interests with regards to submitted work.

REFERENCES

1. Dumanski SM, Ahmed SB. Fertility and reproductive care in chronic kidney disease. J Nephrol. 2019;32(1):39-50.
2. Organ Procurement and Transplantation Network. National data. [online] Available from https://optn.transplant.hrsa.gov/data/view-data-reports/national-data/.[Last accessed May, 2024]
3. Saha MT, Saha HHT, Niskanen LK, Salmela KT, Pasternack AI. Time Course of serum prolactin and sex hormones following successful renal transplantation. nephron. 2002;92(3):735-7.
4. McKay DB, Josephson MA. Reproduction and Transplantation: Report on the AST Consensus Conference on Reproductive Issues and Transplantation. Am J Transplant. 2005;5(7):1592-9.
5. Curtis KM, Tepper NK, Jatlaoui TC, Berry-Bibee E, Horton LG, Zapata LB, et al. US Medical Eligibility Criteria for Contraceptive Use, 2016. MMWR Recomm Rep. 2016;65(3):1-103.
6. Irani RA, Coscia LA, Chang E, Lappen JR. Society for Maternal-Fetal Medicine Consult Series #66: Prepregnancy evaluation and pregnancy management of patients with solid organ transplants. Am J Obstet Gynecol. 2023;229(2):B10-32.
7. Levea SLL. Pregnancy and kidney transplantation. Kidney News. 2023;15(8):13-6.
8. Agarwal KA, Pavlakis M. Sexuality, contraception, and pregnancy in kidney transplantation. Kidney Med. 2021;3(5):837-47.
9. Davison JM, Dunlop W. Renal hemodynamics and tubular function in normal human pregnancy. Kidney Int. 1980;18(2):152-61.
10. Shah S, Verma P. Overview of pregnancy in renal transplant patients. Int J Nephrol. 2016;2016:e4539342.
11. Davison JM. The effect of pregnancy on kidney function in renal allograft recipients. Kidney Int. 1985;27(1):74-9.
12. Chewcharat A, Kattah AG, Thongprayoon C, Cheungpasitporn W, Boonpheng B, Gonzalez Suarez ML, et al. Comparison of hospitalization outcomes for delivery and resource utilization between pregnant women with kidney transplants and chronic kidney disease in the United States. Nephrol Carlton Vic. 2021;26(11):879-89.
13. Yadav A, Salas MAP, Coscia L, Basu A, Rossi AP, Sawinski D, et al. Acute kidney injury during pregnancy in kidney transplant recipients. Clin Transplant. 2022;36(5):e14668.
14. Ong SC, Kumar V. Pregnancy in a kidney transplant patient. Clin J Am Soc Nephrol. 2020;15(1):120-2.
15. Weir MR, Burgess ED, Cooper JE, Fenves AZ, Goldsmith D, McKay D, et al. Assessment and management of hypertension in transplant patients. J Am Soc Nephrol. 2015;26(6):1248-60.
16. Cabiddu G, Spotti D, Gernone G, Santoro D, Moroni G, Gregorini G, et al. A best-practice position statement on pregnancy after kidney transplantation: focusing on the unsolved questions. The Kidney and Pregnancy Study Group of the Italian Society of Nephrology. J Nephrol. 2018;31(5):665-81.

17. EBPG Expert Group on Renal Transplantation. European Best Practice Guidelines for Renal Transplantation. Section IV: Long-term management of the transplant recipient. IV.10. Pregnancy in renal transplant recipients. Nephrol Dial Transplant. 2002; 17 (Suppl 4):50-5.
18. Cyganek A, Pietrzak B, Kociszewska-Najman B, Grzechocińska B, Songin T, Foroncewicz B, et al. Intrauterine growth restriction in pregnant renal and liver transplant recipients: risk factors assessment. Transplant Proc. 2014;46(8):2794-7.
19. Bramham K, Nelson-Piercy C, Gao H, Pierce M, Bush N, Spark P, et al. Pregnancy in renal transplant recipients: A UK National Cohort Study. Clin J Am Soc Nephrol. 2013;8(2):290-8.
20. Yin O, Kallapur A, Coscia L, Kwan L, Tandel M, Constantinescu SA, et al. Mode of obstetric delivery in kidney and liver transplant recipients and associated maternal, neonatal, and graft morbidity during 5 decades of clinical practice. JAMA Netw Open. 2021;4(10):e2127378.
21. Mishra Vineet V, Sakshi N, Kavita M, Rohina A, Sumesh C, Khushali G. Pregnancy outcome in renal transplant recipients: Indian scenario. Indian J Transplant. 2016;10(3):57-60.

CHAPTER

18 Urinary Tract Infection in Pregnancy

Divya Bajpai, Manjusha Yadla

HIGHLIGHTS

- Urinary tract infections (UTIs) are a frequent renal complication affecting up to 8% of pregnancies.
- They are divided into three main categories: Asymptomatic bacteriuria, acute cystitis, and acute pyelonephritis.
- Asymptomatic bacteriuria occurs in up to 2–7% of pregnancies. If left untreated, it progresses to symptomatic UTI in 25–30% of pregnant women.
- Symptomatic UTIs can be divided into acute cystitis (infection of bladder and urethra) and acute pyelonephritis (infection of kidneys).
- Pyelonephritis can lead to complications like anemia, septic shock, acute kidney injury, acute respiratory distress, renal abscess, emphysematous pyelonephritis, and preterm labor.
- Severe pyelonephritis warrants urgent treatment with parenteral empiric antibiotics, which can be switched to appropriate oral antibiotics after 24–48 hours once the patient is symptomatically better.
- All patients with pyelonephritis need regular monitoring of kidney function. Urological intervention might be required if there is urinary tract obstruction or renal abscess.

INTRODUCTION

Urinary tract infection (UTI) is the frequent perinatal infection complicating up to 8% of pregnancies.[1] It is an underemphasized preventable risk factor to prevent adverse maternal and fetal outcomes in lower-middle-income country settings, as routine screening for asymptomatic bacteriuria (ABU) is not a recommendation in antenatal care programs due to cost and other logistic issues. However, it is recommended in Infectious Diseases Society of America (IDSA) guidelines of the United States, the Canadian Task Force on Preventive Care, and the National Institute of Health and Clinical Excellence of the United Kingdom.[1]

Urinary tract infections are categorized based on clinical presentation as lower tract (acute cystitis), upper tract (acute pyelonephritis), and ABU **(Fig. 1)**. ABU is seen in 2–7% of pregnancies, with most cases presenting in early gestation.[2,3] A history of prior UTI, diabetes mellitus, and low socioeconomic status increases the chances of ABU. ABU will progress to symptomatic UTI in up to 20–35% of pregnant women without treatment.[4] Acute cystitis is documented in 1–2%, but it is difficult to assess the exact incidence of acute cystitis as many women are treated empirically. Acute pyelonephritis commonly occurs in the second or third trimester in up to 2% of pregnancies.[5] Risk factors of acute

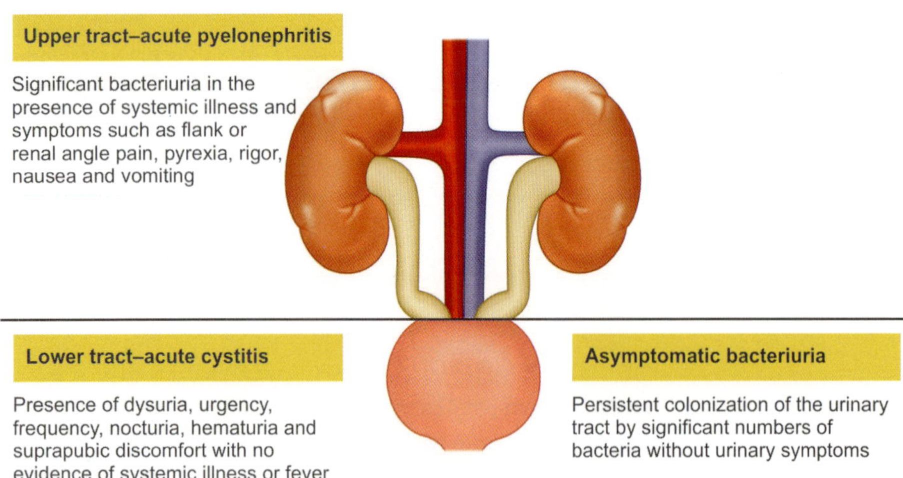

Fig. 1: Classification of urinary tract infections.

pyelonephritis include untreated ABU, age <20 years, nulliparity, sickle cell trait, smoking, delayed presentation to care, and preexisting diabetes mellitus. Recurrence of UTI is seen in up to 20% of pregnancies.[6]

Pregnancy outcomes: Untreated bacteriuria has been linked to a higher likelihood of preterm birth, low birth weight, and perinatal mortality in the majority of studies, although not all. For instance, in a meta-analysis done on women who did not have bacteriuria, the chances of experiencing preterm birth and having a low-birth-weight baby were 50% and 66% lower, respectively, compared to those with ABU.[7] A case-control study including more than 15,000 pregnant women discovered a higher likelihood of preeclampsia when either ABU or symptomatic UTI was present.[8] There is no definitive evidence to suggest a direct link between acute cystitis during pregnancy and an elevated likelihood of low birth weight, premature delivery, or pyelonephritis. Pregnancies of women with pyelonephritis compared to those without were more likely to be complicated by anemia, septicemia, acute pulmonary insufficiency, acute renal dysfunction [0.4% vs. 0.03%; odds ratio (OR), 16.5; 95% confidence interval (CI), 8.8–30.7], and spontaneous preterm birth. Most of the preterm births occurred between 33 and 36 weeks.[6]

PATHOGENESIS

In health, the sterility of the urogenital tract is maintained by acidic pH, high osmolality, and antegrade flow of urine. During pregnancy, the urogenital tract undergoes significant physiological changes which facilitate colonization with pathogens. There is a decrease in detrusor tone and an increase in bladder volume. Also, progesterone-mediated ureteric dilatation increases and detrusor tone decreases. Additionally, 90% of pregnant women develop ureteric smooth muscle relaxation, and pressure from the gravid uterus leads to dilatation of ureters. This results in urinary stasis, compromised ureteric valves, and retrograde flow (vesicoureteric reflux), facilitating bacterial colonization. Pregnancy-induced glycosuria, aminoaciduria, and reduced urinary osmolality favor bacterial growth.

The bacteria ascend to the uterus, causing an inflammatory reaction, which leads to uterine contractions and chorio-amniotic membrane degradation causing preterm rupture of membranes and preterm deliveries.

MICROBIOLOGY

Immunomodulation during pregnancy leads to a less efficient response against the bacterial cell surface antigens facilitating pathogenicity. However, the organisms causing UTI in pregnancy are of the same species and virulence as those in the non-pregnant state. *Escherichia coli* accounts for up to 70–90% of infections.[9] *Enterobacter* species, *Proteus* (2%), and *Klebsiella* are other gram-negative organisms responsible for UTIs.

Gram-positive organisms, including group B *Streptococcus* and *Staphylococcus saprophyticus*, are less frequent but clinically significant. Vaginal infection with group B streptococcal infection is significantly associated with preterm rupture of membranes, preterm delivery, and neonatal sepsis. Treatment of the same is timely warranted. Other causes like *Mycobacterium tuberculosis*, *Chlamydia* species, and fungal infections, such as *Candida albicans*, must be considered when bacterial causes are ruled out.

Clinical case capsule 1

Mrs XYZ, 29-year-old lady, is a primigravida with singleton pregnancy at 3 months' gestation. She is normotensive and nondiabetic. She remains asymptomatic.

On a routine antenatal visit, her urine culture showed growth of *Escherichia coli* (10^5 colony-forming unit/mL). What is the next best step in her management?

ASYMPTOMATIC BACTERIURIA

Diagnosis and Screening

Asymptomatic bacteriuria is diagnosed when there is isolation of the same bacterial strain in two consecutive voided urine samples with quantitative counts of $\geq 10^5$ colony-forming units/mL (CFU/mL) or a single catheterized urine specimen with a count of $\geq 10^2$ CFU/mL in the absence of symptoms consistent with UTI.[2] However, in clinical practice, the diagnosis is usually made with a single positive sample, and a confirmatory sample is usually needed only when the organism is not a typical uropathogen (like lactobacillus). The IDSA recommends screening all pregnant women for ABU once in early pregnancy.[2] Women at high risk for infection (diabetes mellitus, urinary tract anomalies, recurrent UTI, sickle cell disease) might require repeat screening subsequently.

Rapid screening tests, such as reagent strip analysis, dipstick, chromogenic limulus amoebocyte lysate assay, semiautomated urine screen (Bac-T-screen®), or interleukin-8 testing must not be used for ABU screening in pregnancy as they have low sensitivity and specificity. Also, urine culture gives information about the antibiotic sensitivity pattern. Hence, culture from clean catch and midstream urine (the second portion of the voided urine after discarding the initial stream) is recommended. Routine catheterization is not advised for ABU screening.

Management

Untreated ABU is strongly associated with adverse maternal and fetal outcomes **(Table 1)**.

Treatment must be tailored to the antibiotic susceptibility pattern of the isolated organism. Preferred drugs include nitrofurantoin, beta-lactams, and fosfomycin **(Table 2)**. Nitrofurantoin is best avoided during the first trimester. Usually, the duration of treatment is 5–7 days. Longer

TABLE 1: Perinatal consequences of bacteriuria in pregnancy.[9-15]

Maternal consequences	***Fetal consequences***
Symptomatic cystitis or pyelonephritis	Fetal growth restriction
Preterm labor (<37 weeks of gestation)	Perinatal mortality
Preeclampsia	Low birth weight (<2.5 kg)
Anemia	Prematurity (<37 weeks of pregnancy)
Postpartum endometritis	Developmental delay/mental retardation
Chorioamnionitis	

TABLE 2: Antibiotics for asymptomatic bacteriuria and cystitis in pregnancy.

Antibiotic	***Dosages***	***Remarks***
Amoxicillin	500 mg PO TID	Resistance may limit its utility among gram-negative pathogens
Amoxicillin–clavulanate	500 mg PO TID/875 mg PO BD	
Cephalexin	500 mg PO QID	
Cefpodoxime	100 mg PO BD	
Fosfomycin	3 g PO Single dose	Might not achieve therapeutic levels in the kidneys. Avoid use if pyelonephritis is suspected
Nitrofurantoin	100 mg PO BD	• Not to be used if pyelonephritis is suspected • Avoid use during the first trimester • Avoid at term • Nitrofurantoin—the risk of fetal hemolytic anemia (if G6PD deficient)
TMP–SMX	800/160 mg PO BD	

(BD: twice a day; G6PD: glucose-6-phosphate dehydrogenase; PO: per oral; TID thrice a day; TMP–SMX: trimethoprim–sulfamethoxazole)

courses lead to increased fetal exposure to antibiotics. Single-dose fosfomycin can also lead to the successful eradication of bacteriuria.

There is insufficient evidence to support the role of repeat screening with urine culture after treatment of ABU. Also, it is unclear whether long-term prevention is required in women with ABU during pregnancy. Due to the scarcity of data, American College of Obstetricians and Gynecologists (ACOG) guidelines do not support the use of repeat culture in these women.

Clinical case capsule 2

Mrs ABC, 26-year-old primigravida, presented with dysuria and increased frequency of micturition at the 26th week of gestation. She denies any history of fever, chills, abdominal discomfort, decreased urine output, or shortness of breath. Clinical examination is unremarkable. Her urine examination showed 20–25 pus cells/HPF (high power field) and no RBCs. Serum creatinine is 0.6 mg/dL with no abnormalities on renal ultrasound. She was treated with oral amoxicillin for a duration of 7 days. Her symptoms resolved with treatment. She was educated about the possible recurrence of symptoms during pregnancy.

ACUTE CYSTITIS

Acute cystitis is symptomatic inflammation of the lower urinary tract, more precisely, the urinary bladder, which can be infectious or noninfectious.

Clinical Features

The typical symptoms of acute cystitis are sudden onset of dysuria, urinary urgency, and frequency. It is sometimes accompanied by suprapubic tenderness. Urinalysis is remarkable for pyuria and occasionally hematuria.

Diagnosis

Urine examination and urine cultures would suggest the diagnosis. Urine nitrite positivity in the presence of symptoms strongly suggests cystitis on the basis of which empiric treatment can be started. Differential diagnosis of acute bacterial cystitis includes gonococcal and nongonococcal (chlamydia, mycoplasma) urethritis. These patients commonly present with urethral discharge and have persistent symptoms despite antibiotic treatment. Other genital infections like vulvitis, vaginitis, or cervicitis must also be considered.

Recurrent episodes of cystitis may need further evaluation with ultrasound of the kidneys, ureters, and bladder for anatomical abnormalities like chronic cystitis changes in the bladder or the presence of postvoid residue.

Management

Antibiotic therapy can be started empirically, which can then be modified based on culture reports. The total duration of therapy is usually 7–10 days, depending on the agent used **(Table 2)**. Due to their broader spectrum of activity, the empiric antibiotics of choice are cefpodoxime, amoxicillin-clavulanate, and fosfomycin. There is no evidence to suggest the superiority of one agent over another. Quinolones and tetracyclines are contraindicated in pregnancy.

Appropriate duration of treatment is crucial as there may be a possibility of recurrent infection if inadequately treated. The benefits of prophylactic antibiotics post therapy are uncertain. However, it is indicated in women with recurrent cystitis (three or more episodes) during pregnancy. The susceptibility pattern on the urine culture guides the choice of suppressive antibiotic.

Clinical case capsule 3

Mrs SKS is a 28-year-old lady, G2 L1, in the 32nd week of gestation. She does not have hypertension or diabetes mellitus. She presented with a fever with chills and rigors associated with flank pain and dysuria for the last 3 days. She noticed oliguria for 1 day. On examination, she was febrile tachycardiac, with BP 90/50 mm Hg. Her urine examination showed plenty of pus cells/HPF. Serum creatinine was 2.4 mg/dL, and an abdomen ultrasound showed enlarged kidneys with a normal pelvicalyceal system. She was initiated on parenteral third-generation cephalosporins. Urine culture showed *Escherichia coli* (10^5 colony-forming unit/mL). Treatment included IV hydration as guided by volume status, antipyretic measures, and close fetal monitoring. After 5 days of parenteral therapy, she improved symptomatically and was shifted to oral antibiotics. Her serum creatinine normalized, and the repeat urine culture was sterile. She was started on amoxicillin low-dose prophylaxis (per culture sensitivity), followed up with close observation until delivery.

ACUTE PYELONEPHRITIS

Acute pyelonephritis results from an acute infection of the upper urinary tract and kidneys, commonly presenting in the second and third trimesters.

Clinical Features

Classic symptoms of acute pyelonephritis (similar to nonpregnant women) include fever (>38°C) with chills and rigors associated with flank pain, anorexia, nausea, and vomiting. On examination, the patient may have flank tenderness or costovertebral angle tenderness. Up to 20% of pregnant women with severe pyelonephritis can develop septic shock with or without acute respiratory distress syndrome (ARDS). It can lead to severe anemia mediated by endotoxin release.[10] Acute pyelonephritis may progress to certain complications, such as renal abscess, perinephric abscess, renal vein thrombosis, papillary necrosis, acute kidney injury, and emphysematous pyelonephritis.

Diagnosis

Diagnosis is based on clinical profile, urine analysis, and urine cultures. All cultures, including blood and urine, are to be obtained before initiating antibiotic therapy. Pyuria is almost always present, and its absence suggests an alternative diagnosis. Timely diagnosis and prompt treatment are warranted, which can be delayed due to diverse clinical features. A wide range of differential diagnoses must be considered, including acute cholecystitis, pneumonia, appendicitis, pancreatitis, premature labor, or even placental abruption. Genitourinary examination for a possible vaginal or cervical focus of infection is warranted.

Imaging is not routinely required for the diagnosis. Still, it is recommended in women who are critically ill with or without symptoms of renal colic or a history of renal stones, diabetes mellitus, urinary tract anomalies, or immunosuppression. Renal ultrasound is the preferred imaging which helps to evaluate for complications. CT abdomen may not be indicated in a pregnant state unless the benefits supersede the risk of fetal radiation exposure.

Management

Unlike nonpregnant women, pregnant patients with acute pyelonephritis should be managed as inpatients. Empirical intravenous antibiotics are recommended until the woman is afebrile for 24–48 hours and is symptomatically better, after which she can be shifted to appropriate oral antibiotics. Broad-spectrum beta-lactams are the mainstay of initial empiric therapy with choice guided by local antibiogram **(Box 1)**. Fluoroquinolones and aminoglycosides are contraindicated in pregnancy. Oral choice is limited to beta-lactams and trimethoprim–sulfamethoxazole (only in the second trimester). Nitrofurantoin and fosfomycin are not the preferred drugs for pyelonephritis.

A carbapenem is preferred in women with extended-spectrum beta-lactamase (ESBL)-producing Enterobacteriaceae (or history of infection with multiresistant

BOX 1: Antibiotics for empiric treatment of pyelonephritis in pregnancy.

Mild or moderate pyelonephritis:
- Ceftriaxone 1 g IV q24h, or
- Cefepime 1 g IV q12h, or
- Cefotaxime 1–2 g IV q8h, or
- Ceftazidime 2 g IV q8h, or
- Aztreonam 1 g IV q8h, or
- Ampicillin 1–2 g IV q6h plus gentamicin IV 1.5 mg/kg q8h (aminoglycosides are associated with fetal ototoxicity. Must be reserved only for patients who are not responding to other antibiotics)

Severe pyelonephritis (or those with urinary tract obstruction or impaired immune system):
- Ticarcillin–clavulanate 3.1 g IV q6h, or
- Ampicillin–sulbactam 1.5 g IV q6h, or
- Piperacillin–tazobactam 3.375 g IV q6h, or
- Meropenem 1 g q8h, or
- Ertapenem 1g q24hr

organisms). Meropenem and ertapenem are the preferred carbapenems (not imipenem) in pregnancy. The total duration of antibiotics is usually 10–14 days and is guided by clinical profile and complications. If there is no symptomatic improvement beyond 48 hours, a repeat urine culture and renal ultrasound must be performed. It is vital to rule out urinary tract anomalies or complications like a renal abscess, emphysematous pyelonephritis, or urinary tract obstruction, which might warrant urosurgical intervention.

PREVENTING RECURRENCE

Recurrent pyelonephritis can occur in 6–8% of pregnant women.[11] Once the therapy is over, low-dose antimicrobial prophylaxis guided by culture sensitivity till delivery is a safer option in women with pyelonephritis. In women who do not receive suppressive prophylaxis, repeated monthly cultures are recommended till delivery for evaluation for recurrent bacteriuria.

OBSTETRIC MANAGEMENT

Severe pyelonephritis is not an indication for emergent delivery. It is recommended to delay the induction of labor or cesarean section (for standard obstetrical indications) till the patient is afebrile or as long as it is relatively safe for the mother and fetus. Some women (who develop preterm labor before 34 weeks) might require tocolysis as pyelonephritis is associated with preterm birth. However, it is best avoided in patients with severe sepsis or those who are critically ill.

CONCLUSION

Urinary tract infections are common occurrences that significantly impact the mother and the fetus. Regular screening and timely management can improve the outcomes.

REFERENCES

1. Lee AC, Mullany LC, Koffi AK, Rafiqullah I, Khanam R, Folger LV, et al. Urinary tract infections in pregnancy in a rural population of Bangladesh: population-based prevalence, risk factors, etiology, and antibiotic resistance. BMC Pregnancy Childbirth. 2019;20(1):1.
2. McCormick T, Ashe RG, Kearney PM. Urinary tract infection in pregnancy. Obstet Gynaecol. 2008;10:156-62.
3. Patterson TF, Andriole VT. Detection, significance, and therapy of bacteriuria in pregnancy. Update in the managed health care era. Infect Dis Clin North Am. 1997;11(3):593-608.
4. Nicolle LE, Gupta K, Bradley SF, Colgan R, DeMuri GP, Drekonja D. Clinical Practice Guideline for the Management of Asymptomatic Bacteriuria: 2019 Update by the Infectious Diseases Society of America. Clin Infect Dis. 2019;68(10):e83-e110.
5. Smaill FM, Vazquez JC. Antibiotics for asymptomatic bacteriuria in pregnancy. Cochrane Database Syst Rev. 2019;2019(11):CD000490.
6. Wing DA, Fassett MJ, Getahun D. Acute pyelonephritis in pregnancy: an 18-year retrospective analysis. Am J Obstet Gynecol. 2014;210(3):219.e1-6.
7. Romero R, Oyarzun E, Mazor M, Sirtori M, Hobbins JC, Bracken M. Meta-analysis of the relationship between asymptomatic bacteriuria and preterm delivery/low birth weight. Obstet Gynecol. 1989;73(4):576-82.
8. Minassian C, Thomas SL, Williams DJ, Campbell O, Smeeth L. Acute maternal infection and risk of pre-eclampsia: a population-based case-control study. PLoS One. 2013;8(9):e73047.
9. Gilstrap LC, Cunningham FG, Whalley PJ. Acute pyelonephritis in pregnancy: an anterospective study. Obstet Gynecol. 1981;57(4):409-13.
10. Hill JB, Sheffield JS, McIntire DD, Wendel GD. Acute pyelonephritis in pregnancy. Obstet Gynecol. 2005;105(1):18-23.
11. Cox SM, Shelburne P, Mason R, Guss S, Cunningham FG. Mechanisms of hemolysis

and anemia associated with acute antepartum pyelonephritis. Am J Obstet Gynecol. 1991;164(2):587-90.
12. Lenke RR, VanDorsten JP, Schifrin BS. Pyelonephritis in pregnancy: a prospective randomized trial to prevent recurrent disease evaluating suppressive therapy with nitrofurantoin and close surveillance. Am J Obstet Gynecol. 1983;146(8):953-7.
13. Savage WE, Hajj SN, Kass EH. Demographic and prognostic characteristics of bacteriuria in pregnancy. Medicine (Baltimore). 1967;46(5):385-407.
14. Mittendorf R, Williams MA, Kass EH. Prevention of preterm delivery and low birth weight associated with asymptomatic bacteriuria. Clin Infect Dis Off Publ Infect Dis Soc Am. 1992;14(4):927-32.
15. Pfau A, Sacks TG. Effective prophylaxis for recurrent urinary tract infections during pregnancy. Clin Infect Dis Off Publ Infect Dis Soc Am. 1992;14(4):810-4.

CHAPTER

19 Kidney Stone Disease in Pregnancy

Dilip Kumar Pal, Subhajit Malakar, Partha Pratim Sinha Roy

HIGHLIGHTS

- Diagnosis and treatment of renal stones during pregnancy is a complex problem.
- Risks to the fetus from ionizing radiation and interventional procedures need to be balanced with optimizing clinical care for the mother.
- Management of such patients requires a clear understanding of available options, with a multidisciplinary team approach.
- We discuss the role of different diagnostic tests including ultrasound, magnetic resonance urography, and computerized tomography. We also provide an update on recent developments in the treatment of renal stones during pregnancy.
- Expectant management remains first-line treatment. Where definitive treatment of the stone is required, new evidence suggests that ureteroscopic stone removal may be equally safe, and possibly better than traditional temporizing procedures.

INTRODUCTION

Pregnancy-related urolithiasis is a serious medical issue that may have an impact on the health of both the mother and the fetus. It is by far the most typical reason why pregnant women have abdominal pain linked to urology. Urolithiasis can lead to serious complications for the mother, including ureteral blockage, upper urinary tract infection, urosepsis, and perinephric abscess, all of which require rapid hospitalization and management. This illness also offers a serious health risk to the fetus by causing preterm labor or interfering with the progression of regular labor.

Urolithiasis in pregnancy presents a diagnostic and therapeutic challenge because of its ability to mimic other acute illnesses such diverticulitis, appendicitis, or placental abruption.[1] A multidisciplinary engagement is frequently required for managing this condition. Additionally, the whole arsenal of diagnostic and therapeutic techniques that are frequently employed in nonpregnant women cannot be used due to the harmful effects on mother and fetus.

Pregnancy causes physiological and structural alterations to the urinary tract, especially in the upper compartment, which may encourage lithogenesis. Urolithiasis risk may also be increased by changes in hormonal dynamics and biochemical characteristics of the urinary tract that are typical of pregnancy.

EPIDEMIOLOGY

Urolithiasis is quite common worldwide with incidence ranging from 1% to 5% in Asia, 7% to 13% in North America, and 5% to 9% in Europe.[2] According to recent data, the prevalence and incidence of urolithiasis in women are both significantly rising. Over the past 30 years, nephrolithiasis in women has generally increased in the United States at a rate of 1.9% yearly, and female hospital admissions for stone-related conditions have climbed by 52%.[3] In contrast to nonpregnant women of comparable age and demography, pregnant women do not generally have an increased risk of developing kidney stones.[4] Although reports in the literature range considerably from 1 out of every 200–800 pregnancies, the real frequency of urolithiasis during pregnancy is still completely unclear. According to published research, the prevalence of stone disease among expectant women has not changed over the previous 20 years.[4]

About 90% of stones form during the second and third trimesters of pregnancy. Ureteral stones are twice as likely to occur as kidney stones and seem to impact both sides similarly, even though the right ureter tends to be more dilated than the left.

IMPACT OF RENAL STONES ON PREGNANCY

Pregnant women with kidney stones may face an increased risk of miscarriage, preeclampsia, and cesarean births. In one study, it was also connected to early membrane rupture. Preterm birth rates have been reported to range between 2.5% and 40%. The majority of studies do not mention any elevated risk for the baby, including risk of congenital abnormalities, low birth weight, low Apgar scores, and perinatal death.[5] However, the exact impact of kidney stones on pregnancy outcomes is difficult to identify due to inconsistent findings across various researches.

ETIOPATHOGENESIS

There are no specific etiological variables in pregnancy that cause stone formation. Various factors contribute to the risk of urolithiasis, including being in the age range of the third to fifth decade of life, inadequate water intake (<1.5 L/day), exposure to elevated environmental temperatures and/or dry climates, a diet rich in calcium, sodium, and red meat, occupation (such as exposure to hot and dry conditions), social class (linked to occupation and diet), and excessive weight or obesity (importantly in women). Etiopathogenesis is summarized in **Table 1**.

PATHOPHYSIOLOGY OF UROLITHIASIS IN PREGNANCY

Pathophysiology of urolithiasis in pregnancy is shown in **Flowchart 1**.

TABLE 1: Etiopathogenesis of stone formation.

Stone promotion (mechanism)	***Stone inhibition (mechanism)***
Urinary stasis (mechanical compression, progesterone)	Hypercitraturia (increased GFR)
Elevated urine pH	
Hypercalciuria (increased GFR, increased vitamin D)	*Increased excretion:* Glycosaminoglycan, uromodulin, and nephrocalcin (increased GFR)
Lithogenic factors	
Increased excretion: Uric acid, sodium and oxalate (increased glomerular filtration rate)	

(GFR: glomerular filtration rate)

Flowchart 1: Pathophysiology of urolithiasis in pregnancy.

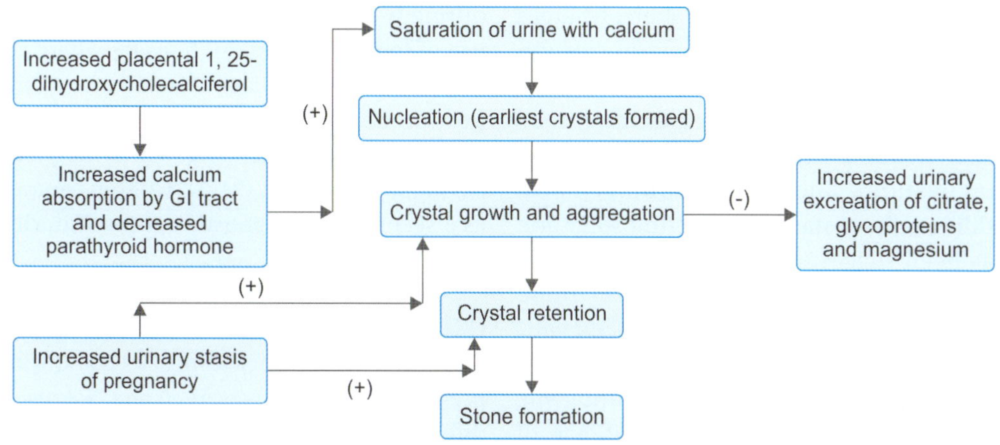

PHYSIOLOGICAL HYDRONEPHROSIS OF PREGNANCY

During pregnancy, up to 90% of women may experience physiological hydronephrosis on the right side and 67% on the left. This condition arises from a combination of mechanical and hormonal factors. The main mechanical cause is the compression of the ureters by the growing uterus at the pelvic brim, which leads to obstruction. Specifically, the right ureter intersects the iliac artery at the pelvic brim, while the left ureter crosses more proximally and laterally, making it less likely to be compressed. This anatomical difference accounts for the higher incidence of right-sided hydronephrosis. Additionally, the uterus's rightward rotation and the protective effect of the sigmoid colon on the left ureter are mechanical factors that further explain the predominance of right-sided hydronephrosis during pregnancy.

URINARY CHANGES IN PREGNANCY

Kidney has propensity to develop hydronephrosis in pregnancy. Increased progesterone levels during pregnancy reduce ureteral peristalsis, which results in ureteral dilatation above the pelvic brim. This physiological hydronephrosis may cause urine to stagnate, thereby increasing the risk of kidney stones' formation. All these usually resolve by 4–6 weeks after delivery.

During pregnancy, the glomerular filtration rate (GFR) physiologically increases by 50% in response; also, there is rise in the excretion of sodium, calcium, and uric acid in the urine. This increase in GFR, along with the placenta's production of 1,25-dihydroxycholecalciferol to meet the growing needs of the fetus, results in hypercalciuria. However, elevated levels of urine oxalate are not observed in pregnant patients until the postpartum period. Notably, urine calcium levels are higher in the second and third trimesters compared to the postpartum period. The pH of urine also rises during pregnancy, which promotes the crystallization of calcium phosphate over calcium oxalate. This shift leads to a higher prevalence of calcium phosphate stones during pregnancy, unlike in the general population where up to 65% of stones are calcium oxalate calculi. Stone analysis shows that 74% of stones in pregnant patients are predominantly calcium phosphate, whereas only 26% are mainly composed of calcium oxalate. The body counters the increase in stone-promoting factors by excreting more crystallization inhibitors, such as citrate, magnesium, and glycosaminoglycans. Additionally, gestational hyperthiosulfaturia has been suggested as a factor that lowers the risk of urolithiasis. The rise in these inhibitory substances may help explain why, despite physiological hydronephrosis and an increase in the concentration of lithogenic factors in urine, the overall incidence of nephrolithiasis does not seem to escalate during pregnancy.

CLINICAL FEATURES

"Renal colic" or severe flank pain that radiates to the groin is the typical clinical presentation. Moreover, nausea and vomiting could happen. Frequent urination and dysuria are common, especially when there is an infection or when the stone has migrated to the lower urinary tract. On examination, there may be renal angle discomfort in addition to microscopic or extensive hematuria. 89–100% of pregnant women with renal stone present with flank pain. Hematuria occurs in 75–95% of cases.[6] Preterm labor or uterine contractions are other possible symptoms of renal stones.

INVESTIGATIONS

Due to its accessibility, low cost, and lack of ionizing radiation, ultrasound (US) is frequently utilized as the initial diagnostic procedure in pregnant patients complaining of abdominal pain.

MRI is the preferred imaging modality when ultrasonography provides conflicting results, as it is effective in investigating the specific causes of abdominal and pelvic pain during pregnancy. Notably, MRI avoids the use of ionizing radiation. In cases where US fails to establish a diagnosis and symptoms persist despite conservative treatment, consideration should be given to magnetic resonance urography (MRU) without contrast as a second-line diagnostic approach during pregnancy.

While low-dose computed tomography (LD-CT) is highly sensitive and specific for detecting urinary tract stones, its use during pregnancy should be reserved as a last resort due to the potential risks associated with radiation exposure. However, standard CT is contraindicated in pregnancy. Intravenous urogram (IVU) should not be used as it leads to radiation exposure.

Ultrasound

When there is a suspicion of stone disease, US is the primary investigation of choice. Without exposing the fetus to radiation, real-time US shows the renal parenchyma, pelvicalyceal system, dilated ureter, and occasionally the calculus. Doppler US can yield strong intensities; therefore, it should be used carefully, minimizing exposure length and acoustic output, especially in the first trimester. The sensitivity of US to identify pregnancy-related nephrolithiasis ranges from 34% to 92.5%.[7]

Additionally, the mechanical compression of the ureter between the gravid uterus and the iliopsoas muscle is highly nonspecific, making it challenging to differentiate between ureteral obstruction caused by calculi and physiological hydronephrosis. Chung SD et al. have demonstrated the utility of transvaginal US in assessing the distal ureter and distinguishing between blockage and physiological hydronephrosis during pregnancy.[8]

In pregnant women, the resistive index (RI), which is calculated as the peak systolic intrarenal blood flow divided by the peak systolic blood flow, has shown some potential. Pregnancy-related physiological hydronephrosis does not seem to have an impact on the RI. An increased RI (>0.70) cannot be attributed to pregnancy, as normal pregnancy often has little effect on the intrarenal RI.

The absence of a "ureteral jet"—the movement of urine at the ureterovesical junction—on the suspected side of an obstruction has a 100% sensitivity rate and a 91% specificity rate. To reduce false-positive results, patients should be scanned in the contralateral decubitus posture.

COMPUTED TOMOGRAPHY SCAN

Due to teratogenic dangers and the chance of a child developing cancer, CT should be avoided in pregnancy. In the general population, LD-CT has been proven effective for the identification of calculi.

Even though low-dose multidetector CT exhibits remarkable accuracy (95% sensitivity and 98% specificity) in detecting calculi in the general population, it is still employed as a last-resort test. The fetal dose from a single-acquisition abdominopelvic CT investigation is typically within the range of 10–50 mGy. While doses below 50 mGy pose minimal risk of pediatric cancer, fetal exposure from pelvic CT within the 20–50 mGy range increases the likelihood of fatal childhood cancer by a factor of 1.4–2, despite modest risks of teratogenesis. Therefore, high-dose ionizing radiation tests, such as CT scans, should only be justified in pregnant women when no other diagnostic option is available, and the study is clearly in the mother's best interests.

Magnetic Resonance Imaging

When accessible, MRU without contrast is now thought of as the second-line pregnancy investigation because it is equally safe and accurate to CT. Without the use of intravenous contrast agents, MRU can quickly collect pictures of the upper urinary tract.

The urinary system and ureters can be found using MRU, which uses strong T2-weighted "water" images with thick slabs to distinguish between normal and aberrant dilatation caused by urolithiasis.

Thin-slice, high-resolution, highly T2-weighted fast spin echo (FSE) sequences can improve the ability of MRU for detection of small stones.

Magnetic resonance urography has been identified as capable of revealing various manifestations in both physiological hydronephrosis and pathologic blockage among pregnant individuals experiencing symptomatic hydronephrosis. Physiologic dilatation typically lacks renal enlargement and perirenal fluid indicative of blockage. Moreover, physiologic dilatation exhibits a distinctive tapering attributed to the extrinsic compression of the uterus in the middle third of the ureter. While stones present as signal voids atop the high signal of urine within a dilated ureter, aiding the visualization of obstructive calculi, MRI may not accurately detect ureteral calculi.

In addition to proximal ureteral dilatation, the presence of a standing column of urine below the level of the pelvic brim ("double kink sign") suggests an obstructing distal ureteral calculus. "Unusual" sites of obstruction, such as the pelvic ureteral junction or the vesicoureteric junction, an abrupt end to the ureter (rather than a smooth taper at the level of the pelvic brim), and perinephric or periureteral edema are additional MRI features pointing to pathologic rather than physiological hydronephrosis. It is worth mentioning that MRI can also reveal complications such as pyelonephritis, visualized as an enlarged edematous kidney. Focal areas of pyelonephritis exhibit lower signal intensity on T2-weighted images and restricted proton diffusion on diffusion-weighted imaging (DWI).[9]

However, MRU has limitations, as small calculi may not be visualized effectively, and the technique is expensive and time-consuming. Other potential drawbacks include the risk of spatial misregistration between slices during normal patient breathing and the development of flow-void aberrations in urine on T2-weighted images in dilated collecting systems, resembling filling defects. These flow artifacts do not layer dependently, as expected in a stone, and are frequently centered, making interpretation challenging.

MANAGEMENT

Prevention

The most effective approach to urolithiasis is prevention, and some studies have suggested proactive strategies to steer clear of the challenges associated with treating urolithiasis during pregnancy. Denstedt and Razvi (1992) recommended preventive measures for asymptomatic caliceal stones in women of reproductive age who are pregnant.[10] Biyani and Joyce (2002) endorsed metabolic testing for individuals with a history of stone formation and suggested preventive treatment for asymptomatic stones before pregnancy.[11]

Diet

Dietary changes are essential for preventing urolithiasis. General guidelines include limiting high-oxalate meals and purines while increasing hydration. Because salt and sodium tend to enhance fluid retention and hypercalciuria, they should be consumed in moderation. Low-calcium diets are often associated with an unexpected increase in calcium stone formation and are therefore discouraged.

A low-oxalate diet helps to avoid the production of calcium oxalate stones. Chocolate, nuts, green leafy vegetables, coffee, spinach, beets, and tea are all high in oxalate.

It is recommended to drink enough fluids to produce a 24-hour urine volume of 2,000 mL each day. Lemon juice contains citrate, a natural inhibitor of kidney stone formation.

A low-methionine diet has been shown to reduce the risk of cystine stone formation.

Conservative

Unless the patient's condition demands emergency decompression via percutaneous nephrostomy (PCN) tube insertion or cystoscopy and ureteral stent placement, conservative therapy is usually the preferred approach. Expectant treatment, which includes rehydration, analgesia, antiemetics, and close observation, successfully induces spontaneous stone passage in 23–84% of cases.[12]

Flowchart 2 shows an algorithm of stone disease management in pregnancy.

Analgesia

While nonsteroidal anti-inflammatory drugs (NSAIDs) are not recommended during pregnancy due to the risk of spontaneous miscarriage, oligohydramnios, and premature ductus arteriosus closure, paracetamol is safe. Low-dose and short-term administration of morphine is deemed safe for pregnant women.

Flowchart 2: Algorithm of stone disease management in pregnancy.

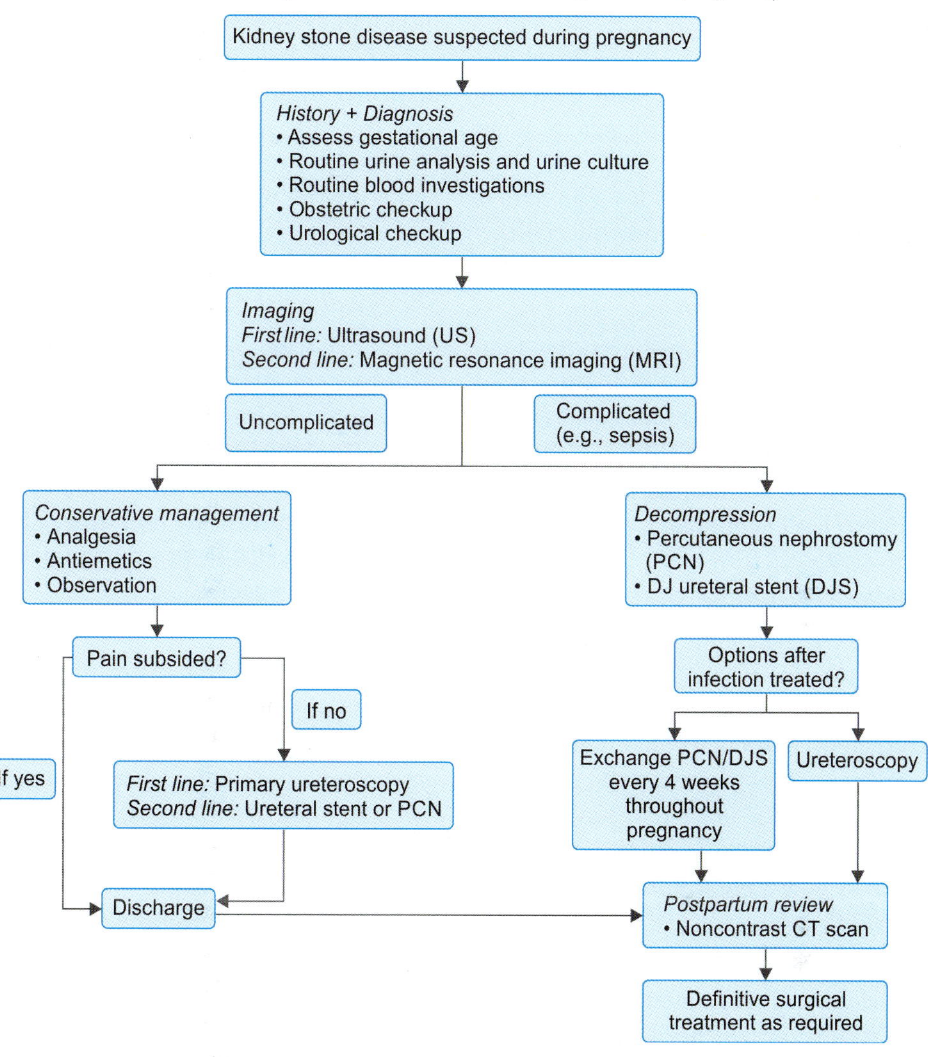

Antiemetics

One of the recognized measures for measuring nausea and vomiting in pregnant women is the Pregnancy-Unique Quantification of Emesis (PUQE) index. The Royal College of Obstetricians and Gynaecologists (RCOG) offers advice on certain drugs that have not been demonstrated to damage the fetus. Dopamine antagonists such as domperidone and metoclopramide, phenothiazines such as prochlorperazine, and antihistamines such as cyclizine and promethazine are such examples. Because the former has extrapyramidal side effects, the latter is recommended as a second-line therapy. There is a lack of information about the use of ondansetron during pregnancy.

Antibiotics

When antibiotics are required, penicillin and cephalosporins are the safest medications to use. Nitrofurantoin and trimethoprim-sulfamethoxazole are two more antibiotics that are routinely utilized. Fluoroquinolones are not indicated as a first-line treatment during pregnancy due to their toxicity. Short courses are unlikely to be harmful to the fetus, and thus, it is reasonable to use this class of drugs with resistant or recurrent infections.

Surgical Intervention

Approximately 30% of pregnant individuals with kidney stones will need some form of intervention. The choice of the final intervention method should consider the patient's specific characteristics and the available treatment options.

Immediate Decompression

For those experiencing renal dysfunction and/or sepsis due to an obstructing calculus, immediate decompression is crucial. This can be achieved through either ureteral stent placement or PCN insertion. US, instead of fluoroscopy, can be utilized to confirm stent placement. The resolution of the stone itself can then be addressed at a later date.

Temporizing Measures

All individuals with symptomatic urolithiasis during pregnancy may need PCN or ureteral stent implantation when conservative approaches have failed. However, it presents a challenge because stent replacement is frequently needed every 4–6 weeks during pregnancy due to the higher rates of encrustation. A negative impact on quality of life can also be caused by PCN and indwelling ureteral stents. Rivera et al. discovered that 47% of patients with ureteral stents needed early induction due to stent intolerance in a 15-year retrospective assessment of all pregnant patients with kidney stone disease (KSD) at their hospital.[13] In situations where conservative methods have failed, this supports the benefits of definitive stone therapy. It is understood that this may not be practical based on the environment and local knowledge, and a referral to a specialist center may be required.

Shockwave Lithotripsy

Extracorporeal shock wave lithotripsy (ESWL) is frequently used in the nongravid population; however, it requires frequent use of ionizing radiation. The potential adverse effects of energy dispersion on the fetus are unknown. At this time, ESWL is contraindicated during pregnancy due to harmful effect on fetus.

Ureteroscopy

Ureterorenoscopic surgery (URS), introduced in pregnancy over two decades ago, has become the preferred surgical method for pregnant women for kidney stone removal. While local anesthetic sedation is deemed safe in carefully selected cases, the majority of facilities still opt for general or spinal anesthesia during URS procedures. Particularly in the first trimester, it is crucial to avoid general anesthesia, as the use of volatile gases during this period may lead to morphogenetic abnormalities in the fetus.

The advent of next-generation laser systems, such as the thulium fiber laser (TFL), offers advantages like a shorter recovery period, potentially enhancing the role of URS in pregnancy even further.

Percutaneous Nephrolithotomy

Even though there have only been a small number of case reports of successful percutaneous nephrolithotomy (PCNL) procedures during pregnancy (fewer than 20 in the world literature to date), pregnancy is typically regarded as a contraindication for PCNL due to the prolonged use of fluoroscopy and general anesthesia, as well as the requirement of the patient to be in a prone position.

Open surgery

Previously, pregnant women who needed urolithiasis treatment had open lithotomy. Modern surgical techniques for urolithiasis, in contrast, can be performed without anesthesia or radiation, resulting in reduced morbidity rates while maintaining comparable or higher success rates. Consequently, open surgery is now reserved as a final option. It is employed when stone removal is necessary before childbirth due to complications arising from conservative or invasive urolithiasis care, or if ureteroscopy is deemed contraindicated.

COMPLICATIONS

Complications from surgical procedures are more likely in pregnant women. Pregnancy-related physiological changes are linked to an increase in perioperative risk. Any surgical operation may result in complications including:

- Pulmonary embolism
- Preterm delivery
- Deep vein thrombosis
- Aspiration

Internal stent insertion complications may include the following:

- Stent encrustation, which could be increased during pregnancy, requires replacement every 3–4 weeks.
- Infection
- Sepsis
- Stent migration

Percutaneous nephrostomy complications may include the following:

- Recurrent obstruction requiring regular flushing or replacement
- Infection or sepsis as a result of tube obstruction
- Fetal damage as a result of prolonged anesthetic requirements and ionizing radiation
- The risk of bleeding from nephrostomy tube implantation, tube dislodgment, and tube erosion

According to current research, in expert hands, complications from ureteroscopy and intracorporeal lithotripsy in pregnancy are uncommon. The risk of complications may be somewhat raised due to the anatomic changes of pregnancy; nonetheless, the potential complications are the same as in the general population. An algorithm of the stone disease management in pregnancy is shown in **Flowchart 2**.

REFERENCES

1. Burgess KL, Gettman MT, Rangel LJ, Krambeck AE. Diagnosis of urolithiasis and rate of spontaneous passage during pregnancy. J Urol. 2011;186(6):2280-4.
2. Ramello A, Vitale C, Marangella M. Epidemiology of nephrolithiasis. J Nephrol. 2000;13:S45-50.
3. Strope SA, Wolf JS, Hollenbeck BK. Changes in gender distribution of urinary stone disease. Urology. 2010;75:543-6.
4. Riley JM, Dudley AG, Semins MJ. Nephrolithiasis and pregnancy: has the incidence been rising? J Endourol. 2014;28:383-6.
5. Swartz MA, Lydon-Rochelle MT, Simon D, Wright JL, Porter MP. Admission for nephrolithiasis in pregnancy, risk of adverse birth outcomes. Obstet Gynecol. 2007;109:1099-104.
6. Butler E, Cox SM, Eberts EG, Cunningham FG. Symptomatic nephrolithiasis complicating pregnancy. Obstet Gynecol. 2000;96:753-6.

7. Rosenberg E, Sergienko R, Abu-Ghanem S, et al. Nephrolithiasis during pregnancy: Characteristics, complications, and pregnancy outcome. World J Urol. 2011;29:743-7.
8. Chung SD, Chen YH, Keller JJ, Lin CC, Lin HC. Urinary calculi increase the risk for adverse pregnancy outcomes: A nationwide study. Acta Obstet Gynecol Scand. 2013;92: 69-74.
9. Mullins JK, Semins MJ, Hyams ES, Bohlman ME, Matlaga BR. Half Fourier single shot turbo spin echo magnetic resonance urography for the evaluation of suspected renal colic in pregnancy. Urology. 2012; 79(6):1252-5.
10. Denstedt JD,Razvi H.Management of urinary calculi during pregnancy. J Urol 1992;148:1072-5.
11. Biyani CS,Joyce AD.Urolithiasis in Pregnancy II:Management. BJU Int.2002:89(8): 819-23
12. Lieske JC, Pena de la Vega LS, Slezak JM, Bergstralh EJ, Leibson CL, Ho KL. Renal stone epidemiology in Rochester, Minnesota: an update. Kidney Int. 2006;69:760-4.
13. Rivera ME, McAlvany KL, Brinton TS, Gettman MT, Krambeck AE. Anesthesic exposure in the treatment of symptomatic urinary calculi in pregnant women. Urology.2014;84(6):1275-8.

Index

Page numbers followed by *b* refer to box, *f* refer to figure, *fc* refer to flowchart, and *t* refer to table.

J

K

L

M

N

Q

R

V

W